S0-CDW-972

Lymphatic Mapping and Probe Applications in Oncology

Lymphatic

Mapping

and Probe

Applications

in Oncology

edited by

Omgo E. Nieweg

The Netherlands Cancer Institute
Amsterdam, the Netherlands

Richard Essner

John Wayne Cancer Institute at Saint John's Health Center
Santa Monica, California

Douglas S. Reintgen

H. Lee Moffitt Cancer Center and Research Institute
University of South Florida
Tampa, Florida

John F. Thompson

Sydney Cancer Centre
Royal Prince Alfred Hospital, Camperdown, and
University of Sydney
Sydney, New South Wales, Australia

RC269.5
L96
2000

MARCEL DEKKER, INC.   NEW YORK · BASEL

ISBN: 0-8247-0267-0

This book is printed on acid-free paper.

Headquarters
Marcel Dekker, Inc.
270 Madison Avenue, New York, NY 10016
tel: 212-696-9000; fax: 212-685-4540

Eastern Hemisphere Distribution
Marcel Dekker AG
Hutgasse 4, Postfach 812, CH-4001 Basel, Switzerland
tel: 41-61-261-8482; fax: 41-61-261-8896

World Wide Web
http://www.dekker.com

The publisher offers discounts on this book when ordered in bulk quantities. For more information, write to Special Sales/Professional Marketing at the headquarters address above.

Copyright © 2000 by Marcel Dekker, Inc.   All Rights Reserved.

Neither this book nor any part may be reproduced or transmitted in any form or by any means, electronic or mechanical, including photocopying, microfilming, and recording, or by any information storage and retrieval system, without permission in writing from the publisher.

Current printing (last digit):
10 9 8 7 6 5 4 3 2 1

PRINTED IN THE UNITED STATES OF AMERICA

Foreword

The single most important prognostic factor for patients with solid neoplasms is the metastatic status of the regional lymph nodes draining the primary tumor. Until recently, the only approach to the identification of regional node metastases was complete lymphadenectomy and pathological examination of each excised node using hematoxylin & eosin staining. This technique underestimates the true frequency of nodal metastases because it samples only a small percentage of the total nodal volume and uses a staining method that is not ideally sensitive. However, despite inadequacies as a staging procedure (and significant morbidity), routine complete lymph node dissection has continued to be popular because of its purported therapeutic value in patients whose tumor may metastasize to the regional nodes before extension to distant sites. Unfortunately, the only patients who derive benefit from elective regional lymph node dissection in early-stage melanoma and breast cancer are the minority with nodal metastases; the majority of patients are exposed to the morbidity of complete lymphadenectomy without possible benefit. Because of dissatisfaction with this traditional approach, we sought to develop an improved technique.

During the 1970s, we conceptualized cutaneous lymphoscintigraphy as a method to identify the lymph basin at risk of receiving cancer cells metastasizing from a primary tumor in the trunk or other sites with ambiguous lymphatic drainage. During the 1980s, we formulated the necessary surgical and pathological concepts and developed sensitive techniques to determine which nodes *within* that nodal basin drained a particular primary cutaneous site. The location of these nodes varied widely depending on the site of the primary tumor and the patient's lymphatic anatomy. We called these nodes the sentinel nodes, unaware that

R. S. Cabañas had previously used this term to refer to a lymph node in a fixed anatomical location adjacent to the inferior epigastric vein, which appeared to be the primary drainage node for lymphatic flow from the penis. We presented the concept of intraoperative lymphatic mapping and sentinel lymphadenectomy for patients with primary cutaneous melanoma at the 1990 meeting of the Society of Surgical Oncology. Since then, acceptance of our approaches has been rapid, and over 250 articles have been published on this subject. The sentinel node is the first lymph node on the direct lymphatic drainage pathway from the primary tumor site. It is the node most likely to receive metastatic cells from the primary tumor. The tumor status of the sentinel node thus indicates the tumor status of the nodal basin. Focused examination of the sentinel node permits more extensive sampling of nodal tissue and ultrastaging for micrometastases by sensitive immunohistochemical and molecular techniques. These techniques would not be cost-effective or practical if it were necessary to examine all nodes removed during a routine lymphadenectomy. Intraoperative lymphatic mapping with sentinel lymphadenectomy currently spares 70–80% of melanoma and breast cancer patients with negative nodes the morbidity of radical lymphadenectomy.

The international interest aroused by sentinel lymphadenectomy in recent years has been extraordinary and suggests that this very simple concept will revolutionize the management of melanoma and breast cancer. Indeed, the concept is likely to be applicable to all solid neoplasms that metastasize via the lymphatics. It is of some concern because lymphatic mapping has been accepted so quickly that there has been no comprehensive guide available to direct those who wish to accept and apply the approach. *Lymphatic Mapping and Probe Applications in Oncology* will correct that situation. O. E. Nieweg, R. Essner, D. S. Reintgen, and J. F. Thompson have compiled an excellent text that surveys the entire field of lymphatic mapping with respect to a variety of neoplasms, including melanoma, breast cancer, vulvar cancer, and penile cancer.

Although the concept is ostensibly simple, the process of mapping, definitive identification, and evaluation of the sentinel node requires the orchestrated effort of several specialists. Lymphatic mapping is a multidisciplinary undertaking, and the well-written chapters of this text consistently emphasize the importance of establishing a committed team of nuclear medicine physicians, surgeons, and pathologists who are expert in the application of their respective specialties to this technique. Much practical information is included that will be of value to multidisciplinary physician groups attempting to apply sentinel node technology in their own practices.

We owe a debt of gratitude to the editors of this comprehensive text describing the application of this new technology. Each of these internationally distinguished surgeons has made significant contributions to the field, and together the reports in their book represent the state of the art in lymphatic mapping.

However, the field continues to evolve rapidly and we believe that our progress to date only scratches the surface of a revolutionary technology that may be applicable to all solid neoplasms. We therefore look forward to the continued evolution of these approaches and to additional publications that maintain the standard of excellence achieved in this book.

Donald L. Morton
Alistair J. Cochran

Preface

Lymphatic mapping with sentinel lymphadenectomy is undoubtedly one of the most interesting developments in oncology today. Use of this minimally invasive procedure can document regional lymph node involvement with a high degree of accuracy. The concept is appealing because it is so simple and logical. In addition, it apparently is applicable to a range of neoplastic diseases, including melanoma, breast cancer, carcinoma of the vulva, carcinoma of the penis, and possibly other types of cancer as well.

The underlying hypothesis goes back a long way. The pioneering surgeon William S. Halsted (1852–1922) proposed that lymph nodes were a barrier to the spread of tumor cells, that lymphatic dissemination of neoplasms progressed in an orderly fashion, and that lymph nodes were a source of distant spread of tumor cells. Over the years ideas have changed, and during most of the latter half of the twentieth century the general opinion was the opposite. Only a few individuals had the vision and courage to challenge the widely held view that Halstedian thinking was obsolete.

R. S. Cabañas, a resident in urology at the Memorial Sloan-Kettering Cancer Center in New York, initially used the term "sentinel node." In 1977, he suggested that squamous cell carcinoma of the penis initially drained to a particular lymph node in the groin that was always in the same position. For penile cancer this appeared to make some sense, because penile cancer is always located in exactly the same part of the body, unlike melanoma or even breast cancer. Cabañas called that node the "sentinel" node.

However, it was D. L. Morton and A. J. Cochran, at the John Wayne Cancer Institute at Saint John's Health Center in Santa Monica and UCLA, respectively, who developed the concepts of *lymphatic mapping* and *selective lymph node biopsy* for melanoma. They reasoned that any node in a particular lymphatic field could be the sentinel node, depending on the location of the primary melanoma and with a certain individual variability.

It is not surprising that Morton played a key role in the inception of lymphatic mapping because he was one of the early proponents of lymphoscintigraphy, and lymphoscintigraphy is a cornerstone of lymphatic mapping. Being a melanoma surgeon, Morton was also wrestling with the question of whether or not to perform elective lymph node dissection, a controversial procedure in that disease. In retrospect, it is understandable that treatment of melanoma was the breeding ground for lymphatic mapping and that Morton was its initiator.

The original definition of a sentinel node has recently become a source of some confusion. Morton stated that a sentinel node is the initial lymph node into which the primary tumor drains. In other words, the sentinel node (first-tier node, first-echelon node) is the lymph node on the direct drainage pathway from the primary tumor. Some investigators have altered this definition and come up with their own interpretations. This is understandable, because everybody is looking at this development from his or her own background and perspective. For instance, some investigators in the field of nuclear medicine define the sentinel node as the first lymph node that becomes visible on the lymphoscintigraphy images. Although there is some truth in that definition, because the first node that lights up *is* a sentinel node, this definition does not acknowledge the fact that there may be more than just one sentinel node. Sometimes there are two lymphatic ducts draining the primary tumor, running to two different lymph nodes in the same basin. Because of a preferential flow, one node may appear on the scintigraphy images earlier than the other, but that does not mean that only the first node is a sentinel node. Tumor cells can travel through either duct and lodge in either node. There may even be more than two sentinel nodes. All these first-tier nodes should be collected by the surgeon and examined by the pathologist. Therefore, this particular definition is too narrow: too few nodes are labeled sentinel node and metastases may be missed.

Other investigators define a sentinel node as either a blue node or a radioactive node. In their opinion, every blue node or radioactive node is a sentinel node. These investigators do not acknowledge the fact that some of the tracer may pass through the first-tier lymph node and lodge in secondary nodes that are not directly at risk of harboring metastatic disease. Thus, this definition is too broad and too many nodes may be removed. In this book we adhere to Morton's original definition to avoid confusion.

Lymphatic Mapping and Probe Applications in Oncology had its inception in the work of B. A. E. Kapteijn at The Netherlands Cancer Institute. She studied various aspects of lymphatic mapping and her findings were reported in a Ph.D. thesis. Her work with its basic information was in such demand that the book was reprinted twice. The apparent interest in the subject prompted Marcel Dekker, Inc., to encourage us to produce the present volume. The feeling proved to be correct because interest in lymphatic mapping continues to grow at a rapid pace, and the number of publications on the subject is increasing exponentially. Lymphatic mapping is the hot topic at many national and international conferences in various fields of medicine. Training courses are frequently oversubscribed. Despite the lack of firm proof from randomized trials that lymphatic mapping is beneficial, one thing is now crystal clear: this development cannot be stopped! These techniques will be incorporated into routine patient care. There is a great demand for information. *Lymphatic Mapping* was produced to fill this need by providing a comprehensive review of the current state of the art.

The sentinel node is identified through elegant applications of techniques that visualize a physiological process. Chapter 1 describes the relevant microanatomy and physiology of the lymphatic system, and Chapter 2 presents the history of lymphatic mapping. Lymphatic mapping is the work of a multidisciplinary team. It cannot be overstated how important it is for the surgeon (or gynecologist or urologist) to have adequate nuclear medicine support. This is lymphatic *mapping*. The nuclear medicine physician provides the road map that guides the surgeon. Chapters 2, 3, and 9 present various aspects of lymphoscintigraphy. The surgical technique is described in Chapter 4. Important features of gamma-ray detectors are discussed in Chapter 5. The current status of knowledge of lymphatic mapping in melanoma is described in Chapter 6. The pathologist is an important member of the lymphatic mapping team, and Chapters 7 and 8 discuss the pathological evaluation of a sentinel node. Chapter 10 deals with breast cancer, Chapter 11 with carcinoma of the vulva, and Chapter 12 with carcinoma of the penis. Chapter 13 deals with radiation protection issues related to the sentinel node procedure. Chapter 14 provides practical information for doctors who intend to implement lymphatic mapping in their hospital. A gamma-ray detection probe can be used for other purposes in addition to lymphatic mapping. These applications are described in Chapters 15, 16, and 17. Practical information on lymphatic mapping can be gathered from the case reports presented in Chapter 18. Chapter 19 speculates about the future role of this procedure. All chapters were written to be understandable to all members of the team. Statements are illustrated by clinical examples where useful. We have endeavored to point out where controversy exists and to present evidence where it exists. We hope that this book will provide practical information for those who intend to include this procedure in their clinical armamentarium.

Omgo E. Nieweg
Richard Essner
Douglas S. Reintgen
John F. Thompson

Contents

Contributors

Jan G. Aalders, M.D., Ph.D. Department of Gynecologic Oncology, Groningen University Hospital, Groningen, the Netherlands

Albert Jan Arends, M.Sc. Department of Medical Physics, Catharina Hospital, Eindhoven, the Netherlands

Shmuel Avital, M.D. Department of Surgery, Tel Aviv Sourasky Medical Center, Tel Aviv, Israel

Claudia G. Berman, M.D. Department of Radiology, University of South Florida, Tampa, Florida

Paul J. Borgstein, M.D., Ph.D. Department of Surgical Oncology, Vrije Universiteit Medical Center, Amsterdam, the Netherlands

Peter Bostick, M.D. Roy E. Coats Research Laboratories, John Wayne Cancer Institute at Saint John's Health Center, Santa Monica, California

Eli Brazovsky, M.D. Department of Pathology, Tel Aviv Sourasky Medical Center, Tel Aviv, Israel

Alistair J. Cochran, M.D. Departments of Pathology, Laboratory Medicine, and Surgery, University of California at Los Angeles, Los Angeles, California

Joanne A. de Hullu, M.D.   Department of Gynecologic Oncology, Groningen University Hospital, Groningen, the Netherlands

Peter H. Dignum, B.Sc.   Department of Radiation Protection, Vrije Universiteit Medical Center, Amsterdam, the Netherlands

Richard Essner, M.D.   Department of Surgical Oncology, John Wayne Cancer Institute at Saint John's Health Center, Santa Monica, California

Gilad Gitstein, M.D.   Department of Pathology, Tel Aviv Sourasky Medical Center, Tel Aviv, Israel

Armando E. Giuliano, M.D.   Joyce Eisenberg-Keefer Breast Center and the Department of Surgical Oncology, John Wayne Cancer Institute at Saint John's Health Center, Santa Monica, California

Riad Haddad, M.D.   Department of Surgery, Tel Aviv Sourasky Medical Center, Tel Aviv, Israel

Nora M. Hansen   Joyce Eisenberg-Keefer Breast Center and the Division of Surgical Oncology, John Wayne Cancer Institute at Saint John's Health Center, Santa Monica, California

Cornelis A. Hoefnagel, M.D., Ph.D.   Department of Nuclear Medicine, The Netherlands Cancer Institute, Amsterdam, the Netherlands

Otto S. Hoekstra, M.D., Ph.D.   Department of Nuclear Medicine, Vrije Universiteit Medical Center, Amsterdam, the Netherlands

Simon Horenblas, M.D., Ph.D.   Department of Urology, The Netherlands Cancer Institute, Amsterdam, the Netherlands

Robert Howman-Giles, M.D.   Nuclear Medicine and Diagnostic Ultrasound, Missenden Medical Centre, Camperdown, New South Wales, Australia

Colleen Jaffray, M.D.   Department of Surgery, University of South Florida, Tampa, Florida

Liesbeth Jansen, M.D., Ph.D.   Department of Surgery, Gelre Hospital, Lukas Site, Apeldoorn, the Netherlands

Peter C. A. Kam, M.D.   Department of Anaesthetics, Royal Prince Alfred Hospital, Camperdown, and University of Sydney, Sydney, New South Wales, Australia

B. Acca E. Kapteijn, M.D., Ph.D.   Department of Surgery, The Netherlands Cancer Institute, Amsterdam, the Netherlands

Bin B. R. Kroon, M.D., Ph.D.   Department of Surgery, The Netherlands Cancer Institute, Amsterdam, the Netherlands

Weigno Li, M.D.   Division of Surgical Oncology, University of South Florida, Tampa, Florida

Sybren Meijer, M.D., Ph.D.   Department of Surgical Oncology, Vrije Universiteit Medical Center, Amsterdam, the Netherlands

Willem Meinhardt, M.D., Ph.D.   Department of Urology, The Netherlands Cancer Institute, Amsterdam, the Netherlands

Donald L. Morton, M.D.   Department of Surgical Oncology, John Wayne Cancer Institute at Saint John's Health Center, Santa Monica, California

Sara H. Muller, Ph.D.   Department of Nuclear Medicine, The Netherlands Cancer Institute, Amsterdam, the Netherlands

Omgo E. Nieweg, M.D., Ph.D.   Department of Surgery, The Netherlands Cancer Institute, Amsterdam, the Netherlands

James Norman, M.D.   Department of Surgery, University of South Florida, Tampa, Florida

Joseph Papo, M.D.   Department of Radiology, Tel Aviv Sourasky Medical Center, Tel Aviv, Israel

Do A. Piers, M.D., Ph.D.   Department of Nuclear Medicine, Groningen University Hospital, Groningen, the Netherlands

Rik Pijpers, M.D., Ph.D.   Department of Nuclear Medicine, Vrije Universiteit Medical Center, Amsterdam, the Netherlands

Douglas S. Reintgen, M.D.   Department of Surgery, H. Lee Moffitt Cancer Center and Research Institute, University of South Florida, Tampa, Florida

Lary A. Robinson, M.D.   Division of Cardiovascular and Thoracic Surgery, H. Lee Moffitt Cancer Center and Research Institute, University of South Florida College of Medicine, Tampa, Florida

D. Michael Rose, M.D.   Department of Surgical Oncology, John Wayne Cancer Institute at Saint John's Health Center, Santa Monica, California

Emiel J. Th. Rutgers, M.D., Ph.D.   Department of Surgery, the Netherlands Cancer Institute and Antoni Van Leeuwenhoek Hospital, Amsterdam, the Netherlands

Tatiana B. Sazonova-Tiourina, M.Sc.   Department of Radiotherapy, Catharina Hospital, Eindhoven, the Netherlands

Schlomo Schneebaum, M.D.   Radioguided Surgery Unit, Department of Surgery, Tel Aviv Sourasky Medical Center, Tel Aviv, Israel

Heimen Schraffordt Koops, M.D., Ph.D.   Department of Surgical Oncology, Groningen University Hospital, Groningen, the Netherlands

Steven Shiver   Department of Surgery, University of South Florida, Tampa, Florida

Yehuda Skornick, M.D.   Department of Surgery, Tel Aviv Sourasky Medical Center, Tel Aviv, Israel

Stacey Stern, M.S.   Statistical Coordinating Unit, John Wayne Cancer Institute at Saint John's Health Center, Santa Monica, California

Gerrit J. J. Teule, M.D., Ph.D.   Department of Nuclear Medicine, Vrije Universiteit Medical Center, Amsterdam, the Netherlands

John F. Thompson, M.D.   Sydney Melanoma Unit, Sydney Cancer Centre, Royal Prince Alfred Hospital, Camperdown, and Department of Surgery, University of Sydney, Sydney, New South Wales, Australia

Anton Troitsa, M.D.   Department of Surgery, Tel Aviv Sourasky Medical Center, Tel Aviv, Israel

Roger F. Uren, M.D.   Department of Nuclear Medicine, University of Sydney, Camperdown, Sydney, New South Wales, Australia

Renato A. Valdés Olmos, M.D., Ph.D. Department of Nuclear Medicine, The Netherlands Cancer Institute, Amsterdam, the Netherlands

Ate G. J. van der Zee, M.D., Ph.D. Department of Gynecologic Oncology, Groningen University Hospital, Groningen, the Netherlands

Arthur van Lingen, M.D., Ph.D. Department of Nuclear Medicine, Vrije Universiteit Medical Center, Amsterdam, the Netherlands

Xiangning Wang, M.D. Department of Surgery, University of South Florida, Tampa, Florida

Duan-Ren Wen, M.D. Departments of Pathology and Laboratory Medicine, University of California at Los Angeles, Los Angeles, California

Microanatomy and Physiology of the Lymphatic System

Peter C. A. Kam and John F. Thompson
Royal Prince Alfred Hospital, Camperdown, and University of Sydney, Sydney, New South Wales, Australia

Roger F. Uren
University of Sydney, Sydney, New South Wales, Australia

INTRODUCTION

It is essential for nuclear medicine physicians, pathologists, and the various specialists who perform operations to have a sound knowledge of the anatomy and physiology of the body regions with which they concern themselves. Imaging and surgery of the lymphatic ducts and lymph nodes thus require a thorough understanding of the lymphatic system. This system is essentially a complex network of channels which drain fluids and proteins from the interstitial spaces of the body's organs and tissues, and an immunological control system involving peripheral lymph nodes and circulating lymphocytes. Lymphatics return the capillary ultrafiltrate and proteins together with bacteria, fat micelles, and immune cells into the general circulation via veins in the neck. Some ultrafiltrate is reabsorbed by the vascular system of lymph nodes. Overall total body lymph flow at rest is approximately 2–4 L/day, but there are large variations in the lymphatic flow within different organs [1]. The purpose of this chapter is to review the anatomy and physiology of the lymphatic system. The lymphatics of body parts that are subject to sentinel lymph node exploration are discussed in detail.

MICROANATOMY OF THE LYMPHATIC SYSTEM

Although there are remarkable similarities in the lymphatic microanatomy within different organs, there are also some essential differences [2]. This review will deal with the common ultrastructural features first and then examine the differences between organs. The lymphatic system (Fig. 1) begins as a network of blind ending capillaries which absorb lymph from the interstitial spaces. These capillaries are called *initial lymphatics* and are also known in the literature as *prelymphatics, lymphatic capillaries*, or *terminal lymphatics* [2,3]. The initial lymphatics then form the *lymphatic collecting vessels* (also known as the *lymphatic collectors, collecting ducts*, or *conducting lymphatics*). These lymphatic collecting vessels in turn feed into *afferent lymph trunks*. Lymph nodes are lo-

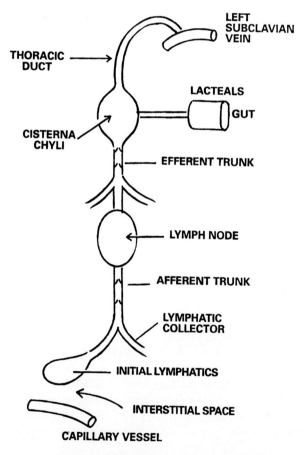

FIGURE 1 Principal elements of the lymphatic system.

cated along the lymphatic system so that one or several afferent lymphatic collecting vessels drain into a node, and the efferent lymphatic collecting vessels leave the nodes and drain toward *major (large central) lymphatic trunks* which transport the lymphatic fluid into large veins in the neck. The lymphatic collectors drain into local or sometimes remote lymph nodes which are arranged in regional groups. Nodes within a regional group are often interconnected. Lymph from most parts of the body finally drains into the venous circulation via the *thoracic duct*, at the junction of the left subclavian and jugular veins. In general, lymph passes through a series of lymph nodes before reaching a major collecting duct. The exceptions to this general arrangement are the lymph vessels of the thyroid gland, the esophagus, and the coronary and triangular ligaments of the liver, which drain directly to the thoracic duct without passing through lymph nodes. The flow rate in the large lymphatic conduits, including the thoracic duct, is approximately 1–3 mL/min. Numerous valves are present along the lymphatic collecting vessels and trunks, and they aid in directing lymphatic drainage from the periphery toward the subclavian vein.

The initial lymphatics exist either as blind terminal sacs or as an anastomosing network of lymphatic capillaries 10–50 μm in diameter in the interstitial space, in close relationship to the blood capillaries and small venules. These are sometimes connected to irregular-shaped sinusoids which have no basement membrane.

The walls of the initial lymphatics are made up of a single layer of endothelial cells with a discontinuous basement membrane, tethered to the surrounding connective tissue by collagen filaments (Fig. 2). Each lymphatic endothelial cell

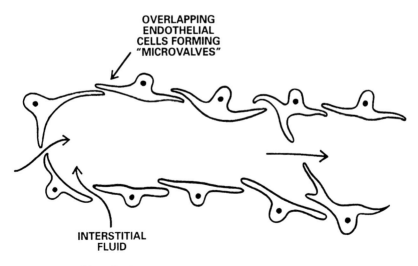

FIGURE 2   Initial lymphatics.

is very thin, measuring 0.1 μm or less at its edge where it meets the adjacent cell and thickens only in the perinuclear area to measure 2–4 μm. It characteristically has sparse rough endoplasmic reticulum scattered throughout the cytoplasm. It also contains fine contractile filaments (40–60 Å in diameter) in the cytoplasm, lying parallel to the long axis of the cell.

The interendothelial junctions are approximately 10–25 nm wide, rendering the initial lymphatics highly permeable to plasma proteins and particulate material though occasionally gaps of several micrometers are present between cells. The overlapping junctions run obliquely and therefore function like flap valves, allowing the entry of fluid but closing when the intraluminal pressure increases above interstitial pressure. There is bulk flow of fluid, proteins, macromolecules, and other substances through these interendothelial junctions into the lumen of the initial lymphatics. Plasma membrane invaginations are present on both the luminal and abluminal surfaces of the endothelial cells, suggesting that pinocytosis may be responsible for vesicular transport of particles larger than 30 nm across the lymphatic endothelium.

The anchoring filaments are microfibrils approximately 8 nm in diameter. They are attached to the walls of the initial lymphatics at one end and to collagen fibers in the interstitium at the other end (Fig. 3). These filaments pull the endothelial walls of the initial lymphatics apart as the matrix of the interstitial space swells with increased interstitial fluid volume.

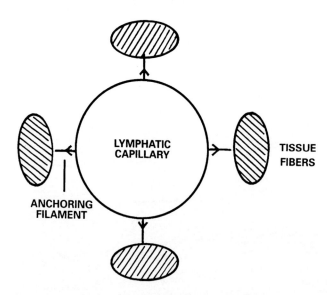

FIGURE 3   Anchoring filaments of initial lymphatics.

Thus, the microanatomy of the initial lymphatics allows the endothelial lining to function as a microvalve system between the interstitium and itself. As the anchoring filaments prevent the collapse of the initial lymphatics, large interendothelial gaps open between the overlapping junctions, allowing the entry of interstitial fluid, cells, bacteria, and solid particles. When the luminal lymphatic pressure is higher than the interstitial pressure, an apposition of the overlapping margins of the endothelial cell results, thereby closing the interendothelial junction and preventing leakage of lymph into the interstitial space. The lymphatic collecting vessels are similar to the initial lymphatics with respect to the structure of their endothelium but, in addition, have bicuspid semilunar valves which promote lymphatic flow toward the central lymphatics and prevent the backflow of lymph. The valves are made up of thin collagen sheets between two endothelial layers. Thus, the valves are funnel shaped and can operate at very low flow rates irrespective of the size or shape of the lumen of the lymphatics. Viscous fluid stresses appear to be the main physical factor influencing the functional status of the valves. The intervalvular distance is 1–3 mm in the small lymphatics and increases to 6–12 mm in the larger lymphatics. There are approximately 30–35 valves in the thoracic duct, where the intervalvular distance is about 12–15 mm.

The walls of the lymphatic collecting vessels consist of an intima lined by endothelial cells and a basement membrane, a media with longitudinal and circular layers of smooth muscle, and an adventitia with connective and elastic fibers, fibroblasts, and nerve endings (Fig. 4). The collecting lymphatics form a series of discrete contractile units, each separated from the next by a valve. Each unit or compartment between two consecutive valves forms a lymphatic ''microheart'' called a *lymphangion*. The lymphangion is the basic functional unit of the lymphatic system, and its length varies between 6 and 20 mm in different organs.

Spontaneous peristalsis of about 10 contractions per minute occurs in lymphangions, producing synchronized opening and closing of the valves which prevent reflux of fluid. The contractility of lymphangions is regulated by their filling pressures, humoral mediators, and neural mechanisms. As the intraluminal pressure increases, the frequency of the peristaltic contractions increases, indicating a myogenic autoregulation. Alpha-adrenergic stimulation due to sympathetic activity increases the rate and force of contractions of lymphangions. Serotonin (5-hydroxytryptamine) is a potent stimulator of lymphatic contractions. Prostaglandins E_1, E_2, and I_2 inhibit lymphatic motility. Anesthetic agents also inhibit the intrinsic contractility of the lymphatic vessels. It has been shown, for example, that halothane decreases the rate of lymph flow by 25–59% [2].

The walls of the major lymphatic trunks essentially have a structure similar to that of lymphatic collectors but with a thicker muscle layer and abundant elastic fibers in the media, and more nerve endings in the adventitia. They contain valves

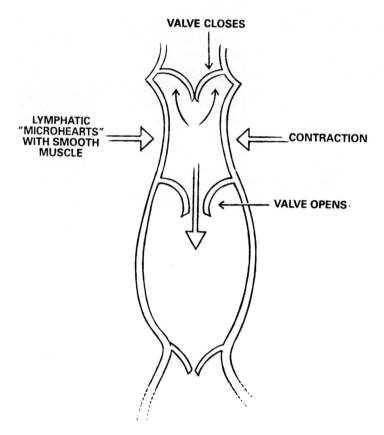

Figure 4   Lymphatic collectors.

which are essential for the forward flow of lymph fluid and for preventing the generation of high hydrostatic forces due to gravity. The intervalvular distance is approximately 6–10 cm. The lymphatic pressures can vary from less than 25 mmHg in the absence of lymphatic obstruction to over 100 mmHg during obstruction.

Large lymphatic conduits from the lower limbs and the abdominal viscera converge, and the lymph (now known as chyle) flows into a large saccular dilatation of the lymphatic trunk called the *cisterna chyli*. This acts as a temporary reservoir for chyle, which then passes onward in the *thoracic duct*. The thoracic duct receives about 75% of the body's lymph and drains into the left subclavian vein at its junction with the jugular vein.

LYMPHATIC SYSTEMS IN DIFFERENT ORGANS AND TISSUES

There is considerable variability in the lymphatic network within different organs. The deep lymphatic trunks usually accompany arteries and veins and almost all reach the thoracic duct. However, additional entry points into the venous system through the inferior vena cava and the renal, suprarenal, azygous, and iliac veins have been reported but are likely to be variable. The brain and the eye lack a conventional lymphatic system.

Skin

Studies of the microlymphatics of the skin have shown a widespread subepithelial network (Fig. 5) [2,4]. A superficial subpapillary layer of prelymphatic capillaries (initial lymphatics) forms a closely interconnected hexagonal network. These initial lymphatics are connected to deeper layers of lymphatic capillaries in the dermis, and lymph is then transported centrally through subcutaneous lymphatic collecting vessels. The subdermal lymphatics communicate with those below the deep fascia [4]. With increased depth, the lymphatic channels become larger, but the density of the network is reduced. The epidermal lymphatics lack intraluminal valves, but the deeper lymphatic collecting vessels and trunks have valves. The lymphatic endothelium in the cutaneous tissue is extremely thin and lacks interen-

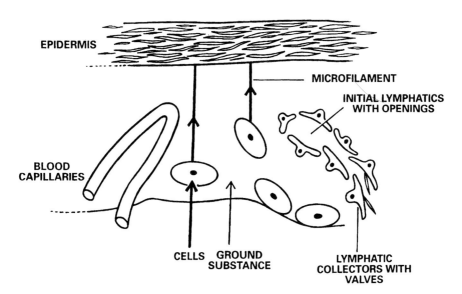

FIGURE 5 Diagrammatic representation of microlymphatics of skin.

dothelial junctions, but has macroscopic openings. There is a large variability in cutaneous lymph flow rates reported. The rate of cutaneous lymph flow as measured by an intradermal injection of radioactively labeled colloids is influenced by the properties of the injected colloid, the site of injection, the vascularity of the underlying tissues, and muscle movement of the part of the body. Using technetium-99m-labeled antimony sulfide colloid (^{99m}Tc–antimony trisulfide, ^{99m}Tc–Sb$_2$S$_3$) [5], the cutaneous lymph flow rates are highest at the periphery of the limbs and slowest in the head and neck regions and the proximal limbs. The mean flow rate of cutaneous lymph flow is 1.5 cm/min in the head and neck region, 2 cm/min in the shoulder, 2.8 cm/min in the anterior trunk, 3.9 cm/min in the posterior trunk, 4.2 cm/min in the thigh, 5.5 cm/min in the forearm and hand, and 10.2 cm/min in the leg or foot.

Kidneys

The kidney has an extensive cortical network of initial lymphatics distributed along blood vessels, tubules, and Bowman's capsule. The lymphatics originate in the cortex and under the renal capsule and drain into interlobular lymphatics, which, in turn, empty into the hilar lymphatic network [2] and these end in the lateral aortic nodes. A third plexus of lymphatic vessels is present in the perirenal fat and drain directly to the lateral aortic nodes.

Small Intestine

The microlymphatics of the small intestine consist of three layers of lymphatics that are located in the villi, the submucosa, and the smooth muscle surrounding the submucosa (Fig. 6) [2,6]. Each villus has a lymphatic ending called a *lacteal*. The lacteals fuse at the base of the villi to form the submucosal network of lymphatics, which has dense interconnection but lacks valves. The lacteals and the submucosal lymphatics lack smooth muscle and therefore cannot contract spontaneously.

The lymphatics in the smooth-muscle layer form a densely interconnected network which is not directly connected to the mucosal and submucosal lymphatic networks. The network of lymphatics in the muscle also has no functional valves. The mucosal, submucosal, and muscular layer lymphatic networks merge to form large collecting lymphatics near the mesenteric border of the intestine. At this site, intrinsic lymphatic contractions may be observed and the first lymphatic valves can be identified. The lymph drains into lymphatic conduits running through the mesentery. These, in turn, empty into the main mesenteric lymph ducts, which are contractile and possess valves to prevent reflux. They are frequently paired with the mesenteric artery and vein.

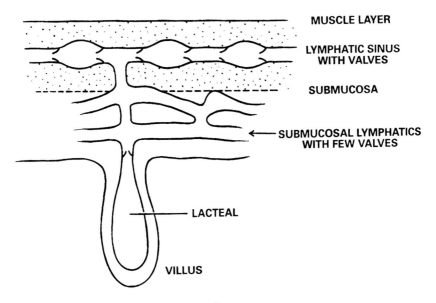

MUSCLE LAYER

LYMPHATIC SINUS
WITH VALVES

SUBMUCOSA

SUBMUCOSAL LYMPHATICS
WITH FEW VALVES

LACTEAL

VILLUS

FIGURE 6 Lymphatic network in the small intestine.

Large Intestine

In the large intestine, lymph vessels begin as minute subepithelial blind sacs which open into a periglandular plexus [7]. From the periglandular plexus, vessels pierce the muscularis mucosae to join a submucosal plexus. Efferents from the submucosal plexus traverse the muscularis and drain into a plexus between the longitudinal and circular layers. Collecting vessels leave the large intestine through the muscle and enter the large lymphatic vessels which follow the mesenteric arteries. Lymphatic vessels from the root of the appendix and the cecum pass anteriorly to the anterior ileocolic nodes and ileocolic nodes, and posteriorly to the posterior and inferior ileocolic nodes.

Lymphatic vessels of the ascending and transverse colon drain into lymph nodes along the right and middle colic arteries and their branches and end in the superior mesenteric nodes. Those of the descending and sigmoid colon drain into small nodes along the left colic arteries and end in the pre-aortic nodes near the origin of the inferior mesenteric artery.

Lymphatic vessels from the wall of the upper half of the rectum ascend with the superior rectal vessels through the pararectal nodes to nodes in the lower sigmoid mesocolon and along the inferior mesenteric artery. From the lower half of the rectum and the anal canal above the mucocutaneous junction, lymph vessels follow the middle rectal vessels to the internal iliac nodes, although some may accompany the inferior rectal and internal pudendal vessels. Lymphatics from the anal canal below the mucocutaneous junction descend to the anal margin and drain into the medial superficial inguinal nodes.

Reproductive Organs

In the male, testicular lymphatic vessels begin as a superficial plexus under the tunica vaginalis, and as a deep plexus within the substance of the testis and the epididymis [7]. These drain into four to eight collecting lymphatics which ascend in the spermatic cord and end in the lateral aortic and pre-aortic nodes. Collecting lymphatic vessels from the ductus deferens end in the external iliac nodes, whereas those from the seminal vesicles drain into both the internal and external iliac nodes. The lymphatic channels from the prostate drain into the internal iliac and sacral nodes. The skin of the scrotum and penis is drained by lymphatic vessels which follow the external pudendal blood vessels to the superficial inguinal nodes. Lymphatic vessels from the tissue inside the glans penis drain into the deep inguinal and external iliac nodes, whereas those from the erectile tissue and the penile urethra pass into the internal iliac lymph nodes.

In the female, lymphatic vessels from the ovary ascend along the ovarian artery to the lateral aortic and pre-aortic lymph nodes. Lymphatic vessels in the uterus are present in the subperitoneal area and deep in the uterine wall. Lymphatic vessels from the upper part of the body, the fundus, and the uterine tubes drain mainly to the lateral aortic and pre-aortic nodes with a few passing to the external iliac nodes. The vessels from the isthmus of the uterus follow the round ligament and drain into the superficial inguinal nodes. Collecting vessels from the cervix pass laterally in the parametrium to the external iliac nodes, posterolaterally to the internal iliac nodes and posteriorly along the sacrogenital fold to the rectal and sacral nodes. The vessels from the upper vagina accompany the uterine artery to the internal and external iliac nodes, and those from the intermediate part of the vagina drain into the internal iliac nodes. Lymph from the lower vagina below the hymen, the vulva, and the perineal skin pass to the superficial inguinal nodes, and those from the clitoris and the labia minora drain into the deep inguinal nodes. Some efferent lymphatic collecting vessels from the clitoris may directly drain into the internal iliac nodes.

Lungs

There are two sets of pulmonary lymphatics [2]: one set located in the connective tissue of the pleura and the other in the connective tissue surrounding the airways and blood vessels, called the peribronchovascular lymphatics. The pleural lymphatic network consists of initial lymphatics, from which collecting lymphatics drain into a system of caudal nodes. The peribronchovascular lymphatics begin as blind sacs within the connective tissue of terminal bronchioles and pulmonary arterioles. Expansion of the lungs reduces the overlap of their endothelial cells. Fluid in the pleural spaces also drains into an extensive network of lymphatics in the parietal pleura and the diaphragm. The lateral parietal lymphatics are located over the intercostal spaces but not over the ribs. The lymphatic vessels of the parietal pleura end in three ways: those in the costal region join the vessels of the internal intercostal muscles to reach the parasternal nodes; those of the diaphragmatic pleura form a plexus on the thoracic surface; and those of the mediastinal pleura end in the posterior mediastinal nodes [7].

Breast

The lymphatic vessels of the mammary gland start in a plexus in the connective tissue and the walls of the lactiferous ducts which communicates with the cutaneous subareolar plexus (of Sappey) around the nipple [7]. A plexus of minute vessels is present on the subjacent deep fascia, but this is not important in normal lymphatic drainage. Lymph from tissue at the lateral quadrants of the breast tends to drain to the axilla, and lymph from the medial quadrants drains to the internal mammary nodes. The efferent vessels from the gland pass around to the anterior axillary border through the axillary fascia to the pectoral lymph nodes. Some vessels may pass directly to the subscapular nodes. Lymphatic vessels from the superior region of the mammary gland pass into the supraclavicular, infraclavicular, or axillary nodes. The axillary nodes receive more than 75% of lymph from the gland. The remainder of the lymph from the mammary gland, especially that from the medial parts of the gland, drain into the internal mammary lymph node chain via lymphatic vessels which accompany the perforating branches of the internal thoracic artery. Occasionally, lymphatic vessels follow the lateral cutaneous branches of the posterior intercostal arteries to the intercostal nodes. The axillary nodes are grouped as the lower or level I nodes (those lying below pectoralis minor), middle or level II nodes (those behind pectoralis minor), and apical (upper) or level III nodes (those between pectoralis minor and the lower border of the clavicle). Drainage to the nodes in the axilla tend to occur first to level I nodes, but direct drainage to level II or III nodes is not uncommon. There may be one or two nodes between the pectoralis major and minor and these are called Rotter's nodes.

LYMPH NODES

The lymph nodes are small, bean-shaped masses of tissue found at variable intervals along the lymphatic system. They contain maturing lymphocytes in germinal centers with many phagocytic cells and are enclosed in a capsule. The main function of the lymph node is to filter the lymph and act as a germinal center for immune responses. Several afferent lymphatic ducts enter each lymph node

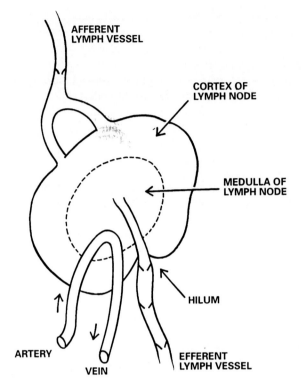

FIGURE 7 The lymph node as a filtration unit.

via its cortex (see Fig. 7). The lymph then flows through sinuses lined by endothelial cells within the lymph node [3]. Lymphocytes are released into the sinuses if the perfusing lymph contains a foreign antigen. Each lymph node is supplied by a network of continuous capillaries which drain into specialized endothelial venules. Lymphocytes in blood can reenter the lymph node via the intercellular spaces between the endothelial venules. The efferent lymph vessels leave the node via the hilum. Within the medulla of the lymph node, mass transfer occurs between the lymph and blood.

PHYSIOLOGY OF LYMPH FORMATION

Lymph formation, which is essentially the filling of the lymphatic capillaries (initial lymphatics), is the main determinant of lymph flow. Once lymphatic fluid enters the lymphatic collecting vessels, it is propelled along either by active contractions or external forces, and flow is unidirectional.

The rate of movement of fluid and protein out of blood passing through capillaries (see Fig. 8) into the interstitial space [1–3] can be summarized by

$$V_c = K_c \left[(P_c - P_T) - R_p (\Pi_c - \Pi_T) \right]$$

where V_c is the volume of the capillary filtrate, K_c is the filtration coefficient, P_c is the capillary hydrostatic pressure, P_T is the interstitial fluid hydrostatic pressure, R_p is the reflection coefficient of plasma protein, Π_c is the oncotic pressure of plasma protein, and Π_T is the oncotic pressure of interstitial fluid. As a result of imbalance between transcapillary hydrostatic and oncotic forces, a driving pres-

BLOOD CAPILLARY

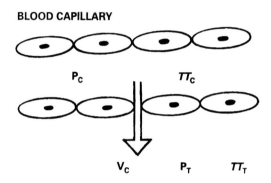

INTERSTITIUM

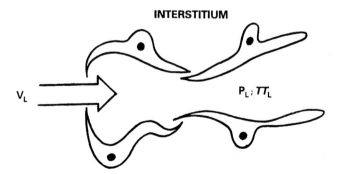

FIGURE 8 Blood capillary forces and lymph formation. V_c is the net volume of fluid out of the capillary; P_c is the capillary hydrostatic pressure; Π_c is the oncotic pressure of plasma protein; P_T is the interstitial fluid hydrostatic pressure; Π_T is the oncotic pressure of interstitial fluid; V_L is the net volume of fluid entering the initial lymphatics; P_L is the hydrostatic pressure of the initial lymphatics; Π_L is the oncotic pressure of the lymphatic fluid.

sure occurs and produces a continuous leakage of fluid from the capillary into the interstitium. This is usually balanced by an equal outflow of fluid from the interstitial space via the lymphatics.

In addition, there is protein movement across the capillary wall caused by bulk flow and diffusion. The transport of large molecules from plasma to lymph depends on their molecular size rather than their molecular weight.

Several mechanisms have been proposed to explain the entry of interstitial fluid into the initial lymphatics [2,3,8]. The most widely held view is that the overlapping interendothelial junctions of the initial lymphatic (lymphatic capillaries) act as valves and promote unidirectional movement of fluid from the interstitial space into the lumen of the lymphatics. The innermost overlapping edges are able to flap back and forth and hence act as flap valves. When the initial lymphatics are compressed by the surrounding tissues, by arterial pulsations or by the action of an active lymphatic pump, the flaplike edges of the endothelial cells are apposed and the contents of the initial lymphatics are squeezed forward (Fig. 9). As the initial lymphatics recoil following compression, the intraluminal pressure falls and the flaps open, promoting filling of the lymphatics. The anchoring filaments may pull on the endothelial cells as a result of recoil of the surrounding tissue, setting up a pressure difference across the lymphatic wall sufficient to remove fluid from the interstitial space.

Another mechanism proposed to explain the filling of initial lymphatics is the osmotic pressure theory (Fig. 10). The protein concentration in the initial lymphatics is about two to three times that in the interstitial space. This produces an inward osmotic pressure gradient which tends to move fluid into the initial lymphatics.

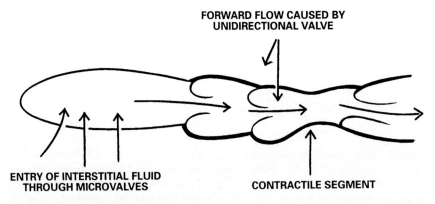

**FORWARD FLOW CAUSED BY
UNIDIRECTIONAL VALVE**

**ENTRY OF INTERSTITIAL FLUID
THROUGH MICROVALVES**

CONTRACTILE SEGMENT

Figure 9   Suction forces aiding lymphatic absorption.

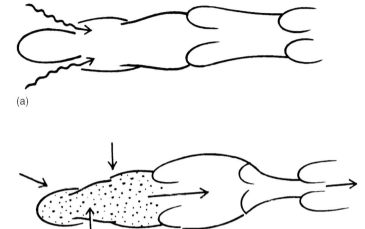

(a)

(b)

FɪɢᴜʀᴇE 10   Osmotic theory of lymphatic absorption: (a) at rest; (b) during tissue compression.

Observations of lymphatic flow patterns in the wing membranes of bats suggest that intraluminal pressures in the initial lymphatics fluctuate due to wall contractions and forward flow of lymph. The intraluminal pressures are negative or are tending toward negative values. The presence of lymphatic valves upstream ensures that retrograde flow does not interfere with the "suction" process.

PROPULSION OF LYMPH

Lymph is moved along the collecting lymphatics to transport lymph ultimately to the left subclavian vein. In their excellent review, Aukland and Reed [1] summarized the important intrinsic and extrinsic factors involved in the propulsion of lymph through lymphatic channels.

Intrinsic rhythmic contractions at a rate of 10–15/min occur in lymph vessels with smooth muscle in their walls, especially in the lower limbs and the thoracic duct. A transmural distending pressure of 2–4 cm H_2O is required to initiate contractions of the lymphangion, the basic functional contractile unit of the lymphatic system. Under normal conditions, the contractions of the lymphangion increase intraluminal pressure by 1–2 mmHg, but this may vary in different regions of the body. Pulse pressures of 20 mmHg have been measured in mesenteric lymphatic channels, and even greater intraluminal pressures of 60–120 mmHg have been recorded in obstructed lymphatics in human legs [2,9].

The lymphangion is known as a lymphatic "microheart" because, like the heart, it has a pacemaker, filling and ejection actions, and contractility which is dependent on extracellular calcium ion concentration and on sympathetic innervation (in the larger vessels). Spontaneous contractions of the collecting lymphatics result from a myogenic pacemaker [2,3,8,9], which is located in the circular muscle layer of each lymphangion immediately downstream from each valve. The contraction spreads at a velocity of 4–5 mm/s within a lymphangion. The contraction of each lymphangion occurs in four phases: a short isometric contraction phase, an ejection phase, a short isometric relaxation phase, and a filling phase. The frequency of contraction and stroke volume of the lymphangion increases as it becomes distended. Catecholamines, in physiological concentrations, increase the frequency and amplitude of spontaneous contractions. β-Agonists (e.g., isoprenaline) reduce both the frequency and strength of spontaneous contractions. Serotonin (5-hydroxytryptamine) increases the basal tone of the lymphangions and increases the amplitude of contractions at higher concentrations. Bradykinin can increase lymph flow as a secondary effect of increasing capillary permeability and interstitial fluid formation. Prostaglandin A_2, B_2, and F_2, thromboxane A_2, and leukotrienes B_4, C_4, and D_4 all increase the frequency and strength of contractions of lymphangions. However, prostaglandins E_1, E_2, and I_2 inhibit lymphatic motility. Calcium ions are important for the control of the pacemaker of the lymphangion and the propagation of the impulse. Acetylcholine enhances contraction, whereas caffeine and anaesthetic agents depress contractions.

Intermittent external pressure on lymphatic channels enhances unidirectional flow within them, whereas sustained external pressure reduces it. Several studies have shown that lymph flow may be increased by active and passive movements of the limbs, massage, gastrointestinal peristalsis, respiratory movements, and transmitted arterial pulsations. Experiments in dogs suggest that passive movements of the limbs increase lymph flow from the skin and connective tissue to a greater extent than muscle lymph flow. Passive movement does not appear to increase the capillary filtration rate [2,10].

In active limb movements, muscle contraction compresses the collecting lymphatics intermittently to produce a rise in lymph pressure. This may facilitate lymph flow in the larger lymphatics, as the valves in the lymphatic channels allow the lymph pressure to rise in a stepwise fashion in successive segments. There is also some evidence that active muscle contractions can cause a rise in net capillary filtration. To what extent muscle contractions facilitate the filling of the initial lymphatics is unknown.

External massage of the drainage area for lymph vessels causes an immediate increase of lymph flow. Experiments suggest that this is due to the propulsion of tissue fluid into the lymphatics [10]. This knowledge may be applied in lymphatic mapping to encourage the flow of the tracer.

Contraction of intestinal smooth muscle during peristalsis has been shown to propel lymph into the lymphatic channels within the mucosal and muscular layers of the small intestine, in spite of the sparse number of valves. Intestinal peristalsis also propels lymph along the mesenteric lymphatic ducts [2,10,11].

Respiratory movements cause intermittent changes in the intrathoracic and intra-abdominal pressures. These pressure changes propel lymph from the lymphatics in the abdomen and also along the thoracic duct. The increase in intra-abdominal pressure, which occurs during coughing or straining, can also increase the propulsion of lymph through the effects of pressure on the cisterna chyli.

PRESSURE, RESISTANCE, AND FLOW IN PERIPHERAL LYMPHATICS

There are considerable variations in the intralymphatic pressures which have been reported, apparently due to differences in methodology. The pressures in the pre-nodal lymphatics depend on the intrinsic contractility of lymphangion and active or passive movements of neighboring muscles (Table 1). Unlike the venous system, hydrostatic pressures are not important in affecting peripheral lymphatic pressures. The pressure in the collecting lymphatics of the leg ranges between 0 and 5 mmHg during the diastolic phase of the lymphangions, whether the leg is erect or supine. During the systolic phase, the mean pressure can reach 50 mmHg and increase to over 100 mmHg if there is any obstruction [10,11].

The resistance to lymph flow in the large lymphatic trunks such as the thoracic duct is low (0.13–0.99 mmHg min/mL in dogs). Resistance in lymph nodes appears to be 50–200 times higher than lymph trunk resistance. Lymph node resistance is reduced by increased inflow pressure and perfusion. Increased pressure in the veins draining a lymph node increases the lymph node resistance to lymph flow.

TABLE 1 Pressure (mmHg) in Peripheral Lymph Vessels

Species	Site	Resting pressure	During intrinsic contractions	During muscle movement
Man	Leg	0–3	25–50	No direct effect
	Foot	8–16	?	?
Dog	Femoral	1–6.5	?	4–33
Guinea pig	Mesenteric	3–15	12–30	

Postnodal lymph flow in the human thoracic duct is approximately 1–3 L/day. The liver contributes 30–50% of this total volume, mainly because the basement membrane of the hepatic capillaries is fenestrated. Intestinal lymph flow is the second greatest contributor to total thoracic duct flow, and this increases with meals. The limbs contribute less than 10% of total lymph flow, their contribution being largely dependent on active and passive movements of the limbs.

There is a marked diurnal variation in lymph output in man [8,9]. During the night, lymph flow is low and the concentrations of protein and enzymes in the lymph are high. Lymph flow can be increased by 83% during muscle contraction seen with ergometer cycling, and by 117% by immersion in a warm-water foot bath [8]. There is an inverse relationship between lymph flow rate and lymph protein concentration. Venous stasis can decrease lymph flow by approximately 50%.

COMPOSITION OF LYMPH

The initial lymphatics appear to permit equilibration of plasma proteins between interstitial fluid and lymph. There is little leakage of proteins from the collecting ducts, as the endothelium lacks open junctions. Under normal conditions, there is little loss of proteins in lymph nodes, but progressive loss of protein by exudation into perinodal tissue can occur if the efferent lymphatic pressure is greater than 8 mmHg. The concentration of protein in lymph varies from region to region due to the variability of the permeability and reflection coefficient of the exchange vessels [11] (Table 2). Lymph from the liver is particularly rich in protein.

Most of the protein in lymph is derived from plasma proteins by filtration, diffusion, and vesicular transport [9]. Studies indicate that lymph contains all the protein fractions of plasma but at a lower concentration and with a higher percentage contributed by lower–molecular-weight proteins. A small contribution of

TABLE 2 Lymph Flow and Composition in Man

Site	Flow (L/day)	Lymph-to-plasma protein ratio
Thoracic duct	1–3	0.66–0.69
Liver	0.3–1	0.66–0.89
GI tract	0.4–1.2	0.50–0.6
Kidney	0.1–0.3	0.47
Limbs	<0.1	0.2–0.5

TABLE 3 Proteins in Human Lymph

Site	Protein	Amount (g/L)	Lymph-to-serum ratio
Thoracic duct	Total	35–48	0.5–0.69
	Albumin	21–34	0.56–0.82
Liver	Total	34–87	0.57
	Albumin	29–42	0.9
Leg	Total	34	0.4
	Albumin	16	0.4

lymphatic proteins may be derived from protein synthesis in tissues. A large proportion of the immunoglobin G (IgG) found in the lymph in the small intestine is derived from the absorption of ingested IgG. The protein concentration of the lymph of the liver is lower than in the serum of liver venous blood, suggesting that newly synthesized protein is released into the blood circulation rather than into the lymph (Table 3).

The lipids in lymph and plasma consist of triglycerides, phospholipids, cholesterol esters, fatty acids, and free cholesterol. Lipid concentrations change markedly after meals. The lipid content of intestinal and liver lymph is much higher than in other lymph. Lymph–serum lipid ratios are similar for most organs but are much higher for liver and intestinal lymph.

Enzymes normally present in plasma are also present in lymph, but generally at lower concentrations than in plasma. The activity of an enzyme in the lymph reflects that in plasma but is also dependent on capillary pressure, the microstructure of the capillary, the molecular size of the enzyme, and the rate of lymph flow from the particular tissue (Table 4). Other substances carried in

TABLE 4 Enzymes in Lymph

Enzyme	Source of lymph	Concentration	Lymph-to-serum ratio
Acid phosphatase	Thoracic duct	0.5 mmol/mL	0.5
	Leg	3.69 mmol/mL	0.57
Aldolase	Thoracic duct	10 mmol/mL	1.66
Alkaline phosphatase	Thoracic duct	1.3–1.9 mmol/mL	0.6–0.8
	Leg	2.76 mmol/mL	0.43
Amylase	Thoracic duct	262 mmol/mL	0.83
Glutamic pyruvic transaminase	Thoracic duct	2 mmol/mL	0.65
Lactic dehydrogenase	Thoracic duct	27 mmol/mL	0.77
Lipase	Thoracic duct	1.6 mg/dL	0.84

low concentrations in lymph compared to serum include hormones and coagulation factors.

The great majority of cells in human peripheral lymph are lymphocytes. In one study, 83% of the cells were small and medium-sized lymphocytes [10,11]; approximately 50% of these were T cells, 10% were B cells, and 6% were phagocytes. There were 0.9% neutrophils, 0.2% eosinophils, and 15% erythrocytes.

REMOVAL OF PARTICULATE MATTER BY LYMPHATICS

Several pathways through the walls of the initial lymphatics (lymphatic capillaries) have been identified. These include pores through the plasma membrane, vesicles, fenestrations of the basement membrane, and interendothelial junctions. The open junctions are the most important pathways in the walls of the initial lymphatics and are most numerous in the lymphatics of the intestine and peritoneal surface of the diaphragm. Vesicular transport across the endothelial cells can occur, but it is limited and slow [2,12].

The uptake of colloidal particles occurs through two pathways [12]: across the endothelium within vesicles and through intercellular clefts or junctions. After an intradermal injection, the transfer of particles across the lymphatic endothelium occurs within a few seconds, as shown by their presence within vesicles in the cytoplasm and invaginations along the endothelial surface. Although vesicular transport is responsible for much of the transport of particles across the lymphatic endothelium, the endothelial cells can retain large amounts of the particles. As the intercellular clefts are continuous with the adjoining tissues, an uninterrupted channel is present between the lymphatic lumen and the interstitial space. Colloidal marker particles (such as ferritin, thorium, carbon, and latex spheres) can be seen within the intercellular clefts within the first few minutes following an intradermal injection.

Lymph from most tissues passes through one or more lymph nodes in its passage from the interstitial space to the bloodstream, although there may be a few exceptions. The lymph node filters the lymph and extracts particulate antigens and aging cells by phagocytosis. When colloidal carbon particles are injected intramuscularly, they travel rapidly in the lymphatics as free-carbon particles to the regional lymph nodes. In the lymph nodes, the carbon particles are phagocytosed and stored by macrophages. A small proportion of the particles are phagocytosed by the lymphatic endothelial cells. Filtration through the lymph can be influenced by a number of factors. Radiotherapy, for example, can markedly decrease nodal filtration capacity because it produces nodal and perinodal fibrosis. In dogs, it has been demonstrated that lymph node filtration can be reduced by the chemotherapeutic agents fluorouracil and thiotepa but not by methotrexate.

CONCLUSIONS

Understanding of the anatomy and physiology of the lymphatic system is important for lymphatic mapping and sentinel lymphadenectomy. The lymphatic system is essentially a complex network of channels which drain fluids and proteins from the interstitial spaces of the body's organs and tissues, and transport them to the lymph nodes. The radioactive tracers and vital dyes that are used for lymphatic mapping follow the same pathways. Overall total-body lymphatic flow at rest is approximately 2–4 L/day, but there are large variations in the lymphatic flow within different organs. Regulation of lymph flow is primarily dependent on the ultrastructure and distribution of lymphatic vessels within different tissues. However, the flow rate can be increased by exercise of the relevant body part or by gentle massage to the advantage of the nuclear medicine physician who is performing lymphoscintigraphy or the surgeon who is seeking to identify lymphatic channels and sentinel lymph nodes after blue dye injection.

REFERENCES

1. K Aukland, RK Reed. Interstitial–lymphatic mechanisms in the control of extracellular fluid volume. Physiol Rev 73:1–78, 1993.
2. GW Schmid-Schonbein. Microlymphatics and lymph flow. Physiol Rev 70:987–1028, 1990.
3. NP Reddy. Lymphatic circulation: physiology, pharmacology and biomechanics. CRC Crit Rev Biomed Eng 14:45–91, 1986.
4. F Ikom, GW Schmid-Schonbein. Lymph transport in the skin. Clin Dermatol 13:419–427, 1995.
5. RF Uren, RB Howman-Giles, JF Thompson, J Roberts, E Bernard. Variability of cutaneous lymphatic flow rates in melanoma patients. Melanoma Res 8:279–282, 1998.
6. JL Unthank, HG Bohlen. Lymphatic pathways and role of valves in lymph propulsion from small intestine. Am J Physiol 254:389–398, 1988.
7. LH Bannister. Lymphatic system. In: LH Bannister, MM Berry, P Collins, M Dyson, JE Dussek, MWJ Ferguson, eds. Gray's Anatomy. 38th ed. Edinburgh: Churchill–Livingstone, 1995, pp. 1605–1626.
8. NL Browse. Lymphoedema: pathophysiology and classification. J Cardiovasc Surg 26:91–106, 1985.

9. WL Olszewski, A Engset. Lymphatic contractions. New Engl J Med 300:316, 1979.
10. WL Olszewski. Lymph pressure and flow in limbs. In: WL Olszewski, ed. Lymph Stasis: Pathophysiology, Diagnosis and Treatment. Boca Raton: CRC Press, 1989, pp. 109–152.
11. WL Olszewski. Pathophysiology. In: WL Olszewski, ed. Peripheral Lymph: Formation and Immune Function. Boca Raton: CRC Press, 1985, pp. 117–125.
12. F Ikomi, GL Hanna, GW Schmid-Schonbein. Mechanism of colloidal particle uptake into the lymphatic system: basic study with percutaneous lymphography. Radiology 196:107–113, 1995.

2

The History of Lymphatic Mapping

Roger F. Uren
University of Sydney, Sydney, New South Wales, Australia

John F. Thompson
*Royal Prince Alfred Hospital, Camperdown, and University of Sydney, Sydney,
New South Wales, Australia*

Robert Howman-Giles
Missenden Medical Centre, Camperdown, New South Wales, Australia

INTRODUCTION

Lymph nodes were first described in the Hippocratic era and the concept of a
system that absorbed any excess fluid pooling in the interstitial space was probably developed soon after. Massa [1a] described lymphatics in the kidney in 1532,
but it was Gasparo Aselli [1b] who, as a professor of anatomy in Pavia, Italy,
first extensively described lymphatic vessels in many different animals. He called
them ''lacteal veins'' because of their milky color. Lymphatic channels in the
abdomen were identified and studied in the seventeenth century. The thoracic
duct was described in 1651 by Von Pecquet of Montpellier [2]. At about the
same time, Bartholin of Copenhagen and Rudbeck of Uppsala wrote about lymphatics in the liver, attributing much of the early knowledge of the lymphatic
system to Galen [1c]. In the eighteenth century, several British authors, including
William Cruikshank and William Hewson, emphasized the important functions
of the lymphatic system and documented differences between the superficial and
internal lymphatics. In the nineteenth century, Sappey made his seminal contributions to the understanding of the lymphatic system.

During the first half of the twentieth century, radiographic methods were
developed which allowed images of the lymphatic system to be recorded in individual patients. In 1939, Gray [1d] used contrast material to make a radiograph
of the lymphatic system, and in 1952 Kinmonth [1e] described the technique of
radiographic contrast lymphangiography. Much of the information in standard

teaching textbooks about lymphatic drainage is still based on the radiographic contrast lymphangiogram. This technique, however, was designed to display as many lymphatic channels and lymph nodes as possible with the aim of detecting tumor involvement of the nodes and, therefore, did not reflect physiological lymphatic drainage.

Lymphatic flow patterns were also examined by using blue dye, a technique first described by Gerota [1f]. In 1950 [1g], Weinberg injected blue dye into the wall of the stomach during surgery and was able to follow the blue lymphatic channels to the draining lymph nodes. In 1951 he used the same approach to locate the draining lymph nodes in lung cancer patients. Eichner, in 1954 [1h], adapted this approach and used it in patients with gynecological cancer.

The technique of lymphoscintigraphy, which was developed in the 1950s, was designed to map patterns of lymphatic drainage without disturbing the physiology of the lymphatics. It is the development and progress of this and related techniques which will therefore occupy most attention in this chapter.

LYMPHATIC MAPPING OF THE SKIN

The first comprehensive descriptions of the lymphatic drainage of the skin were based on the elegant work of the anatomist Sappey, who in the nineteenth century injected mercury into the lymphatics of cadavers to display the lymph channels [3,4]. He reported drainage to the axilla and groin from the skin of the trunk (Figs. 1–3) and showed a vertical midline zone anteriorly and posteriorly where drainage tended to overlap. A similar zone was identified passing horizontally around the waist from the umbilicus to the region of the second lumbar vertebra posteriorly. In these zones, called ''Sappey's lines'' by others, drainage was said to be possible to either side in the case of the vertical zone or to either the groin or the axilla in the case of the horizontal zone. Outside these zones, however, Sappey stated that lymphatic drainage was always to the ipsilateral groin or axilla, depending on whether the skin site of interest was above or below the horizontal band around the waist.

In the early 1950s, Walker was the first to use radiotracers to map lymphatic drainage [5]. Following this, Sherman et al. developed the concept of lymphoscintigraphy [6], demonstrating that colloidal gold could be traced from the point of intradermal injection to the draining lymph nodes. This was the advent of cutaneous lymphoscintigraphy as we know it today. Initially, colloidal gold-198 (^{198}Au) was used. This tracer has a very small particle size of about 5 nm. The disadvantage of colloidal ^{198}Au is that it is a beta emitter and thus tissues around the site of injection receive a high radiation dose. Technetium-99m (^{99m}Tc)-labeled colloids were developed to deal with this problem.

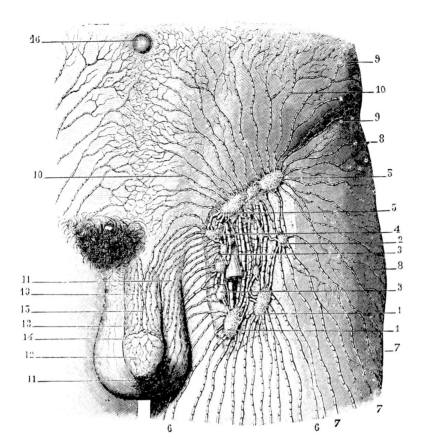

Figure 1   Lymphatics draining to groin lymph nodes. (From Ref. 4.)

The Zones of Ambiguity

Sappey's concept of the lymphatic drainage of the trunk was accepted as correct for 130 years until modified somewhat by Haagensen et al. [7], who enlarged the ambiguous zone to a 5-cm band down the midline and around the waist. Sugarbaker and McBride confirmed that drainage was ambiguous from these areas, but it continued to be thought that lymph drainage from skin of the trunk outside these ambiguous zones would be predictable to the axilla or groin [8].

Colloidal [198]Au was used by Fee et al. in 1978 when they studied 32 patients with melanoma [9]. This study confirmed that lymphoscintigraphy could accurately predict the node fields that potentially contained metastatic melanoma.

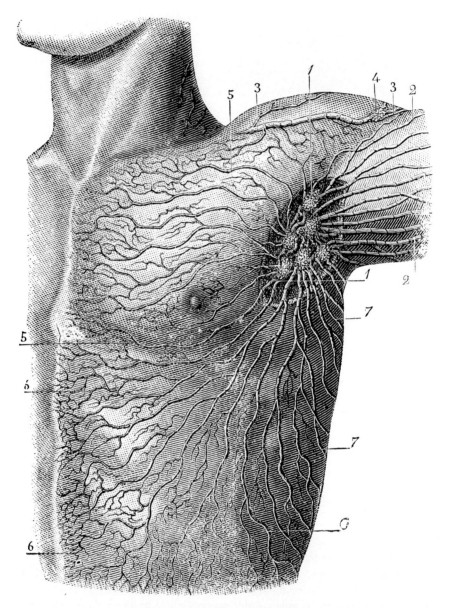

FIGURE 2 Lymphatics draining to the axillary lymph nodes. (From Ref. 4.)

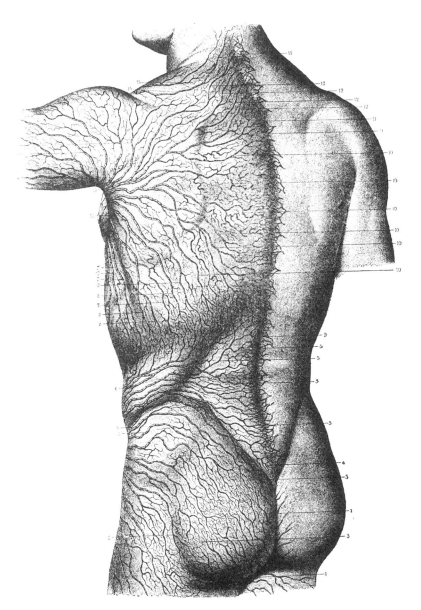

Figure 3   Lymphatics draining the posterior trunk. (From Ref. 4.)

Nine of their patients had nodal metastases, and in every case, lymph drainage from the primary site to this node field was demonstrated on lymphoscintigraphy. Around this time, other investigators were also using scintigraphy to map lymph drainage in patients with melanomas located on the trunk and elsewhere when drainage was considered uncertain (i.e., in Sappey's zones of uncertainty or in the head and neck [10,11]). It was emphasized that lymphoscintigraphy could not predict whether lymph nodes contained metastases, but that it could identify which node fields were at greatest risk of harboring occult metastases [12].

More studies began to appear which expanded the zone of uncertainty around Sappey's lines and also demonstrated that drainage in the head and neck was quite variable [13]. The results of lymphoscintigraphy began to be used as a guide to determine which lymph node fields were to be subjected to elective lymphadenectomy [14–16]. It also became increasingly apparent that drainage could sometimes be identified with node fields, which would not be considered potential metastatic sites on clinical grounds [17].

For many years, cutaneous lymphoscintigraphy was thus used to identify which node fields received lymphatic drainage from the primary melanoma site on the skin and, therefore, which node fields were potential sites of occult metastases. With experience, it became clear that lymphoscintigraphy should be performed before wide local excision or lymphadenectomy, as it was shown that these procedures disrupted the normal lymphatic drainage pathways [18,19]. As such studies proceeded, the zones of ambiguity on the trunk and elsewhere were continually expanded as more and more exceptions to the expected patterns of lymphatic drainage were demonstrated [20,21]. Nevertheless, lymphoscintigraphy continued to be performed only when some clinical doubt was present about the pattern of drainage. The threshold of doubt varied considerably from surgeon to surgeon, with the end result that there was considerable variation in the sites subjected to lymphadenectomy by different surgeons for lesions at the same site on the skin. Lymphoscintigraphy was not performed if the primary site was on a limb or close to an individual node field.

The Sentinel Node Concept

The term ''sentinel node'' to describe the lymph nodes receiving lymphatic drainage from a lesion site was first used by Cabañas in 1977 [22]. However, he used the term to describe a group of nodes that regularly drained the penis and did not use any intraoperative mapping technique to locate the relevant one or two nodes in individual patients. The current use of the term must be attributed to Morton, Cochran, and colleagues at the John Wayne Cancer Institute in Santa Monica, California. In 1992, they described a method of mapping the lymphatic drainage from a primary melanoma site using intradermal injections of blue dye [23]. The stained lymphatic was followed surgically until the blue channel was seen entering a blue-stained node in the draining node field. This node was called the "sentinel node." It was found that if this node was free of metastatic disease, then the node field was almost invariably free of disease. The disadvantage of this approach was that the surgical technique was difficult to learn, requiring about 50 operations before a surgeon achieved reliable results. It was this study, however, which demonstrated that the metastatic melanoma status of a whole node field could be accurately determined by selectively removing and carefully examining one or two sentinel nodes. It is of interest that blue dye injection had long been used to identify lymphatics peripherally and had also been used as an aid to permit canulation for radiological lymphangiography (Fig. 4). However, the concept of tracing it to a specific lymph node or nodes had not previously been considered.

Facilitating the Search for the Sentinel Node

The discovery by Morton and co-workers caused others to search for more rapid and less technically demanding methods of locating sentinel lymph nodes. Alex and Krag [37] described the use of a labeled colloid in combination with a gamma-detecting probe to locate the sentinel node in patients with melanoma. This technique was much simpler than the original method described by Morton and colleagues. Uren and colleagues showed that the standard lymphoscintigraphy technique, which had been in routine use to determine which node fields drained melanoma primary sites, could be modified to allow the exact location of the sentinel nodes to be marked on the skin. This information could then be used to aid in rapid surgical location of sentinel nodes [24,25]. Digital gamma cameras were found to be important in this process as they allowed dynamic studies to be performed, with lymph channels followed until they were seen entering the sentinel nodes. Because some tracer may pass onward quite rapidly to second-tier nodes, not all radioactive nodes are sentinel nodes and only the dynamic phase of the study allows the true sentinel nodes to be identified. A second advantage of the dynamic acquisition is that an estimate of the speed of lymph flow can be obtained [26,27], which helps the surgeon time the injection of blue dye prior to surgery, as well as allowing the surface location of all sentinel nodes to be marked on the skin. It is very important that this marking procedure occur with the patient lying in the same position that they will be in at the time of surgery, otherwise the mark will not overlie the node. The depth of the node from the skin surface can also be measured, which is a further aid to its surgical identification. Unusual drainage pathways are defined and any interval nodes between the primary melanoma site and the draining node field can be marked. When the patient presents to the operating theater following lymphoscintigraphy with an "X" marking the location of the sentinel node on the skin and a depth measurement, it facilitates the operative procedure and, in most patients, the senti-

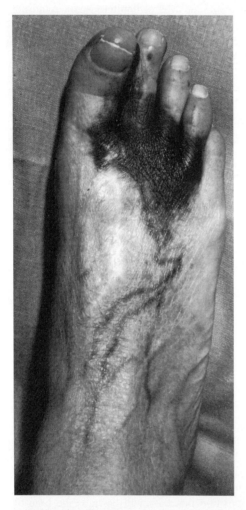

FIGURE 4   Blue dye injected into interdigital clefts to demonstrate lymphatic channels passing proximally in the foot toward the groin, thus facilitating cannulation for radiological lymphangiography.

nel node is rapidly found at the appropriate depth, staining blue with a blue channel entering one side of the node. Surgeons require a shorter training period to accurately excise the sentinel node using this method.

Unexpected Lymphatic Drainage Pathways

Using lymphoscintigraphy in this way meant that patients with lesion sites previously thought to have unambiguous drainage were also studied, and this led to the discovery of several unusual and previously unknown pathways for lymphatic drainage of the skin [28–33]. It is now clear that when faced with an individual patient with a melanoma, there are, in fact, very few, if any, places on the skin of the human body which have completely unambiguous drainage, and in any event, this concept is now redundant because the location of the sentinel node has become the main application of lymphatic mapping of the skin. Several large surgical studies have now confirmed that sentinel node status is an accurate reflection of node field status in melanoma patients [34–36].

Intraoperative Use of a Gamma Probe

Studies appeared describing the use of an intraoperative gamma probe to locate sentinel lymph nodes during surgery [36–38]. Most now accept that the best method of locating the sentinel nodes at surgery is to use a combination of preoperative lymphoscintigraphy, blue dye injection just before anesthesia, and intraoperative use of a gamma probe to assist in locating the blue node or nodes and show that the node field returns to background levels of activity after the sentinel nodes are removed [39,40]. The delay between the injection of tracer and surgery will vary with different protocols; however, there is enough radioactivity remaining in the sentinel nodes to allow the gamma probe to be used up to 24 h after injection of the tracer. In fact, there are some advantages in this next-day surgical approach. There is less radiation safety concern for operating theater staff and no requirement for radiation licensing of the surgeon. Further, the node-to-background ratio rises with time, which facilitates the location of ''hot'' nodes using the gamma detection probe intraoperatively [39].

Radiopharmaceuticals Used for Lymphatic Mapping

Many different colloidal tracers have been used for cutaneous lymphoscintigraphy over the years, and it appears that several of them are adequate in clinical practice. The main requirement is easy entry of the labeled colloidal particles into the lymphatic capillaries and good retention in sentinel lymph nodes, with minimal movement onward to second tier lymph nodes. This occurs best with colloids which have particle sizes in the 10–50 nm range. These include ^{99m}Tc–antimony trisulfide colloid, microfiltered ^{99m}Tc sulfur colloid, and ^{99m}Tc albumin colloid. Of these three, ^{99m}Tc–antimony trisulfide colloid has the most ideal characteristics for a lymphoscintigraphy imaging tracer [41]. In the future, other agents may be preferred and there are some promising tracers currently under investigation. One theoretically attractive approach is to use receptor-binding nonparticulate tracers which move rapidly from the injection site through the lymph channels to the sentinel nodes but then bind strongly to the node as a result of the receptor binding to lymphoid tissue [42]. This approach may also lead to less tracer passing on to second tier lymph nodes.

Conclusion

Cutaneous lymphatic mapping using lymphoscintigraphy has come of age and is now finding routine application in patients with melanoma. Defining the patterns of lymphatic drainage and locating the sentinel lymph nodes is having a direct impact on the surgical management of these patients. It can be used in the same way for other skin cancers that may show spread to local lymph nodes, such as squamous cell carcinoma and Merkel cell cancer.

LYMPHATIC MAPPING OF THE BREAST

Lymphatic drainage from the four quadrants of the breast was studied by Vendrell-Torne and colleagues in 1972 using colloidal gold [43]. This study demonstrated that the pattern of lymphatic drainage from the breast varied when different breast quadrants were injected with tracer. This fact has subsequently been confirmed by many researchers.

Over the next 20 years, lymphatic mapping of the breast focused on one of two strategies. The first aimed at determining if lymph nodes draining the breast of patients with breast cancer contained metastatic deposits, and the second was intended to define the distribution of internal mammary nodes as a guide to radiation treatment planning.

Internal Mammary Lymphoscintigraphy

This technique, first described by Rossi and shortly after by Schenck, was championed by Ege of the Princess Margaret Hospital in Toronto [44–46]. The method involved injection of radiocolloid into the space between the anterior and posterior rectus sheaths in the upper abdomen and then imaging of the tracer as it passed up via the internal mammary lymph node chain. The images were interpreted with a view to diagnosing the presence of metastases in this lymph node chain. Although several studies were published which showed promising results using this technique to diagnose metastases [47,48] and many studies were published which suggested a significant role for internal mammary lymphoscintigraphy in the management of patients with breast cancer [49–53], it never became widely used and is now rarely performed for this purpose.

Many other investigators used the technique to provide an accurate map of node distribution which could be used as an aid to radiation treatment planning [54–57]. In this role, internal mammary lymphoscintigraphy proved reasonably successful and it is still used for this purpose in some centers.

Axillary Lymphoscintigraphy

This technique involves the interdigital injection of radiocolloid in the hand to image the axillary lymph nodes in a search for nodal metastases [58] or to check the axilla intraoperatively or postoperatively to confirm that an adequate axillary lymph node dissection had been performed [59,60]. The technique did not prove to be an accurate method of staging the axilla for metastases and is no longer used in this role.

Mammary Lymphoscintigraphy

A variety of studies were performed using mammary lymphoscintigraphy with the aim of diagnosing nodal metastases in patients with breast cancer. Tracers were administered in various parts of the breast.

In 1981, Gabelle and colleagues studied intratumoral injection of the tracer in 100 patients with breast cancer and counted the number of nodes seen 4 h later on scan [61]. They found that patients with nodal metastases had fewer nodes visualized on average than those who were free of metastases, but the results were not useful in individual patients.

Serin and colleagues studied 51 patients to determine the accuracy of mammary lymphoscintigraphy with intratumoral injection in diagnosing nodal metastases, comparing the scans with clinical examination of the axilla and pathology [62]. They found this technique to be of no value.

Gasparini and colleagues used periareolar injection of radiocolloid in 26 patients with breast cancer and again scans were performed in the search for metastases [63]. The number of nodes visualized in the axilla was compared to pathology, but no useful data were obtained.

A modification of the above technique was used by Mazzeo and co-workers, who administered subareolar injections in 32 patients and scanned the axilla for metastases [64]. The method proved inadequate.

Terui and Yamamoto studied 100 patients with breast cancer using subperiosteal injections of radiocolloid and demonstrated both internal mammary and axillary drainage in most patients [65]. They used the test to roughly locate the lymph nodes and to evaluate them for metastases. However, it is unclear how the observed lymph drainage patterns were expected to relate to the lymphatic drainage of the actual breast tumors.

Intradermal injection around the surgical wound following surgical removal of a breast cancer was used by Matsubara and colleagues [66]. They found that the contralateral axillary nodes were often visualized as well as nodes in the ipsilateral axilla. These data seem of doubtful relevance to the breast tumor lymphatic drainage, as the method was clearly evaluating dermal lymphatic drainage, not the breast lymphatics. In any case, the dermal lymphatic pathways are likely to have been altered significantly by the prior surgery on the breast.

Saeki and colleagues studied 12 patients with breast tumors and injected labeled microspheres into the breast tissue at unspecified locations [67]. They observed tracer in axillary, subclavian, and parasternal lymph nodes in 10 patients 1 h after injection.

Progress So Far

To this point, lymphatic mapping in the breast had essentially been used in patients with breast cancer in an attempt to diagnose the presence of metastases in draining lymph nodes. In this role, it had not proved sufficiently accurate to be used in making individual patient management decisions. Internal mammary lymphoscintigraphy, axillary lymphoscintigraphy, and mammary lymphoscintigraphy had all been used in this way. This approach to lymphatic mapping of the breast was not addressing the strength of lymphoscintigraphy, that is, the ability to accurately map physiological lymphatic drainage. Instead, these studies had focused attention on one of the limitations of lymphoscintigraphy and that is its poor spatial resolution. It is implausible that lymphoscintigraphy using conventional radiocolloids will ever be able to diagnose the presence of micrometastases in lymph nodes. If labeled antibodies to specific tumor antigens can be developed, then this objective may be achievable in the future.

The Next Phase

Following the revelation by Morton and colleagues in 1992 that a lymph node field in patients with melanoma could be accurately staged by surgically removing only the sentinel lymph node or nodes [23], interest quickly developed to determine if this also held true in patients with breast cancer. For many years these patients had routinely been subjected to a much more extensive elective dissection of the axillary lymph nodes on the side of the breast cancer to determine the nodal status of the axilla, with considerable associated morbidity.

Krag accurately located the sentinel lymph node in the axilla of 18 of 22 patients who had received peritumoral injections of radiocolloid preoperatively [68]. Seven of seven patients with proven metastases were identified, and in three of them, the sentinel node was the only positive node.

Giuliano and colleagues documented the accuracy of the original blue dye method in locating the sentinel node in breast cancer patients, and in the latter part of their study, a sentinel node in the axilla was found in 78% of their patients [69].

Uren and colleagues showed that peritumoral injections of ^{99m}Tc–antimony trisulfide allowed the pattern of lymphatic drainage for individual breast cancers to be determined in over 90% of patients [70]. They demonstrated unexpected drainage across the center line of the breast to internal mammary or axillary nodes in 32% of patients with outer and inner quadrant tumors, respectively. Upper quadrant lesions drained directly to the supraclavicular or infraclavicular nodes in 20% of patients, and in 85% of all patients, drainage occurred to the ipsilateral axilla. In the three patients who had the sentinel node removed with the aid of blue dye injection preoperatively, it was negative in one patient who had no metastases in other nodes (0/11 nodes) and positive in the other two patients, both of whom did have metastases in other nodes (2/23 and 8/14 nodes).

Other studies have subsequently confirmed the accuracy of sentinel lymphadenectomy in the axilla for patients with breast cancer [71–73].

The Future

It is known that the presence of nodal metastases in the axilla of breast cancer patients has an adverse effect on their prognosis. If metastases occur in lymph node basins in proportion to the incidence of lymphatic drainage to that area as shown on lymphoscintigraphy, then in about a third of patients, there is the possibility of micrometastases in the internal mammary or supraclavicular lymph nodes [70]. Because it is possible to obtain an accurate map of peritumoral lymphatic drainage in most patients, it seems illogical to ignore the sentinel nodes in these node fields. We believe that in the future, these sentinel nodes will be resected so that the true nodal status of each patient with breast cancer will be determined [74]. With this knowledge, more precise therapeutic decision making should be possible.

LYMPHATIC MAPPING IN GENITO-URINARY CANCER

Canabas described the pattern of lymphatic drainage from the penis using radiographic lymphangiography [22]. He found that this drainage occurred to "sentinel lymph nodes" in the superficial inguinal area. He was the first to use the term "sentinel nodes" in reference to lymph nodes draining a particular part of the body. His contention was that metastasis would occur first to this group of superficial inguinal nodes, so that if these nodes were normal, then all other nodes would also be normal. Subsequent studies showed a false-negative rate of 25% for this approach [75]. Work is continuing using radiocolloid or blue dye or both to map lymphatic drainage in patients with penile cancer to locate the actual

sentinel node or nodes, just as has been done in melanoma and breast cancer
[76].

   Some early experience in patients with vulva cancer has been encouraging
and suggests that this technique can be successfully applied to patients with this
malignancy [77,78]. There have also been promising descriptions of the application of lymphatic mapping techniques in the abdominal cavity in patients with
high-risk endometrial cancer which have shown that the sentinel nodes in the
pelvis, common iliac, and para-aortic area can be identified [79]. Other studies
are proceeding to confirm the accuracy of this method in uterine cancer. It is
hoped that sentinel lymphadenectomy can in this way replace the current approach of random node sampling. It might also be possible in the future to map
the lymphatic drainage pathways from malignancies in other intra-abdominal
sites such as the bladder and prostate, and even the large bowel.

CONCLUSIONS

At this time, lymphatic mapping has an important and firmly established role in
the surgical management of patients with melanoma by allowing the location
and surgical removal of sentinel lymph nodes. It is on the threshold of a similar
application in breast cancer patients, which in the future is likely to expand to
the removal of all sentinel nodes, including those in the internal mammary and
supraclavicular lymph node fields. It appears inevitable that similar success will
occur by the rigorous application of this lymphatic mapping technique to patients
with vulval and penile cancer. There is also likely to be utility in applying this
to patients with aggressive squamous cell carcinomas in other parts of the body.
Early work in mapping lymphatic drainage in the abdominal cavity raises the
prospect of an expanding role for sentinel lymphadenectomy in patients with a
variety of intra-abdominal malignancies which have a predilection for lymphatic
spread.

REFERENCES

1.   (a) N Massa. N Lib Introd Anat 1532; (b) G Aselli. De Lactibus Sire Lacteis Venis.
     Milan: JB Biellius, 1627; (c) WL Marmelzat. Galen on ''glands'' and ''spongy
     flesh'' with special references to an ancient mechanico-biophysical theory for super-
     ficial lymph node function. J Hist Med Allied Sci 46:419–440, 1991; (d) JH Gray.
     The relation of lymphatic vessels to the spread of cancer. Br J Surg 26:462, 1939; (e)
     JB Kinmonth. Lymphangiography in man; a method of outlining lymphatic trunks at
     operation. Clin Sci II:13–20, 1952; (f) Gerota. Zur technik der lymphgefassinjection.
     Eine neue injections masse fur lymphgefasse. Polychrom. Injection. Anat Anzeiger
     12:216, 1896; (g) Weinberg, 1950; (h) Eichner, 1954.

2. TJ Ryan. Landmarks in the understanding of lymphatic function and the management of edema. Clin Dermatol 13:417–418, 1995.

3. MPC Sappey. Injection, preparation et conservation des vaisseaux lymphatic. Thesis Paris, 1843.

4. MPC Sappey. Anatomie, physiologie, pathologie des vaisseaux lymphatiques consideres chez l'homme at les vertebres. In: A DeLahaye, E Lecrosnier, eds. Paris, 1874.

5. L Walker. Localization of radioactive colloids in lymph nodes. J Lab Clin Med 36: 440–449, 1950.

6. AI Sherman, M Ter-Pogossian, EC Tocus. Lymph node concentration of radioactive colloidal gold following interstitial injection. Cancer 6:1238–1243, 1953.

7. CD Haagensen, CR Feind, FP Herter, CA Slanetz Jr, JA Weinberg. Lymphatics of the trunk. In: CD Haagensen, ed. The Lymphatics in Cancer. Philadelphia: WB Saunders, 1972, pp. 437–458.

8. EV Sugarbaker, CM McBride. Melanoma of the trunk: the results of surgical excision and anatomic guidelines for predicting nodal metastases. Surgery 80:22–30, 1976.

9. HJ Fee, DS Robinson, WF Sample, LS Graham, EC Holmes, DL Morton. The determination of lymph shed by colloidal gold scanning in patients with malignant melanoma: a preliminary study. Surgery 84:626–632, 1978.

10. CM Meyer, ML Lecklitner, JR Logic, CE Balch, PQ Bessey, WM Tauxe. Technetium-99m sulfur–colloid cutaneous lymphoscintigraphy in the management of truncal melanoma. Radiology 131:205–209, 1979.

11. DC Sullivan, BP Croker, CC Harris, P Deery, HF Seigler. Lymphoscintigraphy in malignant melanoma: 99m-Tc antimony sulfur colloid. Am J Roentgenol 137:847–851, 1981.

12. DL Munz, P Altmeyer, MJ Sessler. Axillary lymph node groups—the center in lymphatic drainage from the truncal skin in man. Clinical significance for management of malignant melanoma. Lymphology 15:143–157, 1982.

13. HJ Wanebo, D Harpole, CD Teates. Radionuclide lymphoscintigraphy with technetium-99m antimony sulfide colloid to identify lymphatic drainage of cutaneous melanoma at ambiguous sites in the head and neck and trunk. Cancer 55:1403–1413, 1985.

14. DS Reintgen, D Sullivan, E Coleman, W Briner, BP Croker, HF Seigler. Lymphoscintigraphy for malignant melanoma—surgical considerations. Am Surg 49: 672–678, 1983.

15. MA Eberbach, RL Wahl, LC Argenta, J Froelich, JE Niederhuber. Utility of lymphoscintigraphy in directing surgical therapy for melanomas of the head, neck, and upper thorax. Surgery 102:433–439, 1987.

16. EL Kramer, JJ Sanger, F Golomb, AW Kopf, A Postel. The impact of intradermal lymphoscintigraphy on surgical management of clinical stage I truncal melanoma. J Dermatol Surg Oncol 13:508–515, 1987.

17. JR Logic, CM Balch. Defining lymphatic drainage patterns with cutaneous lymphoscintigraphy. In: CM Balch, GW Milton, HM Shaw, S-I Soong, eds. Cutaneous Melanoma: Clinical Management and Treatment Results Worldwide. Philadelphia: JB Lippincott Company, 1985; pp. 159–170.

18. WV Rees, DS Robinson, EC Holmes, DL Morton. Altered lymphatic drainage following lymphadenectomy. Cancer 45:3045–3049, 1980.
19. A Jonk, BBR Kroon, WJ Mooi, CA Hoefnagel. Contralateral inguinal lymph node metastasis in patients with melanoma of the lower extremities. Br J Surg 76:1161–1162, 1989.
20. MA Eberbach, RL Wahl. Lymphatic anatomy: functional nodal basins. Ann Plast Surg 22:25–31, 1989.
21. J Norman, CW Cruse, C Espinosa, C Cox, C Berman, R Clark, H Saba, K Wells, D Reintgen. Redefinition of cutaneous lymphatic drainage with the use of lymphoscintigraphy for malignant melanoma. Am J Surg 162:432–437, 1991.
22. RM Cabañas. An approach for the treatment of penile cancer. Cancer 39:456–466, 1977.
23. DL Morton, D Wen, JH Wong, JS Economou, LA Cagle, FK Storm, LJ Foshag, AJ Cochran. Technical details of intraoperative lymphatic mapping for early stage melanoma. Arch Surg 127:392–399, 1992.
24. RF Uren, R Howman-Giles, HM Shaw, JF Thompson, WH McCarthy. Lymphoscintigraphy in high risk melanoma of the trunk: predicting draining node groups, defining lymphatic channels and locating the sentinel node. J Nucl Med 34:1435–1440, 1993.
25. RF Uren, R Howman-Giles, JF Thompson, HM Shaw, JM Quinn, CJ O'Brien, WH McCarthy. Lymphoscintigraphy to define sentinel nodes in patients with melanoma. Melanoma Res 4:395–399, 1994.
26. SD Nathanson, L Nelson, KC Karvelis. Rates of flow of technetium 99m-labelled human serum albumin from peripheral injection sites to sentinel lymph nodes. Ann Surg Oncol 3:329–335, 1996.
27. RF Uren, RB Howman-Giles, JF Thompson. Variation in cutaneous lymphatic flow rates. Ann Surg Oncol 4:279–280, 1997.
28. RF Uren, R Howman-Giles, JF Thompson, HM Shaw, WH McCarthy. Lymphatic drainage from peri-umbilical skin to internal mammary nodes. Clin Nucl Med 20:254–255, 1995.
29. RF Uren, R Howman-Giles, JF Thompson, MJ Quinn, C O'Brien, HM Shaw, CMJ Bosch, WH McCarthy. Lymphatic drainage to triangular intermuscular space lymph nodes in melanoma on the back. J Nucl Med 37:964–966, 1996.
30. RF Uren, RB Howman-Giles, JF Thompson, MJ Quinn. Direct lymphatic drainage from the skin of the forearm to a supraclavicular node. Clin Nucl Med 21:387–389, 1996.
31. RF Uren, RB Howman-Giles, JF Thompson, J Roberts. Direct lymphatic drainage from the skin of the elbow to an interpectoral node. Regional Cancer Treat 9:100–102, 1997.
32. RF Uren, R Howman-Giles, JF Thompson. Lymphatic drainage from the skin of the back to retroperotoneal and paravertebral lymph nodes in melanoma patients. Ann Surg Oncol 5:384–387, 1998.
33. CJ O'Brien, RF Uren, HM Shaw, JF Thompson, RB Howman-Giles, K Petersen-Schaefer, MJ Quinn, WH McCarthy. Prediction of potential metastatic sites in cutaneous head and neck melanomas using lymphoscintigraphy. Am J Surg 170:461–466, 1995.

34. JF Thompson, WH McCarthy, CMJ Bosch, CJ O'Brien, MJ Quinn, S Paramaesvaran, K Crotty, SW McCarthy, RF Uren, R Howman-Giles. Sentinel lymph node status as an indicator of the presence of metastatic melanoma in regional lymph nodes. Melanoma Res 5:255–260, 1995.

35. MI Ross, D Reintgen, CM Balch. Selective lymphadenectomy: emerging role for lymphatic mapping and sentinel node biopsy in the management of early stage melanoma. Semin Surg Oncol 9:219–223, 1993.

36. DN Krag, SJ Meijer, DL Weaver, BW Loggie, SP Harlow, KK Tanabe, EH Laughlin, JC Ales. Minimal-access surgery for staging of malignant melanoma. Arch Surg 130:654–658, 1995.

37. JC Alex, DN Krag. Gamma probe guided localization of lymph nodes. Surg Oncol 2:137–143, 1993.

38. JC Alex, DL Weaver, JT Fairbank, BS Rankin, DN Krag. Gamma-probe-guided lymph node localization in malignant melanoma. Surg Oncol 2:303–308, 1993.

39. JF Thompson, P Niewind, RF Uren, CMJ Bosch, RB Howman-Giles, BC Vrouenraets. Single dose isotope injection for both preoperative lymphoscintigraphy and intraoperative sentinel lymph node identification in melanoma patients. Melanoma Res 6:500–506, 1997.

40. R Pijpers, PJ Borgstein, S Meijer, OS Hoekstra, LH van Hattum, GJJ Teule. Sentinel node biopsy in melanoma patients: dynamic lymphoscintigraphy followed by intraoperative gamma probe and vital dye guidance. World J Surg 21:788–793, 1997.

41. WD Kaplan, MA Davis, CM Rose. A comparison of two technetium-99m-labeled radiopharmaceuticals for lymphoscintigraphy: concise communication. J Nucl Med 20:933–937, 1979.

42. DR Vera, ER Wisner, RC Stadalnik. Sentinel node binding via a nonparticulate receptor-binding radiotracer. J Nucl Med 38:530–535, 1997.

43. E Vendrell-Torne, J Setain-Quinquer, FM Domenech-Torne. Study of normal lymphatic drainage using radioactive isotopes. J Nucl Med 13:801–805, 1972.

44. R Rossi, O Ferri. La visualizzazione della catena mammaria interna con 198Au. Presentazione di una nuova metodica: la linfoscintigrafia. Minerva Med 57:1151–1155, 1966.

45. P Schenck. Scintigraphische darstellung des parasternalen lymphsystems. Strahlentherapie 130:504–508, 1966.

46. GN Ege. Internal mammary lymphoscintigraphy. Radiology 118:101–107, 1976.

47. S Matsuo. Studies of the metastasis of breast cancer to lymph nodes—II. Diagnosis of metastasis to internal mammary nodes using radiocolloid. Acta Med Okayama 28:361–371, 1974.

48. GN Ege. Internal mammary lymphoscintigraphy in breast carcinoma: a study of 1072 patients. Int J Radiat Oncol Biol Phys 2:755–761, 1977.

49. P Bourgeois, JG Fruhling. Internal mammary lymphoscintigraphy: current status in the treatment of breast cancer. Crit Rev Oncol Hematol 1:21–47, 1983.

50. L Dionne, J Friede, R Blais. Internal mammary lymphoscintigraphy in breast carcinoma—a surgeon's perspective. Semin Nucl Med 13:35–41, 1983.

51. GN Ege, T Elhakim. The relevance of internal mammary lymphoscintigraphy in the management of breast carcinoma. J Clin Oncol 2:774–781, 1984.

52. GN Ege, RM Clarke. Internal mammary lymphoscintigraphy in the conservative

management of breast carcinoma: an update and recommendations for a new TNM staging. Clin Radiol 36:469–472, 1985.

53. G Inga, G Pepe, M Caruso, S Sportelli, F Pepe, P Panella. The detection of internal mammary lymph nodal chain metastases in breast cancer using radiolabelled colloids. Eur J Gynecol Oncol 8:105–109, 1987.

54. PH Van der Giessen. Parasternal lymphoscintigraphy as an aid in radiation treatment planning. Strahlentherapie 159:422–426, 1983.

55. BD Collier, DW Palmer, JF Wilson, M Greenberg, R Kumaki, JD Cox, TL Lawson, PM Lawlor. Internal mammary lymphoscintigraphy in patients with breast cancer. Correlation with computed tomography and impact on radiation therapy planning. Radiology 147:845–848, 1983.

56. WD Kaplan, JW Andersen, RL Siddon, BT Connolly, CA McCormick, SM Laffin, EM Rosenbaum, CA Jennings, A Recht, JR Harris. The three dimensional localization of internal mammary lymph nodes by radionuclide lymphoscintigraphy. J Nucl Med 29:473–478, 1988.

57. MA Hunt, B Shank, B McCormick. The use of lymphoscintigraphy in treatment planning of primary breast cancer. Int J Radiat Oncol Biol Phys 17:597–606, 1989.

58. RG McLean, GN Ege. Prognostic value of axillary lymphoscintigraphy in breast carcinoma patients. J Nucl Med 27:1116–1124, 1986.

59. E Gitsch, K Philipp, E Kubista. Intraoperative lymphoscintigraphy in radical surgery of cancer. Geburtshilfe-Frauenheilkd 43:112–115, 1983.

60. P Bourgeois, J Fruhling, J Henry. Postoperative axillary lymphoscintigraphy in the management of breast cancer. Int J Radiat Oncol Biol Phys 9:29–32, 1983.

61. P Gabelle, M Comet, JP Bodin, A Dupre, E Carpentier, M Bolla, P Swiercz. Mammary lymphatic scintiscans by intratumoral injection in the assessment of breast cancer. Nouv Presse Med 10:3067–3070, 1981.

62. D Serin, JM Vinot, P Martin, F Reboul, M Robin, J Chevallier. The value of breast lymphoscintigraphy in the definition of axillary staging in cancer of the breast. Bull Cancer 73:299–304, 1986.

63. M Gasparini, C Andreoli, A Rodari, A Costa, GL Buraggi. Lack of efficacy of lymphoscintigraphy in detecting axillary lymph node metastases from breast cancer. Eur J Cancer Clin Oncol 23:475–480, 1987.

64. F Mazzeo, A Accurso, G Petrella, S Capuano, L Maurelli, L Celentano, G Squame, M Salvatore. Pre-operative axillary lymphoscintigraphy in breast cancer: experience with sub-areolar injection of 99Tcm-nanocolloidal albumin. Nucl Med Commun 7: 5–16, 1986.

65. S Terui, H Yamamoto. New simplified lymphoscintigraphic technique in patients with breast cancer. J Nucl Med 30:1198–1204, 1989.

66. S Matsubara, I Umehara, H Shibuya, T Okuyama, J Horiuchi, S Suzuki, H Suzuki, M Ebuchi. Radionuclide lymphoscintigraphy performed on the mastectomized chest wall. Cancer 58:1225–1230, 1986.

67. T Saeki, Y Karaki, M Maeda, T Honda, M Fujmaki. Development of Tc-99m labeled activated carbon microspheres and clinical application. Nippon Geka Gakkai Zasshi 91:729–740, 1990.

68. DN Krag, DL Weaver, JC Alex, JT Fairbank. Surgical resection and radiolocaliza-

tion of the sentinel lymph node in breast cancer using a gamma probe. Surg Oncol 2:335–340, 1993.

69. AE Giuliano, DM Kirgan, JM Guenther, DL Morton. Lymphatic mapping and senti-nel lymphadenectomy for breast cancer. Ann Surg 220:391–401, 1994.

70. RF Uren, RB Howman-Giles, JF Thompson, D Malouf, G Ramsey-Stewart, FW Niesche, SB Renwick. Mammary lymphoscintigraphy in breast cancer. J Nucl Med 36:1775–1780, 1995.

71. AE Giuliano, PS Dale, RR Turner, DL Morton, SW Evans, DL Krasne. Improved axillary staging of breast cancer with sentinel lymphadenectomy. Ann Surg 222: 394–401, 1995.

72. JJ Albertini, GH Lyman, C Cox, T Yeatman, L Balducci, N Ku, S Shivers, C Ber-man, K Wells, D Rapaport, A Shons, J Horton, H Greenberg, S Nicosia, R Clark, A Cantor, DS Reintgen. Lymphatic mapping and sentinel node biopsy in the patient with breast cancer. JAMA 276:1818–1822, 1996.

73. AE Giuliano, AM Barth, B Spivack, PD Beitsch, SW Evans. Incidence and pre-dictors of axillary metastasis in T1 carcinoma of the breast. J Am Coll Surg 183: 185–189, 1996.

74. RF Uren, RB Howman-Giles, JF Thompson. The value of pre-operative lymphoscin-tigraphy in breast cancer treatment. Eur J Cancer 34:203–204, 1998.

75. CA Pettaway, LL Pisters, CPN Dinney, FE Jularbal, DA Swanson, AC Von Eschen-bach, A Ayala. Sentinel lymph node dissection for penile carcinoma: the MD Ander-son Cancer Center experience. J Urol 154:1999–2003, 1995.

76. BAE Kapteijn. Biopsy of the sentinel node in melanoma, penile carcinoma and breast carcinoma. The case for lymphatic mapping. Thesis, University of Amsterdam, Am-sterdam, 1997.

77. C Levenback, TW Burke, DM Gershenson, M Morris, A Malpica, MI Ross. Intraop-erative lymphatic mapping for vulvar cancer. Obstet Gynecol 84:163–167, 1994.

78. C De Cicco, M Sideri, M Bartolomei. Sentinel node detection by lymphoscintigraphy and gamma detecting probe in patients with vulvar cancer (abstr). J Nucl Med 38: 33, 1997.

79. TW Burke, C Levenback, C Tornos, M Morris, JT Wharton, DM Gershenson. In-traabdominal lymphatic mapping to direct selective pelvic and paraaortic lymphade-nectomy in women with high-risk endometrial cancer: Results of a pilot study. Gyne-col Oncol 62:169–173, 1996.

3

Cutaneous Lymphoscintigraphy

Omgo E. Nieweg, Renato A. Valdés Olmos, B. Acca E. Kapteijn, and Cornelis A. Hoefnagel
The Netherlands Cancer Institute, Amsterdam, the Netherlands

Liesbeth Jansen
Gelre Hospital, Lukas Site, Apeldoorn, the Netherlands

INTRODUCTION

Research in imaging is driven by the need for knowledge of anatomy and physiology, as well as the desire to better understand pathophysiology, in order to improve diagnostic methods. Technical developments and advances in computer science have enabled the spectacular development of imaging techniques that we have witnessed over the past 25 years, but the developments in imaging of the lymphatic system have not been so dramatic. Lymphangiography with a contrast medium containing an organic iodine compound has been an established technique since the 1950s [1]. The viscid contrast medium is injected into a lymphatic duct that has been identified with the aid of intradermal administration of a blue dye. The radiopaque medium opacifies lymphatic ducts and lymph nodes. The medium remains in the nodes for a long period of time and can be visualized by radiography. Lymphangiography is particularly suitable for depicting the anatomy of the lymphatic system. Disadvantages are that the technique is time-consuming and requires considerable technical expertise. The contrast medium can damage lymphatic ducts and may induce an allergic reaction. The radiography also leads to a considerable radiation exposure of patients. Newer techniques in diagnostic radiology such as ultrasound, computed tomography (CT), and magnetic resonance imaging (MRI) currently play no role in imaging of the lymphatic system.

Lymphoscintigraphy is a nuclear medicine technique that shows the transport of a tracer through the lymphatic system. Direct intralymphatic administration of the radiolabeled tracer is not required. Radiology excels in depicting anatomy. Nuclear medicine, on the other hand, is superior in the visualization of physiological processes. These features are exemplified in imaging of the lymphatic system. Lymphangiography depicts the lymphatic ducts and the lymph nodes in detail but shows little of the lymph flow. Lymphoscintigraphy, on the other hand, shows uptake in the lymphatic ducts, visualizes the lymph flow and the phagocytic function of the lymph nodes, but provides far less anatomic detail than lymphangiography.

Lymphoscintigraphy was first described in 1953 [2]. Work in the past has been directed toward visualization of the lymphatic drainage in melanoma patients scheduled to undergo elective lymph node dissection [3,4], to delineate the internal mammary lymph nodes for the purpose of adjuvant radiotherapy in patients with breast cancer [5], to identify iliopelvic lymph nodes in patients with genitourinary cancers [6], and in the assessment of patients with lymphedema [7]. This chapter is focused on lymphoscintigraphy in the context of lymphatic mapping and selective lymphadenectomy. Although its main use relates to melanoma patients, the technique can also be applied to other types of skin neoplasms like squamous cell carcinomas and Merkel's cell tumors. For a more extensive discussion of lymphoscintigraphy, the reader is referred to the appropriate textbooks and review articles [8–12]. Lymphoscintigraphy in the context of lymphatic mapping for breast cancer patients is discussed in Chapter 9.

The purpose of the present chapter is to review the experience of The Netherlands Cancer Institute in cutaneous lymphoscintigraphy and to discuss the results published by others. The technique that is described has proven to be of value at our institution and is similar to the technique used at other institutions. Strengths and weaknesses of lymphoscintigraphy are analyzed, pitfalls are pointed out, and the place of this technique in lymphatic mapping and sentinel lymphadenectomy for neoplasms of the skin is discussed.

DEFINITIONS

Strictly speaking, the terms ''scintigraphy'' and ''scanning'' do not refer to the same technique. Scanning is the technique where a gamma-ray detector is moved over the field of interest in a linear fashion as used in the 1960s and 1970s. These scans were made up of a large series of dots. Modern scintigraphy with the aid of a gamma camera is much quicker and a ''scintigram'' provides a markedly more detailed image than the older ''scan.'' Scanning can be compared to what one does with a gamma detection probe that can be moved over the lymphatic field to determine the site with the increased radioactivity. Despite these distinctions, the terms scan and scintigram are often interchanged, particularly in English-speaking countries. Lymphoscintigraphy is the imaging technique that visualizes with the aid of a gamma camera the drainage of a radiopharmaceutical that is taken up by the lymphatic system.

In this chapter, we adhere to the original definition of a sentinel node as given by Morton: A sentinel node (first-tier node, first-echelon node) is the initial lymph node to which the primary tumor drains [13]. It is the lymph node on the direct drainage pathway from the primary tumor. We do not define the sentinel node as either a blue node, a radioactive node, or as the first lymph node that becomes visible on the lymphoscintigraphy images, as some investigators do [14–17]. For a more detailed discussion of the pros and cons of the various definitions of the sentinel node, the reader is referred to the Preface.

UNDERLYING PHYSIOLOGICAL MECHANISMS

Radiolabeled colloids, when administered interstitially, enter the lymphatic system at the lymphatic termini. Particles of the appropriate size migrate into the lumen through the endothelial cells by pinocytosis or through junctions between the cells. Once inside, they do not move back out. Along with the lymphatic fluid, such particles flow through a system of ducts with enlarging diameter toward the sentinel node. When they reach the sentinel node, the radiolabeled particles are trapped. The colloidal structure of the radiopharmaceutical causes the particles to be absorbed through phagocytosis by the reticuloendothelial cells in the lymph node. The radiopharmaceuticals for this purpose are fairly stable and are retained in the node for the time that gamma rays are emitted.

It should be emphasized that these tracers are not *tumor*-seeking agents, but rather *lymph-node*–seeking agents. They are accumulated in lymph nodes whether these contain metastatic disease or not. So, uptake is nonspecific and does not infer nodal metastasis *per se*. In fact, nodes largely replaced by tumor may not accumulate the tracer and remain undetected. Furthermore, gamma cameras have a limited resolution. That implies that the lymphoscintigraphy images usually do not allow the visualization of sufficient anatomic detail to distinguish a tumor-containing node either through abnormal shape or structure. Macrophages have a great avidity for colloidal radiopharmaceuticals, although that does not ensure that all of the tracer that reaches the sentinel node is retained there. Some of it may pass through to efferent lymphatics, only to be absorbed by subsequent nodes.

PURPOSES OF LYMPHOSCINTIGRAPHY, PREPARATIONS, AND INJECTION TECHNIQUE

The wound edges following a wide excision do not necessarily drain to the same lymph node or even same basin as the original lesion [3,18,19]. The relevant cutaneous lymphatics may be disrupted. Studies have shown that if lymphatic mapping is performed after wide local excision, the mean number of sentinel lymph nodes removed is increased. The number of patients where two or more basins have to be dissected is also increased to suggest that more extensive surgery is performed when compared to mapping prior to wide local excision [19]. Because this risk is likely to be much smaller after diagnostic excision with a narrow margin, it is important to perform lymphoscintigraphy and sentinel lymphadenectomy preceding therapeutic wide excision.

The purpose of lymphoscintigraphy for lymphatic mapping is to demonstrate the lymphatic drainage pathway of the neoplasm; to be more precise: to indicate the drainage basin, to determine the number of lymph nodes that are on a direct drainage pathway, to differentiate these first-tier nodes from subsequent nodes, and to locate sentinel nodes outside the usual nodal basins. The request form for lymphoscintigraphy should describe the disease, its location, and prior management. Relevant parts of the medical history of the patient should be mentioned. For instance, prior inguinal hernia surgery may prevent drainage of a lower abdominal wall melanoma to that groin. The purpose of the study is stated on the form. The surgeon should inform the patient of the reason for the scintigraphy and outline how it is done so that the patient knows what to expect.

Lymphoscintigraphy can be performed in any nuclear medicine department, using the standard equipment. The nuclear medicine physician asks the patient about allergic reactions in the past because anaphylaxis can occur, albeit rarely. A number of radiopharmaceuticals is available for lymphoscintigraphy. They all have the same radionuclide: technetium-99m (^{99m}Tc). Advantages and disadvantages of the well-known tracers are discussed under the next section. The amount of radioactivity is determined by the need for good quality images without exposing the patient to unnecessarily large doses of radioactivity. A dose of around 20 MBq (approximately 0.5 mCi) is sufficient. Intraoperative gamma-ray detection is often done utilizing the same dose of the tracer that was used for the lymphoscintigraphy. If the operation is to take place the next day, the dose should be increased taking into account the 6.2-h physical half-life of ^{99m}Tc. A dose of 40–80 MBq (approximately 1–2 mCi) allows reliable gamma probe detection the following day.

We are interested in the route of drainage of a cutaneous lesion. Therefore, the tracer is injected intradermally, raising a wheal. Subcutaneous administration is simpler to accomplish but may not delineate the route of drainage from an overlying cutaneous site. Also, drainage from the dermis is a lot faster than drainage from subcutaneous tissue. Intradermal injection of the tracer is painful. This is especially true for sulfur-containing agents because of the low pH. The injection site may be prepared with a local anesthetic in the form of an ointment. Alternatively, the tracer may be mixed with a local anesthetic. The volume of the tracer should be such that it can be evenly distributed around the skin lesion or the biopsy wound. A volume of 0.2–1.0 mL is sufficient. A thin needle is used. The tracer is administered in close proximity to the lesion or biopsy site. It is enticing to inject the entire volume in one deposit—at the end of the lesion nearest to the lymphatic field. However, a sentinel node may be missed with this approach. We have seen the tracer injected at opposite ends of the lesion go to different sentinel nodes. Uptake of the tracer by the lymphatic system usually happens instantly. Within 1 min, it may flow through lymphatic ducts to the drainage basin. Because this early flow needs to be observed, the tracer is injected with the patient on the scintigraphy table and imaging is started immediately.

RADIOPHARMACEUTICALS

The agents come in kits and are labeled with the radionuclide just before use. Noncolloidal macromolecules such as ^{99m}Tc-labeled human serum albumin (HSA) or dextran can be used to delineate lymphatic channels and to study flow kinetics. In lymphatic mapping, lymphatic *channels* as well as lymph *nodes* need to be visualized. Labeled colloids are used when lymph nodes need to be depicted. Colloid particles are 5–1000 nm in size. The behavior of colloids injected interstitially is dependent on their particle size. Very large particles fail to migrate and remain in the interstitium at the injection site. Very small particles travel so quickly that only a fraction is retained in the first lymph node. The ideal particle size for cutaneous lymphoscintigraphy has been suggested to be between 1 and 100 nm [12,20,21]. This seems a surprisingly wide range, but one has to realize that these numbers were suggested before selective lymphadenectomy gained momentum. Also, there is a trade-off. When quick accumulation and nice flow images are considered to be important, a smaller particle size agent is preferred. A larger particle size will limit the number of "hot" nonsentinel nodes depicted on the images.

A number of different radiopharmaceuticals are used for lymphoscintigraphy worldwide. A ^{99m}Tc–antimony trisulfide colloid (^{99m}Tc–Sb$_2$S$_3$) became available in 1972 [22]. This agent is taken up into the lymphatics much more rapidly than the older tracers [23]. The particle size is 3–40 nm [20,21]. Lymphatics are depicted within a few minutes after intradermal injection. Lymph nodes are visualized within 10–15 min. There are no changes in the drainage pattern on the delayed images after 2–4 h [18]. Although at one time widely used, the ^{99m}Tc–antimony trisulfide was never approved by the U.S. Food and Drug Administration and has been withdrawn from the market in that country.

Another well-known tracer is the ^{99m}Tc sulfur colloid. The unfiltered ^{99m}Tc sulfur colloid has a large particle size of 300–600 nm and therefore migrates slowly from the injection site [20,21]. The ^{99m}Tc sulfur colloid filtered with a 0.1-μm pore size filter has a small particle size: average 38 nm, with 90% of particles less than 50 nm [24]. The preparation technique is also a factor that can affect the size of the particles [25]. Lymphatics and nodes are quickly depicted with this tracer. It is cleared from the injection site with a half-time of 13.9 h [26].

The [99m]Tc (Nanocolloid-Nanocoll®, Amersham Cygne, Eindhoven, the Netherlands) consists of microaggregated albumin. This agent is used throughout Europe. More than 95% of the labeled nanocolloid particles are below 80 nm in size [27]. The clearance half-time is approximately 4 h in healthy tissue [28].

The ^{99m}Tc-labeled HSA is not a colloid. The molecular weight of albumin is 60,000. This tracer travels quickly through the lymphatics with an average speed of 10 cm/min. Good quality images are obtained. The sentinel node is reached 1–12 min (average 4 min) following the injection [29,30]. Despite its small-sized particles, this tracer does not depict more secondary nodes than labeled colloids [26]. Many other agents have been used but have failed to gain widespread acceptance [3,7,21,31,32].

Which agent is to be preferred? Compared to the filtered ^{99m}Tc sulfur colloid, the ^{99m}Tc-nanocolloid is extracted faster from the injection site [28]. Other comparative studies revealed that ^{99m}Tc-labeled HSA travels more rapidly than the ^{99m}Tc sulfur colloid [33] but is less well concentrated in the sentinel node [34]. A recent study compared the filtered (0.2-μm pore size) ^{99m}Tc albumin colloid, the filtered ^{99m}Tc sulfur colloid, and the ^{99m}Tc-labeled HSA [26]. The ^{99m}Tc-labeled HSA had the shortest transit time and best visualized the channels, but also seemed to result in a lower sentinel node-to-background ratio. All three agents demonstrated similar numbers of nodes. Other recent studies showed no relevant differences among the ^{99m}Tc–antimony trisulfide colloid, the filtered ^{99m}Tc sulfur colloid the colloidal albumin, and the ^{99m}Tc-labeled HSA [35,36–38]. However, one study suggested that the filtered ^{99m}Tc sulfur colloid travels faster than the ^{99m}Tc antimony colloid in lymphedema patients [24]. More comparative studies need to be done, focusing on these practical aspects that are important in lymphatic mapping.

IMAGING TECHNIQUE

Lymphoscintigraphy for lymphatic mapping involves dynamic imaging (flow imaging) and static (late) imaging. The dynamic part of the study visualizes the flow of the radioactive tracer through the lymphatic duct to the first lymph node it encounters. Dynamic imaging is essential because of the above-mentioned fact that some of the tracer may pass through to end up in second-tier or even subsequent nodes. Visualization of higher-echelon nodes is useful in some circumstances—for example, when the purpose of lymphoscintigraphy is to identify all internal mammary nodes for adjuvant radiotherapy in breast cancer patients, but it is troubling in lymphatic mapping. The surgeon does not want to remove all radioactive nodes but only those that receive drainage directly from the primary tumor site. Without the visible lymphatic duct identifying nodes that receive drainage directly from the injection site, the first-tier (sentinel) nodes cannot reliably be distinguished from the secondary (nonsentinel) nodes in which the surgeon is not interested.

A large-field-of-view gamma camera is used with a low-energy, high-resolution, parallel-hole collimator. For most tumor locations, the patient lies supine in a comfortable manner. The gamma camera is positioned in front of the patient so that an anterior view is obtained. The camera is positioned over the most likely drainage basin so that the lymphatic duct coming from the primary lesion site will be depicted. A double-headed gamma camera enables one to obtain a simultaneous lateral or oblique view.

There are several ways to perform the dynamic imaging. The principle is that a number of serial images of short duration are obtained. A satisfactory approach is the following. Dynamic acquisition of 60 frames of 20 s in a matrix of $128 \times 128 \times 16$ is begun immediately after injection of the tracer. In this fashion, one obtains a stack of sequential images over a period of 20 min, three images per minute. Each image contains the information on the lymphatic flow over a time frame of 20 s. The computer can then play back these consecutive images quickly one after the other, like a movie. On the computer display, one can see the tracer flow through the lymphatic duct. Within a few minutes, the sentinel node is visualized. The consecutive images can also be projected on top of each other, combined into one 20-min image. This approach allows a better identification of lymphatic ducts. A duration of 20 min is usually sufficient to collect the required information [29,39,40]. Massaging the skin at the injection site or in-between the injection site and the nodal basin stimulates the flow of the tracer when a lymphatic channel is not immediately apparent. Acquisition may be continued when the sentinel node is not identified within 20 min.

Static imaging is performed after completion of the dynamic imaging and is repeated a few hours later (Fig. 1). Anterior and lateral views are obtained, preferably in a total-body mode. These can be complemented by oblique views if necessary. An acquisition time of 5 min in a $256 \times 256 \times 16$ matrix is satisfactory. The first set of static images usually shows both the lymphatic duct and the sentinel node. The second set of static images is obtained at 2–4 h postinjection when the radioactivity has settled down [23,41,42]. By this time, it has cleared the lymphatic channel. These late images depict radioactivity remaining at the primary lesion site, the radioactivity in the sentinel node, and sometimes radioactivity in second-tier nodes. Images obtained even later rarely show a different pattern.

The tracer is accumulated in the sentinel lymph node(s), but most of it stays behind at the injection site. Very little goes to other tissues. The images show a number of hot spots in a dark background. Therefore, it is difficult to determine exactly where the radioactive nodes are located in the body. The body

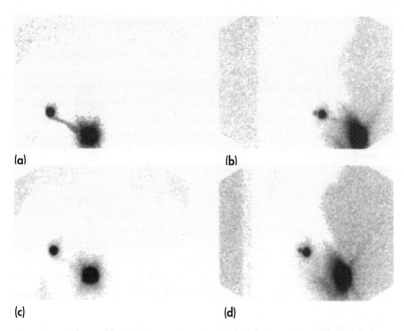

(a)   (b)

(c)   (d)

FIGURE 1   Early and late static images of a 43-year-old man with a melanoma in the right parasternal region. The early images (a, b) show the lymphatic channel running from the primary lesion site to the sentinel node in the right axilla. On the late images (c, d), the radioactivity has largely cleared the lymphatic duct. The sentinel node and remaining radioactivity at the injection site are depicted. The lateral views (b, d) also depict a second-tier node.

contour can be displayed by moving a radioactive point source along the outline of the body during data acquisition (Fig. 2). This will outline anatomic landmarks on the images. A more elegant technique to visualize the body contour involves placement of a cobalt-57 flood source behind the patient during data acquisition [40,43]. A flood source is a large radioactive disk with the size of the gamma camera head. Imaging with the flood source behind the patient is comparable to photography with backlighting: The patient attenuates radioactivity from the flood source and the body contour is outlined. Simultaneous transmission imaging

FIGURE 2   Anterior lymphoscintigraphy of a 47-year-old man with a melanoma on the back. Indication of the body contour greatly facilitates orientation: (a) image without contour; (b) body contour outlined with radioactive marking pen; (c) contour outlined with flood source backlighting.

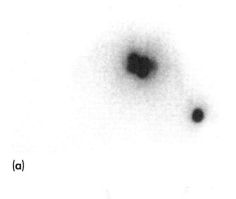

(a)

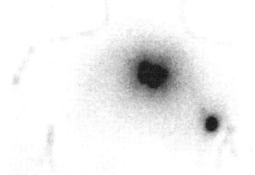

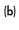

(b)

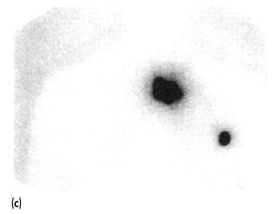

(c)

with the flood source yields images with both the lymph nodes depicted and the body contour outlined (Fig. 2). Orientation is greatly facilitated in this manner.

The location of a sentinel node can also be indicated on the patient. The nuclear medicine physician can mark the course of the lymphatic duct and the exact location of a sentinel node on the overlying skin. The marking procedure is performed with the patient in the same position as during the operation. With the gamma camera in the real-time view mode and the sentinel node within the field of view, a radioactive marker is moved over the skin. Its hot spot coincides with the hot spot representing the sentinel node when the marker is directly over the node. The location of a sentinel node can also be established with a gamma-ray detection probe. This technique works particularly well in the axilla. A skin mark is applied with an indelible ink in that exact location. The sentinel node location can also be indicated by an intradermal tattoo [41]. The skin mark provides the surgeon with valuable information about where to pick up the lymphatic duct and where to expect the sentinel node. The marking procedure requires careful attention to detail and should be done by a dedicated nuclear medicine physician with special expertise. Each patient should be assessed with regard to his or her individual requirements.

The nuclear medicine report should indicate the type of tracer used, its volume, the amount of radioactivity, and the injection site. Both the dynamic and static study should be described. The report should state the lymphatic field(s) of drainage and the number of sentinel nodes. It should mention whether second-tier nodes were visualized and explain which nodes should be considered as such. The skin marks applied by the nuclear medicine physician should be described. Uncertainty with regard to the true number of sentinel nodes should be admitted. It is of crucial importance for the nuclear medicine physician and the surgeon to review the images together. It is equally important for the surgeon to report the operative findings back to the nuclear medicine physician. It is even better for the nuclear medicine physician to come to the operating room to see for himself.

RESULTS

The images are usually easy to interpret. The above-described technique depicts the lymphatic duct(s) in 80–98% of patients. In our hands, it hardly ever fails to visualize the sentinel node(s) [42,44–48]. Lymphatic drainage is complex in the neck and this is the most difficult lymphatic field for the interpretation of lymphoscintigraphy. We could not identify a sentinel node in 3 of 25 (12%) patients with a melanoma in the head and neck region [49]. O'Brien and co-workers faced this problem in 2 out of 97 patients (2%) [23], Alex and co-workers in 2 out of 22 (9%) [50]. In 34% to 84% of the patients, drainage in the neck is discordant with clinical prediction [5,23]. A lymph channel can traverse the upper neck node group and pass directly to a sentinel node in the lower neck. Bilateral drainage is seen in approximately 10% of the patients [52]. Multiple sentinel nodes are depicted in the majority of the patients, on average 2.5 per patient [23,49,53]. A total of five sentinel nodes in the neck is not rare [23,53]. The primary lesion site is often close to where one would expect the sentinel node. The bulk of the radioactive tracer stays behind at the injection site and may obscure a nearby sentinel node. In a patient with a melanoma on the cheek, for instance, a sentinel node in the underlying parotid gland is often not identifiable on the images. In this regard, lateral images may be important to maximize separation between the primary site and the sentinel node. The neck contains more than 100 lymph nodes packed in a small area. Frequently, it is difficult to distinguish first-tier nodes from secondary nodes because more than one sentinel node is often present and because nonsentinel nodes may pick up radioactivity as well (Fig. 3).

The axilla is the easiest lymphatic field for the nuclear medicine physician. Usually there is only one sentinel node [47]. Nonsentinel nodes are depicted less frequently in the axilla than in the neck and groin. When the groin receives drainage from a trunk melanoma, there is often one sentinel node above the level of the inguinal ligament. A melanoma on the leg usually drains to two superficial sentinel nodes below the inguinal ligament. Exceptions to these rules occur rather

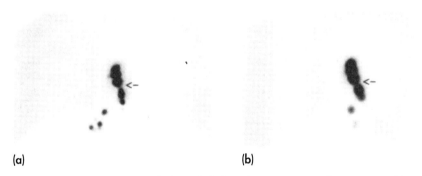

(a)   (b)

FIGURE 3 Anterior (a) and right lateral (b) lymphoscintigrams of a 37-year-old man with a melanoma behind the right ear. A string of lymph nodes is visualized within 2 min. From these images, it is not clear how many sentinel nodes and how many nonsentinel nodes are depicted. The dynamic images were not helpful either. Intraoperative mapping with patent blue dye (Blue Patenté V, Guerbet, Aulney-Sous-Bois, France) revealed lymphatic ducts coming from the primary lesion going to a sentinel node at the anterior margin of the sternocleidomastoid muscle, to a second sentinel node in the parotid gland, and to a third sentinel node immediately underneath the primary lesion site. The other depicted nodes were higher-echelon nodes. The second sentinel node (arrow) contained the highest level of radioactivity and was the only one with metastatic disease.

frequently. We and others have seen up to five sentinel nodes in the groin [54]. Sometimes, the lymph flow goes directly to Cloquet's node, or, rarely, may bypass the superficial groin to drain directly to the hypogastric or iliac nodes. Nonsentinel nodes are often depicted in the groin and may render the images difficult to interpret.

In the neck, the skin mark can usually be placed exactly overlying the target. Occasionally, the mark is somewhat off target, presumably because the position of the head is different during the operation compared to what it was during lymphoscintigraphy. In the axilla, it is difficult to indicate the location of the sentinel node because this is much more a three-dimensional lymphatic basin than the groin or the neck. Also, the position of the arm may not be exactly the same during scintigraphy and during the operation, so layers of axillary fat containing a sentinel node may shift. What one can do is place the skin mark on the anterior chest wall and then calculate the depth on a lateral view [54]. The gamma detection probe is helpful when marking the axilla. The skin mark can always be positioned exactly overlying the target node in the groin.

Although only a small percentage of the radioactivity ends up in the sentinel node, its uptake far exceeds the uptake in the surrounding normal tissue. The accumulation of the ^{99m}Tc-nanocolloid in sentinel nodes and surrounding normal tissues was investigated in a study of 60 consecutive patients with clinically localized melanoma [42]. Sentinel nodes and nearby nonsentinel nodes were removed for examination. All excised nodes as well as small samples of skin and subcutaneous fat were measured in a gamma well counter. The uptake of the tracer as a percentage of the injected dose per gram of tissue and per node was calculated, with a correction for physical decay. The uptake in the whole sentinel node averaged 0.36% of the injected dose, with a range of 0.0013–6.8%. The average uptake per gram of tissue in the sentinel node was 1.0% of the administered dose, with a range of 0.003–17.4%. Lymph nodes are surrounded by fat, which is covered by skin. Uptake in these surrounding tissues was found to be far less than in sentinel nodes. The average uptake of radioactivity in a gram of overlying skin was 0.01% of the injected dose (range: 0.0–0.22%). In a gram of fat, the average uptake was 0.0035% (range: 0.0–0.081%). The visibility of a hot spot depends on the uptake in that location compared to the uptake in the surrounding tissues: the target-to-background ratio. Measured with a gamma detection probe in the open wound, the sentinel node-to-background ratio was calculated to be 36 on average (range: 2–722) when using the ^{99m}Tc nanocolloid [42]. In studies using the ^{99m}Tc-labeled sulfur colloid, ratios are somewhat lower, on average 8.5 with ranges of 1.0 to 65 and 30 to 300 [41,55].

If lymphoscintigraphy were to be repeated, would it show the same drainage pattern? Its reproducibility was the subject of two studies. The first study was performed at our institution and concerned 25 patients with clinically localized melanoma [40]. The same investigator performed two scintigraphic studies in an identical fashion in each patient with a 2–4-week interval. The ^{99m}Tc-nanocolloid was the tracer used. Both dynamic and static imaging were performed. Both scintigraphy series showed drainage to the same lymphatic fields in all patients. However, a difference in number of sentinel nodes depicted on the first and second study was noted in three patients (12%). So, the reproducibility was 88%. Otherwise, the images were identical for number and location of nodes. In the second study, the ^{99m}Tc sulfur colloid was used [55]. The result was similar with a reproducibility of 85%. The reason for this limited reproducibility is unknown, but a number of causes can be considered either related to the tracer, to the technique, or to the patient. Unnoticed variations in the technique of injection or the site of injection and variations in the composition of the radiopharmaceutical are possible explanations. Perhaps lymphatic drainage may vary in time within an individual. Factors like previous exertion, body hydration, variation in tissue oncotic, and hydrostatic pressure of blood may play a role [56]. Lymphoscintigraphy reflects drainage and may show such a variability in the physiologic process. In most patients in our own study, the first scintigraphy study was done a few weeks after the primary lesion had been excised [40]. All patients underwent their second preoperative scan a maximum of 4 weeks after the first scan. During the wound-healing process, granulation tissue is gradually replaced by more dense and compact fibrous tissue. It is conceivable that such alterations influence to some extent the lymphatic drainage of the area concerned. No matter what the reasons for the discrepancies are, the limited reproducibility is a matter of concern. This variability may explain some of the false-negative sentinel node procedures that have been reported.

The reproducibility of the reporting of lymphoscintigraphy studies has also been investigated [44]. There is a concordance rate of 98% when different nuclear medicine physicians interpret the lymphoscintigraphy images of the same patient.

Despite paying attention to every detail of the lymphoscintigraphy, there is sometimes a discrepancy between the number of sentinel nodes that is indicated by lymphoscintigraphy and the number of sentinel nodes found during the operation. This observation prompted us to review the nuclear medicine reports and operative notes of our first 150 patients [57]. The primary lesion was situated in the head and neck region in 13 patients, on the trunk in 52, on the arm in 23, and on a lower extremity in 62 patients. Dynamic and static lymphoscintigraphy were performed as described earlier in this chapter.

Compared to lymphoscintigraphy, a different number of sentinel nodes was found during the operation in 33 of the 189 lymphatic fields (17%). Scintigraphy suggested too few nodes in 26 basins and too many in 6. Only one of the discrepancies was felt to be due to inadequate surgical exploration. The majority of discrepancies in the number of sentinel nodes was apparently caused by the limited resolution of the gamma camera (i.e., its limited discriminating power). A typical scenario was the failure of flow images to distinguish two parallel lymphatic channels that were running to two separate nodes. Occasionally, a single hot spot on the static images proved on exploration to be, in fact, made up by two adjacent sentinel nodes, each with a separate blue lymphatic duct leading to it (Fig. 4). In a few patients, two separate lymphatic channels drained to opposite ends of a single elongated lymph node, giving the false impression that two sentinel nodes were present.

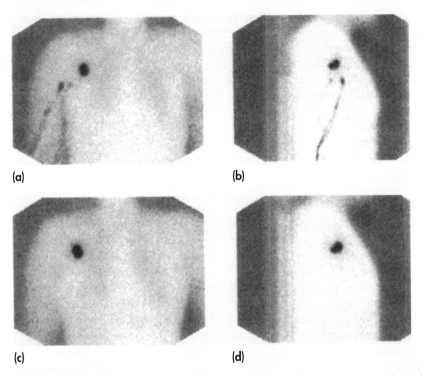

(a)   (b)

(c)   (d)

FIGURE 4   Lymphoscintigraphy of a 48-year-old woman with a melanoma on the right forearm. (a) Anterior view 30 min; (b) right lateral view 30 min; (c) anterior view 2 h; (d) right lateral view 2 h. To the casual observer, the late images (c, d) may show one hot spot. With careful observation of the early lateral view (b), however, there may be two adjoining sentinel nodes. During the operation, we identified two lymphatic ducts and removed two sentinel nodes adjacent to each other. Both were radioactive. Subsequent scanning of the wound for residual radioactivity revealed a definite hot focus right underneath the site where the two sentinel nodes had been removed. Exploring deeper down, a third blue lymphatic channel was found, coming from the direction of the arm, leading to a third node that was both blue and radioactive. The limited resolution of the gamma camera made it impossible to identify the third sentinel node on the images.

LIMITATIONS

There are several reasons why sometimes no sentinel node is identified on the lymphoscintigraphy images. Rarely, there is no drainage of the agent from the injection site [11,23,49]. This risk is greater after a wide therapeutic excision has been performed [3,58], and it is the rule after a skin graft has been applied to cover the defect [59]. Injection of the radiocolloid into the scar of the excisional biopsy may also be associated with no flow from the primary site. Visualization of the liver usually means that some of the tracer was injected intravenously and removed from the circulation by the Kupffer cells.

When the injection site is close to the sentinel node, a different camera angle or a different position of the patient may be needed in order to obtain the required information. For instance, an injection site over the scapula may obscure a sentinel node in the axilla. Dynamic imaging from a lateral angle will then visualize the injection site and the lymphatic duct going around the latissimus dorsi muscle to the sentinel node. An injection site high on the inside of the arm requires the arm to be swung upward in order to avoid overprojection of the injection site and the sentinel node. A primary tumor site on the cheek is best imaged with the head turned to the opposite side. Another option for minimizing the bulk of the radioactivity at the injection site is to cover it with a lead shield.

Lymphatic channels containing obvious tumor can result in blockage of the lymph flow [5,60]. Nodes that are largely replaced by tumor accumulate less of the tracer or sometimes do not accumulate tracer at all [5,12,18,44]. On the other hand, lymphatic channels and nodes are sometimes well delineated despite clinically obvious metastatic tumor deposits [61].

Experience with lymphoscintigraphy has taught us that lymphatic drainage is highly variable. It is now abundantly clear that watershed areas of ambiguous lymphatic flow are much wider than was previously assumed [60]. Drainage sometimes occurs to lymphatic regions other than those expected on the basis of the classic anatomic studies. Drainage across the midline or Sappey's line is not unusual for primary lesions up to 10 cm away. It has been suggested that lymphoscintigraphy is not needed when the primary lesion is located on an extremity because the drainage pattern is predictable [62], but melanomas of the arm can drain directly to a supraclavicular node [63], to an interpectoral node [64], or even to the opposite axilla [65]. Lesser known small lymphatic basins can contain a sentinel node. Hot epitrochlear nodes are sometimes seen in patients with a melanoma of the forearm [66]. A melanoma on the skin of the calf may drain to a sentinel node in the popliteal fossa (Fig. 5). A strong point in favor of lymphoscintigraphy is that such—occasionally bizarre—drainage patterns can be identified.

We find sentinel nodes in strange places, outside the known lymphatic basins. It is understandable that melanoma surgeons call these nodes ''in-transit''

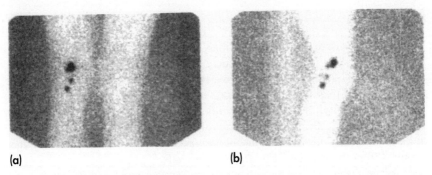

(a)   (b)

FIGURE 5   Anterior (a) and right lateral (b) static images of a 67-year-old woman with a melanoma of the right foot. Three sentinel nodes are depicted in the popliteal fossa.

nodes. They are also known as "interval nodes" or "extra-anatomic" nodes. No matter what name they are given, they *are* sentinel nodes. The work of Uren and co-workers at the Sydney Melanoma Unit deserves to be mentioned [67]. They encountered actual sentinel nodes outside the recognized lymphatic fields in 22% of their patients [44]. A review of our own series revealed this phenomenon in 12%. Certain sites turn up repeatedly and patterns are beginning to emerge. In a number of patients, we have seen sentinel nodes just lateral to the areola of the breast receiving drainage from lesions in the epigastric region. A sentinel node is sometimes found high in the flank, as if having dropped from the axilla (Fig. 6). This can be seen in patients with melanoma on the abdominal wall, on the back, or lower down on the flank [68,69]. Melanomas in the epigastric region and periumbilical skin sometimes drain directly to the internal mammary nodes [44,70]. Lymphatic ducts from melanomas on the back occasionally go directly to the mediastinum [14,44]. Drainage to nodes in the triangular intermuscular space occurs in 30% of the patients with melanomas on the upper part of the back [71,72]. This anatomical entity is situated just lateral to the scapula. It is formed inferiorly by the teres major muscle, medial-superiorly by the infraspinatus and teres minor muscles, and laterally by the long head of the triceps muscle. A static posterior view can give the misleading impression that such a node is located in the axilla. The dynamic study and the lateral view will declare its true location (Fig. 7). More abnormal routes of drainage to watch out for have been described [73]. Without lymphoscintigraphy, these in-transit nodes would elude us.

As has been indicated, it is important to appreciate that not all nodes showing tracer uptake are sentinel nodes. The images can be most difficult to interpret when multiple nodes light up (Fig. 3). One cannot always clearly distinguish first-tier nodes from subsequent (nonsentinel) nodes, even with dynamic imaging. This problem is faced fairly frequently. Despite the fact that the average number of counts in a first-tier node is four to five times as high as the average uptake

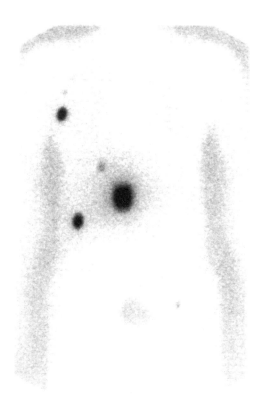

FIGURE 6 Anterior lymphoscintigraphy in a 43-year-old man with a melanoma on the back in the midline. Sentinel nodes are shown in the right axilla, the left groin, and the right flank. A second-tier node is depicted in the right epigastric region.

in a secondary node [40], it is not true that the node with the highest number of counts is *always* the sentinel node. We have occasionally seen a large second-tier node accumulate more of the radioactive tracer than a small first-tier node. Also, it has been suggested that the lymph node closest to the primary lesion site is always the sentinel node [74]. This notion has proven to be wrong [75]. Uncertainty about the hierarchy of hot nodes is best expressed in the lymphoscintigraphy report and discussed with the surgeon. Intraoperative mapping will usually solve the problem. The lymphatic channel can be exposed with the aid of blue dye to actually prove whether a node is a first-tier node, receiving drainage directly from the site of the primary lesion, or a second-tier node, receiving drainage from a first-tier node.

Not every hot spot represents a lymph node. A hot spot may be caused by a drop of the tracer spilled on the skin (Fig. 8). Surgical exploration of a hot spot

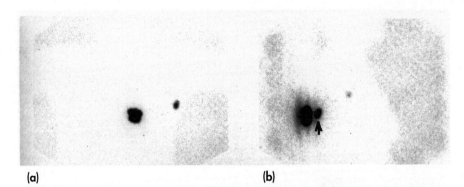

(a)   (b)

FIGURE 7   Posterior (a) and right lateral (b) lymphoscintigram of a 49-year-old woman with a melanoma on the back just to the right of the midline. The posterior image at 30 min shows a lymphatic duct and a sentinel node that could be situated in the right axilla. The lateral image establishes that the sentinel node is situated in the triangular intermuscular space on the back (arrow). A second-tier node is located in the right axilla.

on a scintigram sometimes reveals what appears to be a lymphangioma (''lymphatic lake'') in a lymphatic channel instead of a lymph node. Circumscribed hyperplasia of lymph vessels is known to occur in major lymphatic trunks in the absence of other morbid changes in the surrounding tissues [76]. For no apparent reason, the radioactive tracer is sometimes retained for more than 24 h in such a lesion. We have encountered this phenomenon in the head and neck region, on the back, and on the thigh (Fig. 9).

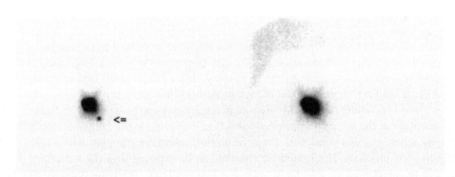

FIGURE 8   Contamination of the skin by a drop of the radiopharmaceutical (arrow) may suggest the presence of a sentinel node (left). This hot spot was easily wiped off (right).

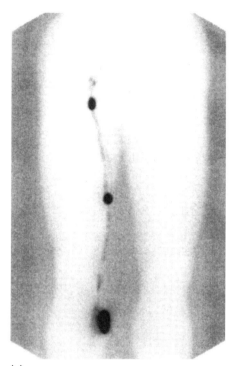

(a)

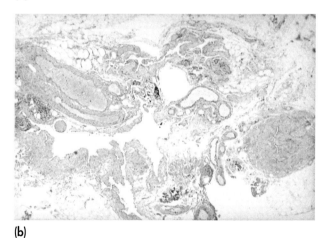

(b)

Figure 9   Lymphoscintigram (a) of a 46-year-old man with a melanoma just below the right knee. A hot spot suggestive of an interval sentinel node is depicted on the right thigh. Surgical exploration revealed a lymphangioma in this location. The true sentinel node was identified in the groin. The pathology slide (b) shows a conglomerate of lymphatic ducts without glandular tissue.

SIDE EFFECTS AND RADIATION DOSE

The radiopharmaceuticals used for lymphoscintigraphy are protein derivatives in some form or other. Consequently, allergic reactions may occur. An allergic reaction may present as a skin rash but also as bronchospasm, anaphylactic shock, and even cardiopulmonary arrest. Fortunately, such events are rare. No complications arose in a study of 160 patients with the ^{99m}Tc sulfur colloid and the ^{99m}Tc-labeled HSA [11]. Over the years, we have seen one allergic reaction (rash) in 25,000 patients undergoing lymphoscintigraphy for various indications. Allergic reactions are treated in the usual fashion depending on the symptoms and severity.

Radiation exposure is another consideration. Use of a radiopharmaceutical inevitably results in exposure of the patient and the hospital personnel to some radiation. Acceptable limits of such exposure are set by government bodies and vary from one region to another. The radiation dose is low for all tracers because of the favorable characteristics of ^{99m}Tc (no beta emission) and the small dose that is needed. However, the exposure is difficult to calculate precisely, because of the variability of the injection site. This subject is discussed in detail in Chapter 13.

THE FUTURE

With increasing experience, interpretation of lymphoscintigrams should become more reliable. For instance, more abnormal drainage patterns will be described in the future [69]. That means that fewer sentinel nodes will go unnoticed by the nuclear medicine physician and the surgeon. Both the strong and weak points of lymphoscintigraphy will become better defined. Because the resolution of gamma cameras is not likely to improve dramatically in the foreseeable future, advances in lymphoscintigraphy will have to come from use of better tracers. What should we be working on to develop better tracers? A typical radiopharmaceutical consists of a radionuclide that emits the radiation that is used for imaging and a second part that determines the biological properties of the molecule. ^{99m}Tc comes close to the ideal radionuclide. It is easy to obtain and to handle in the radiopharmacy laboratory. It emits gamma rays with an energy of 140 keV, particularly suitable for present-day gamma cameras. It has a physical half-life of 6.2 h, long enough for the purposes of lymphoscintigraphy and next-day gamma probe detection, but short enough for contamination, should that happen, to be of a limited duration.

What about the other part that makes up the tracer molecule? What are the properties of the ideal tracer for lymphatic mapping of cutaneous lesions? The ideal tracer is easy to prepare in the radiopharmacy laboratory and remains stable. After administration into the interstitium, it is accumulated in the lymphatic system and travels to the first lymph node. Ideally, within a few hours there should be no residual activity at the injection site. Complete clearance eliminates the problem of remaining radioactivity at a nearby injection site obscuring a sentinel node. The ideal tracer is avidly accumulated and retained in the first node without some of it passing through and moving on to subsequent nodes: a radioactive node is a sentinel node. This obviates the need for dynamic imaging and also eliminates the need for the surgeon to use the blue dye technique. The radiation dose to the patient and hospital personnel is low and there are no other side effects.

Because macrophages have such a great affinity for the protein derivatives that are currently used, it seems logical to take advantage of this fact. Modifications of the shape of the particles or their surface characteristics may improve clearance from the injection site and may make them more appetizing for macrophages [77]. Different protein products with varying size particles also need to be investigated. In the groin, additional (second-tier) nodes are depicted more often than in the axilla. Therefore, it may well be that we will use different tracers for different lymphatic fields in the near future. However, within a few years there may be nonparticulate tracers that are accumulated in a lymph node through other mechanisms. ^{99m}Tc-labeled polydiethylenetriamine pentaacetic acid poly-mannosyl polylysine (DTPA-*man*-PL) may be a step in that direction [78]. An animal experiment showed that this tracer is irreversibly bound to lymphocytes through a receptor-specific interaction. What about tracers that are targeted directly against tumor cells? Will there be tumor-seeking agents that accumulate in lymph nodes with metastatic disease while leaving healthy nodes alone? Such a tracer could be injected either at the tumor site or even into the bloodstream. The surgeon could then remove all radioactive nodes (and visceral metastases for that matter) and be sure to have cured the patient. If no nodes light up, there would be no need to explore the lymphatic field. The problem with this train of thought is that there must be a certain amount of radioactivity in a cancer deposit for it to be detected. That means that such a deposit must have a certain size. That size is currently 3 mm with the best available tracer and the tumor cell type that has the highest avidity for that agent. Monoclonal antibodies against tumor-specific antigens have potential in this respect. However, although the specificity of monoclonal antibodies may be 100%, what is lacking are truly tumor-specific antigens that are consistently present in various tumor subtypes. These antigens need to be tumor-specific, distributed uniformly among tumor cells with a high density, and must be accessible to the antibody that is used. Clinical diagnosis with labeled antibodies has had limited value until now because tumor deposits smaller than 3 mm cannot be detected and such micrometastases need to be identified because they may ultimately kill the patient. Far smaller tumor deposits *can* be detected with current pathological techniques. This also rules out scintigraphy with agents like thallium-201 [79], ^{99m}Tc sestamibi [80], iodine-123 iodobenzamide [81], and indium-111 pentetreotide [81] to name but a few, and also other techniques like ultrasonography for staging and positron emission tomography (PET) [82–84]. Although PET with 2-fluorine-18-fluoro-2-deoxy-D-glucose (FDG) is a highly sensitive technique for detecting metastatic melanoma, it cannot detect metastases smaller than approximately 5 mm [85,86]. So, these tracers and these techniques will not replace (the tracers currently used in) lymphatic mapping, but they may play a future role in identifying patients with metastases 3–10 mm in size that cannot be detected by physical examination. Such patients can then be spared a sentinel node biopsy before a formal regional node dissection. Lymphatic mapping and a more detailed examination of the sentinel lymph node can identify micrometastatic disease with a sensitivity of being able to identify a single melanoma cell in a background of a million lymphocytes. There will not be a PET scan, MRI, or CT scan that has that kind of sensitivity.

CONCLUDING REMARKS

Lymphatic mapping with selective lymph node biopsy has created a renewed interest in lymphoscintigraphy. This development increases our knowledge of the anatomy and physiology of the lymphatic system. Old dogmas continue to be modified. The result is a better understanding of the process of lymphatic dissemination. Lymphoscintigraphy is a crucial link in lymphatic mapping with selective lymphadenectomy. It is an elegant and simple diagnostic technique that can readily be performed in any nuclear medicine department. Lymphoscintigraphy is well tolerated by patients. A number of satisfactory tracers are available for this procedure. Combined dynamic and static imaging with attention to detail yields high-quality images that provide important information. With this technique, the nuclear medicine physician provides a road map that guides the surgeon to the sentinel node. Lymphoscintigraphy flawlessly identifies all basins at risk for metastatic disease. Unusual routes of drainage and sentinel nodes outside the generally recognized lymphatic basins are indicated. The location of a sentinel node can be marked on the skin. This aids the surgeon with the decision of where and in what direction to make the incision. Despite these strong points, the surgeon must be aware of the fact that the images do not necessarily always indicate the true number of sentinel nodes and that a sentinel node can be difficult to distinguish from secondary nodes. We nevertheless feel that lymphatic mapping cannot be done in a responsible fashion without high-quality lymphoscintigraphy in every patient.

REFERENCES

1. JB Kimmonth, GW Taylor, RK Harper. Lymphangiography: a technique for its clinical use in the lower limb. Br Med J 1:940–942, 1955.

2. AI Sherman, M Ter-Pogossian. Lymph node concentration of radioactive colloidal gold following interstitial injection. Cancer 6:1238–1240, 1953.

3. LR Bennett, G Lago. Cutaneous lymphoscintigraphy in malignant melanoma. Semin Nucl Med 13:61–69, 1983.

4. HJ Wanebo, M Chung. Radionuclide lymphoscintigraphy to identify lymphatic drainage patterns of cutaneous head and neck melanoma. Diagn Oncol 3:258–262, 1994.

5. GN Ege. Lymphoscintigraphy–techniques and applications in the management of breast carcinoma. Semin Nucl Med 13:26–34, 1983.

6. WD Kaplan. Iliopelvic lymphoscintigraphy. Semin Nucl Med 13:42–53, 1983.

7. G Stewart, JI Gaunt, DN Croft, NL Browse. Isotope lymphography: a new method of investigating the role of lymphatics in chronic limb oedema. Br J Surg 72:906–909, 1985.

8. MN Croll, LW Brady, S Dadparvar. Implications of lymphoscintigraphy in oncologic practice: principles and differences vis-a-vis other imaging modalities. Semin Nucl Med 13:4–8, 1983.

9. RW McConnell, BG McConnell, EE Kim. Other applications of interstitial lymphoscintigraphy. Semin Nucl Med 13:70–74, 1983.

10. EL Kramer. Lymphoscintigraphy: radiopharmaceutical selection and methods. Nucl Med Biol 17:57–63, 1990.

11. LM Lamki, JR Logic. Defining lymphatic drainage patterns with cutaneous lymphoscintigraphy. In: CM Balch, AN Houghton, GW Milton, AJ Sober, SJ Soong, eds. Cutaneous Melanoma. 2nd ed. Philadelphia: J.B. Lippincott Company, 1992, pp. 367–375.

12. GN Ege. Lymphoscintigraphy in oncology. In: RE Henkin, MA Boles, GL Dillehay, et al., eds. Nuclear Medicine. St. Louis, MO: Mosby, 1996, pp. 1504–1523.

13. DL Morton, D Wen, JH Wong, JS Economou, LA Cagle, FK Storm, LJ Foshag, AJ Cochran. Technical details of intraoperative lymphatic mapping for early stage melanoma. Arch Surg 127:392–399, 1992.

14. DN Krag, SJ Meijer, DL Weaver, BW Loggie, SP Harlow, KK Tanabe, EH Laughlin, JC Alex. Minimal-access surgery for staging of malignant melanoma. Arch Surg 130:654–658, 1995.

15. U Veronesi, G Paganelli, V Galimberti, G Viale, S Zurrida, M Bedoni, A Costa, C De Cicco, JG Geraghty, A Luini, V Sacchini, P Veronesi. Sentinel-node biopsy to avoid axillary dissection in breast cancer with clinically negative lymph-nodes. Lancet 349:1864–1867, 1997.

16. C De Cicco, M Sideri, M Bartolomei, A Maggioni, N Colombo, L Bocciolone, M Chinol, L Leonardi, C Mangioni, G Paganelli. Sentinel node detection by lymphoscintigraphy and gamma detecting probe in patients with vulvar cancer (abstr). J Nucl Med 38:33P, 1997.

17. SPL Leong, I Steinmetz, FA Habib, A McMillan, JZ Gans, RE Allen Jr, ET Morita, M El-Kadi, HD Epstein, M Kashani-Sabet, RW Gagebiel. Optimal selective sentinel node dissection in primary malignant melanoma. Arch Surg 132:666–673, 1997.

18. DC Sullivan, BP Croker Jr, CC Harris, P Deery, HF Seigler. Lymphoscintigraphy in malignant melanoma: ^{99m}Tc antimony sulfur colloid. Am J Radiol 137:847–851, 1981.

19. KE Wells, E Joseph, M Ross, CW Cruse, DP Rapaport, F Glass, J Messina, C Berman, A Cantor, DS Reintgen. Lymphatic mapping for melanoma before and after wide local excision (abstr). Melanoma Res 7:S105, 1997.

20. S Strand, BRR Persson. Quantitative lymphoscintigraphy I: basic concepts for optimal uptake of radiocolloids in the parasternal lymph nodes of rabbits. J Nucl Med 20:1038–1046, 1979.

21. L Bergqvist, SE Strand, BRR Persson. Particle sizing and biokinetics of interstitial lymphoscintigraphic agents. Semin Nucl Med 13:9–19, 1983.

22. VF Fairbanks, WN Tauxe, JM Kiely, WE Miller. Scintigraphic visualization of abdominal lymph nodes with ^{99m}Tc-pertechnetate-labeled sulfur colloid. J Nucl Med 13:185–190, 1972.

23. CJ O'Brien, RF Uren, JF Thompson, RB Howman-Giles, K Petersen-Schaefer, HM Shaw, MJ Quinn, WH McCarthy. Prediction of potential metastatic sites in cutaneous head and neck melanoma using lymphoscintigraphy. Am J Surg 170:461–466, 1995.

24. JC Hung, GA Wiseman, HW Wahner, BP Mullan, TR Taggart, WL Dunn. Filtered technetium-99m-sulfur colloid evaluated for lymphoscintigraphy. J Nucl Med 36: 1895–1901, 1995.

25. NP Alazraki, D Eshima, LA Eshima, SC Herda, DR Murray, JP Vansant, AT Taylor. Lymphoscintigraphy, the sentinel node concept, and the intraoperative gamma probe in melanoma, breast cancer, and other potential cancers. Semin Nucl Med 27:55–67, 1997.

26. EC Glass, R Essner, DL Morton. Kinetics of three lymphoscintigraphic agents in patients with cutaneous melanoma. J Nucl Med 39:1185–1190, 1998.

27. Sorin Biomedica Diagnostics S.p.A. V, Italy. Solco product information, 1998.

28. J Frühling. Comparative study of four ^{99m}Tc-labelled microcolloids, used for lymphoscintigraphy (abstr). Eur J Nucl Med 9:A43, 1984.

29. E Ohtake, K Matsui, Y Kobayashi, Y Ono. Dynamic lymphoscintigraphy with Tc-99m human serum albumin. Radiat Med 1:132–136, 1983.

30. SD Nathanson, L Nelson, KC Karvelis. Rates of flow of technetium-99m-labeled human serum albumin from peripheral injection sites to sentinel lymph nodes. Ann Surg Oncol 3:329–335, 1996.

31. PH Cox. The use of radiocolloids for the evaluation of lymph node function. Thesis, University of Utrecht, The Netherlands, 1974.

32. E Henze, HR Schelbert, JD Collins, A Najafi, JR Barrio, LR Bennett. Lymphoscintigraphy with Tc-99m-labeled dextran. J Nucl Med 23:923–929, 1982.

33. LM Lamki, TP Haynie, CM Balch, VA Bhadkamkar, DA Podoloff, EE Kim. Lymphoscintigraphy in the surgical management of patients with truncal melanoma: Comparison of Tc sulfur colloid with Tc human serum albumin (abstr). J Nucl Med 30:844, 1989.

34. SD Nathanson, P Anaya, L Eck. Sentinel lymph node uptake of two different radionuclides (abstr). Society of Surgical Oncology, 49th Annual Meeting, Atlanta 1996, p. 64.

35. P Sharkey, C Berman, DS Reintgen. Comparison of radiopharmaceuticals utilized in lymphoscintigraphy (abstr). Melanoma Res 7(Suppl 1):S87, 1997.

36. JH Wong, K Terada, P Ko, MN Coel. Lack of effect of particle size on the identi-

fication of the sentinel node in cutaneous malignancies. Ann Surg Oncol 5:77–80, 1998.

37. I Bedrosian, AM Scheff, R Mick, LS Callans, LP Bucky, FR Spitz, C Helsabeck, DE Elder, A Alavi, DF Fraker, BJ Czerniecki. 99m Tc-Human serum albumin: an effective radiotracer for identifying sentinel lymph nodes in melanoma. J Nucl Med 40:1143–1148, 1999.

38. R Pijpers, PJ Borgstein, S Meijer, DN Krag, OS Hoekstra, HNJM Greuter, GJJ Teule. Transport and retention of colloidal tracers in regional lymphoscintigraphy in melanoma: influence on lymphatic mapping and sentinel node biopsy. Melanoma Res 8:413–418, 1999.

39. HJ Pijpers, GJ Collet, S Meijer, OS Hoekstra. The impact of dynamic lymphoscintigraphy and gamma probe guidance on sentinel node biopsy in melanoma. Eur J Nucl Med 22:1238–1241, 1995.

40. BAE Kapteijn, OE Nieweg, RA Valdes Olmos, IH Liem, RKL Baidjnath Panday, CA Hoefnagel, BBR Kroon. Reproducibility of lymphoscintigraphy for lymphatic mapping in patients with cutaneous melanoma. J Nucl Med 37:972–975, 1996.

41. JJ Albertini, CW Cruse, D Rapaport, K Wells, M Ross, R DeConti, CG Berman, K Jared, J Messina, G Lyman, F Glass, N Fenske, D Reintgen. Intraoperative radiolymphoscintigraphy improves sentinel node identification for patients with melanoma. Ann Surg 223:217–224, 1996.

42. BAE Kapteijn, OE Nieweg, SH Muller, IH Liem, CA Hoefnagel, EJT Rutgers, BBR Kroon. Validation of gamma probe detection of the sentinel node in melanoma. J Nucl Med 38:362–366, 1997.

43. JH West, JC Seymour, WE Drane. Combined transmission-emission imaging in lymphoscintigraphy. Clin Nucl Med 18:762–764, 1993.

44. RF Uren, RB Howman-Giles, HM Shaw, JF Thompson, WH McCarthy. Lymphoscintigraphy in high-risk melanoma of the trunk: predicting draining node groups, defining lymphatic channels and locating the sentinel node. J Nucl Med 34:1435–1440, 1993.

45. CG Berman, J Norman, CW Cruse, DS Reintgen, RA Clark. Lymphoscintigraphy in malignant melanoma. Ann Plast Surg 28:29–32, 1992.

46. D Berger, B Feig, D Podoloff, J Norman, W Cruse, D Reintgen, M Ross. Lymphoscintigraphy accurately predicts lymphatic drainage from cutaneous melanomas of the head, neck and trunk (abstr). Soc Surg Oncol 47:103, 1994.

47. BAE Kapteijn, OE Nieweg, IH Liem, WJ Mooi, AJM Balm, SH Muller, JL Peterse, RA Valdes Olmos, CA Hoefnagel, BBR Kroon. Localizing the sentinel node in cutaneous melanoma: gamma probe detection versus blue dye. Ann Surg Oncol 4:156–160, 1997.

48. J Lock-Andersen, N Rossing, KT Drzewiecki. Preoperative cutaneous lymphoscintigraphy in malignant melanoma. Cancer 63:77–82, 1989.

49. L Jansen, H Schraffordt Koops, OE Nieweg, BAE Kapteijn, AJM Balm, A Vermey, CA Hoefnagel, DA Piers, MHE Doting, BBR Kroon. Sentinel node biopsy in head and neck melanoma (abstr). World Federation of Surgical Oncology Societies and Society of Surgical Oncology Joint Meeting, San Diego, 1998.

50. JC Alex, DN Krag, SP Harlow, S Meijer, BW Loggie, J Kuhn, M Gadd, DL Weaver.

Localization of regional lymph nodes in melanomas of the head and neck. Arch Otolarangol Head Neck Surg 124:135–140, 1998.

51. KE Wells, CW Cruse, S Daniels, C Berman, J Norman, DS Reintgen. The use of lymphoscintigraphy in melanoma of the head and neck. Plast Reconstr Surg 93:757–761, 1994.

52. P Bostick, R Essner, T Sarantou, M Kelley, E Glass, L Foshag, S Stern, D Morton. Intraoperative lymphatic mapping for early-stage melanoma of the head and neck. Am J Surg 174:536–539, 1997.

53. KE Wells, DP Rapaport, CW Cruse, W Payne, J Albertini, C Berman, GH Lyman, DS Reintgen. Sentinel lymph node biopsy in melanoma of the head and neck. Plast Reconstr Surg 100:591–594, 1997.

54. RF Uren, R Howman-Giles, JF Thompson, HM Shaw, MJ Quinn, CJ O'Brien, WH McCarthy. Lymphoscintigraphy to identify sentinel lymph nodes in patients with melanoma. Melanoma Res 4:395–399, 1994.

55. A Mudun, DR Murray, SC Herda, D Eshima, LA Shattuck, JP Vansant, AT Taylor, NP Alazraki. Early stage melanoma: lymphoscintigraphy, reproducibility of sentinel node detection, and effectiveness of the intraoperative gamma probe. Radiology 199:171–175, 1996.

56. RL Wahl, O Geatti, M Liebert, B Wilson, P Shreve, BA Beers. Kinetics of interstitially administered monoclonal antibodies for purposes of lymphoscintigraphy. J Nucl Med 28:1736–1744, 1987.

57. L Jansen, OE Nieweg, BAE Kapteijn, RA Valdés Olmos, CA Hoefnagel, BBR Kroon. Accuracy of lymphoscintigraphy in indicating the number of sentinel lymph nodes in patients with melanoma (abstr). World Federation of the Surgical Oncology Society and the Society of Joint Meeting, San Diego, 1998.

58. D Reintgen. More rational and conservative surgical strategies for malignant melanoma using lymphatic mapping and sentinel node biopsy techniques. Curr Opin Oncol 8:152–158, 1996.

59. CM Meyer, ML Lecklitner, JR Logic, CM Balch, PQ Bessey, WN Tauxe. Technetium-99m sulphur-colloid cutaneous lymphoscintigraphy in the management of truncal melanoma. Radiology 131:205–209, 1979.

60. J Norman, CW Cruse, C Espinosa, C Cox, C Berman, R Clark, H Saba, K Wells, D Reintgen. Redefinition of cutaneous lymphatic drainage with the use of lymphoscintigraphy for malignant melanoma. Am J Surg 162:432–437, 1991.

61. D Kamath, A Brobeil, A Stall, G Lyman, CW Cruse, F Glass, N Fenske, J Messina, C Berman, D Reintgen. Cutaneous lymphatic drainage in patients with grossly involved nodal basins. Ann Surg Oncol 6:345–349, 1999.

62. JH North, JE Spellman. Role of sentinel node biopsy in the management of malignant melanoma. Oncology 10:1237–1242, 1996.

63. RF Uren, R Howman-Giles, JF Thompson, MJ Quinn. Direct lymphatic drainage from the skin of the forearm to a supraclavicular node. Clin Nucl Med 21:387–389, 1996.

64. RF Uren, J Roberts, R Howman-Giles, JF Thompson. Direct lymphatic drainage from the skin of the elbow to an interpectoral node. Reg Cancer Treat 9:100–102, 1996.

65. T Das Gupta, G McNeer. The incidence of metastasis to accessible lymph nodes

from melanoma of the trunk and extremities—its therapeutic significance. Cancer 17:897–911, 1964.

66. KK Tanabe. Lymphatic mapping and epitrochlear lymph node dissection for melanoma. Surgery 121:102–104, 1997.

67. JF Thompson, RF Uren, HM Shaw, WH McCarthy, MJ Quinn, CJ O'Brien, RB Howman-Giles. Location of sentinel lymph nodes in patients with cutaneous melanoma: new insights into lymphatic anatomy. J Am Coll Surg 189:195–204, 1999.

68. CV Godellas, CG Berman, G Lyman, CW Cruse, D Rapaport, R Heller, X Wang, F Glass, N Fenske, J Messina, C Puleo, M Ross, DS Reintgen. The identification and mapping of melanoma regional nodal metastases: minimally invasive surgery for the diagnosis of nodal metastases. Am Surg 61:97–101, 1995.

69. JH Wong, K Truelove, P Ko, MN Coel. Localization and resection of an in transit sentinel lymph node by use of lymphoscintigraphy, intraoperative lymphatic mapping, and a hand-held gamma probe. Surgery 120:114–116, 1996.

70. RF Uren, RB Howman-Giles, JF Thompson, HM Shaw, WH McCarthy. Lymphatic drainage from peri-umbilical skin to internal mammary nodes. Clin Nucl Med 20: 254–255, 1995.

71. HJ Wanebo, D Harpole, CD Teates. Radionuclide lymphoscintigraphy with technetium 99m antimony sulfide colloid to identify lymphatic drainage of cutaneous melanoma at ambiguous sites in the head and neck and trunk. Cancer 55:1403–1413, 1985.

72. RF Uren, R Howman-Giles, JF Thompson, MJ Quinn, C O'Brien, HM Shaw, CMJ Bosch, WH McCarthy. Lymphatic drainage to triangular intermuscular space lymph nodes in melanoma on the back. J Nucl Med 37:964–966, 1996.

73. RF Uren, RB Howman-Giles, JF Thompson, J Roberts, E Bernard, WH McCarthy. Lymphatic mapping with lymphoscintigraphy: unusual pathways to watch for (abstr). Melanoma Res 7:S29, 1997.

74. MK Lingam, RM Mackie, AJ McKay. Intraoperative identification of sentinel lymph node in patients with malignant melanoma. Br J Cancer 75:1505–1508, 1997.

75. AT Taylor, D Murray, S Herda, J Vansant, N Alazraki. Dynamic lymphoscintigraphy to identify the sentinel and satellite nodes. Clin Nucl Med 21:755–758, 1996.

76. PJ Koblenzer, MJ Bukowski. Angiomatosis (hamartomatous hem-lymphangiomatosis). Report of a case with diffuse involvement. Pediatrics 28:65–76, 1961.

77. M Frier. Radiopharmaceuticals for sentinel node detection. Nucl Med Commun 20: 306–308, 1999.

78. DR Vera, ER Wisner, RC Stadalnik. Sentinel node imaging via a nonparticulate receptor-binding radiotracer. J Nucl Med 38:530–535, 1997.

79. T Miyazaki, T Ohnishi, H Hoshi, S Jinnouchi, S Futami, S Nagamachi, K Watanabe, R Hamasuna, T Ueda, S Wakisaka. TI-201 uptake in an intracranial primary malignant melanoma. Clin Nucl Med 21:572–586, 1996.

80. C Perre, JE Rütter, PAFM Vos, P Hooge. Technetium-99m-sestamibi uptake in axillary lymph node metastases in breast cancer patients. Eur J Surg Oncol 23:142–144, 1997.

81. CA Hoefnagel, EM Rankin, RA Valdés Olmos, SP Israëls, S Pavel, AGM Janssen. Sensitivity versus specificity in melanoma imaging using iodine-123 iodobenzamide and Indium-111 pentetreotide. Eur J Nucl Med 21:587–588, 1994.

82. JN Bruneton, E Caramella, M Hery, D Aubanel, JJ Manzino, JL Picard. Axillary lymphnode metastases in breast cancer: preoperative detection with US. Radiology 158:325–326, 1986.
83. L Prayer, H Winkelbauer, N Gritzmann, F Winkelbauer, M Helmer, H Pehamberger. Sonography versus palpation in the detection of regional lymph-node matastases in patients with malignant melanoma. Eur J Cancer 26:827–830, 1990.
84. AC Kole, J Pruim, OE Nieweg, RJ Ginkel van, HJ Hoekstra, H Schraffordt Koops, W Vaalburg. PET with L-[1-carbon-11]-tyrosine to visualize tumors and measure protein synthesis rates. J Nucl Med 38:191–195, 1997.
85. OE Nieweg. Potential applications of positron emission tomography in surgical oncology: a review. Eur J Surg Oncol 20:415–424, 1994.
86. HC Steinert, RA Huch Boni, A Buck, R Boni, T Berthold, B Marincek, G Burg, GK Von Schulthess. Malignant melanoma: staging with whole-body positron emission tomography and 2-[F-18]-fluoro-2-deoxy-D-glucose. Radiology 195:705–709, 1995.

4

Operative Technique for Sentinel Lymphadenectomy

Blue Dye Identification and Use of a Gamma Probe

John F. Thompson

Royal Prince Alfred Hospital, Camperdown, and University of Sydney, Sydney, New South Wales, Australia

INTRODUCTION

Unless great care is taken to ensure that sentinel lymph nodes are identified with complete accuracy and that every sentinel node is found and examined when more than one is present in a node field, the sentinel lymphadenectomy technique will provide misleading information. By basing management decisions on information which is incorrect or incomplete, the likelihood of node field recurrence will be greatly increased and the chance of cure for the patient with melanoma may be jeopardized.

Three methods are currently available to locate sentinel nodes and confirm their identity. These are preoperative lymphoscintigraphy, blue dye injection at the time of surgery, and intraoperative use of a gamma probe. There is accumulating evidence that the three methods are best used in a complementary fashion rather than independently [1]. If this is done, the greatest possible accuracy will be achieved when performing sentinel lymphadenectomy, and it appears that reliable identification rates approaching 100% can be achieved by a surgeon with appropriate training and experience when all three modalities are employed [2].

PREOPERATIVE LYMPHOSCINTIGRAPHY

The techniques and results of cutaneous lymphoscintigraphy are discussed in detail in Chapter 3, but several aspects of the procedure need to be emphasized here because they are directly relevant to the planning and execution of surgery to identify and remove sentinel nodes. High-quality preoperative lymphoscintigraphy is invaluable to ensure that sentinel lymphadenectomy is accomplished expeditiously and to minimize the amount of dissection of the relevant lymph node field (or fields) which must be performed. As well, lymphoscintigraphy provides preoperative identification of drainage pathways to unexpected node fields [3–5]. Some have suggested that preoperative lymphoscintigraphy is necessary only for melanomas in sites from which the lymphatic drainage might be ambiguous. It has now become clear, however, that there are few, if any, sites in the body from which lymphatic drainage pathways are able to be predicted with complete confidence [6,7]. Even in sites that appear to have predictable drainage such as the extremities, occasional ectopic lymph nodes will be identified by lymphoscintigraphy.

If preoperative lymphoscintigraphy is performed, information about the exact number and location of sentinel lymph nodes which must be found and removed is known to the surgeon before the operative procedure of sentinel node biopsy commences (Fig. 1). This means that the patient can be made aware of the site or sites of the proposed surgery and can give appropriately informed consent for the operation. The information obtained from the preoperative lymphoscintigram further facilitates the sentinel lymphadenectomy procedure by identifying patients in whom the rate of lymphatic flow from the primary melanoma site to the draining lymph nodes is unusually slow [8–10]. This allows modification of the standard blue dye injection protocol, with earlier dye injection to increase the probability that it will have reached the node field by the time of surgical exposure.

Yet another benefit of carefully performed preoperative lymphoscintigraphy is that if the images are acquired with the patient in the planned operative position and appropriate lateral and/or oblique views are obtained, the depth of each sentinel node beneath the skin surface can be indicated with precision, and its location in relation to the mark previously made on the overlying skin by the nuclear medicine physician will be accurate [5]. This is particularly useful for biopsy of axillary sentinel nodes in obese patients, where locating them can otherwise be particularly difficult and time-consuming. With the patient supine and the arm positioned at a 90° angle to the body for both preoperative lymphoscintigraphy and surgery, operative sentinel node localization is greatly facilitated.

If lymphoscintigraphy is performed the day before a planned sentinel lymphadenectomy procedure, there will be sufficient residual radioactivity in sentinel lymph nodes to allow them to be identified at the time of surgery using a

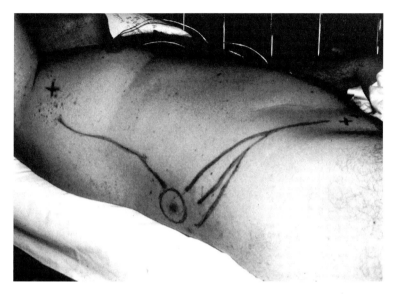

FIGURE 1 Patient with primary melanoma site in right loin showing lymphatic draining pathways to a single sentinel node in the right axilla and three sentinel nodes in the right groin. The skin markings were made at the time of preoperative lymphoscintigraphy.

hand-held gamma probe [11,12]. This can greatly simplify logistics and reduce radiation exposure to both patient and operating theater staff by avoiding the need for a second injection of a radioisotope in the immediate preoperative period. It also provides better discrimination between sentinel and nonsentinel nodes and is particularly useful when the primary injection site is close to the draining lymph node field (as is often the case for head and neck melanoma) [12].

BLUE DYE MAPPING

The Concept

The use of colored substances to demonstrate lymphatic vessels and lymph nodes is not a new concept. It was the technique employed by a number of the earliest anatomists who sought to map human cutaneous lymphatic drainage pathways (see Chapter 2). By injecting materials such as Prussian Blue dye and Chinese ink, they confirmed that lymphatics and blood vessels were distinctly separate entities and produced the first recorded maps of cutaneous lymphatic drainage pathways. In more recent times, blue dye was used extensively to demonstrate lymphatic channels in the foot and hand, allowing them to be cannulated for radiological lymphography (see Fig. 4 in Chapter 2). In the mid-1980s, Morton and his colleagues at the John Wayne Cancer Institute began studies using blue dye which were destined to provide new insights into the clinical relevance of lymphatic drainage pathways for malignancies such as melanoma and breast cancer. First in animal experiments and then in man, it was shown that blue dye traveled rapidly from any given injection site in the skin to a ''sentinel'' lymph node [13,14]. It was postulated that tumor cells would travel along the same lymphatic channels and lodge first in a sentinel node. If a sentinel node was found to be free of micrometastatic disease, it could therefore be assumed that the entire node field was likely to be disease-free and that full regional lymph node dissection was unnecessary. The accuracy of sentinel node status as an indicator of regional lymph node status has since been confirmed by several other histological studies involving sentinel lymphadenectomy with immediate full regional node clearance and careful examination of all the other nodes in the operative specimen [15–17].

Injection Technique

Two blue dyes are in common use for lymphatic mapping and sentinel lymphadenectomy. The more satisfactory agent is probably patent blue dye, but this is not currently available in the United States, where isosulfan blue is normally used. The blue dye is injected intradermally at several points around the melanoma if it remains *in situ*, or on either side of the central part of the biopsy scar if excision–biopsy has been performed previously (Fig. 2). Great care must be taken to ensure that the injection is truly intradermal and not subcutaneous, to avoid the possibility of mapping a lymphatic pathway leading to a node that is not the true sentinel node draining the melanoma site on the skin. If lymphatic mapping using either blue dye or a radiolabeled colloid is attempted after a wide local excision of the primary melanoma, inaccurate sentinel node identification is even more likely to occur. This is because there is evidence that the originally existing lymphatic pathways draining the melanoma are disrupted by the excisional surgery [11] so that lymphatic drainage from the area may be diverted to a lymph node that is not the true sentinel node. If a simple excision–biopsy has been performed with margins of no more than a few millimeters around the melanoma, however, it is thought that subsequent lymphatic mapping will reliably indicate the true sentinel node or nodes. Most of the literature on lymphatic mapping in melanoma is from mapping after an excisional biopsy.

Systemic Effects of Blue Dye Injection

Administration of blue dye produces some effects that can cause concern if not anticipated and understood. The patient's skin can take on an ashen gray, almost cadaveric appearance, and a pulse oximeter may indicate desaturation of the

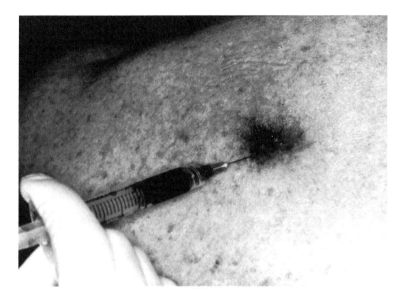

FIGURE 2 Intradermal patent blue dye injection at a primary melanoma site on the leg, prior to sentinel lymph node biopsy.

blood even when arterial oxygen tensions are well above normal. The urine shows blue-green discoloration for up to 24 h postoperatively. More serious side effects are rare. Very occasionally, however, an allergic reaction to the blue dye can occur, with the rapid development of widespread large, watery vesicles filled with pale blue fluid. Standard treatment for an acute allergic reaction, including parenteral antihistamines and corticosteroids, is usually effective in dealing with this potentially serious clinical situation.

Timing of Blue Dye Injection

It is normally satisfactory to inject the blue dye 5–10 min before anesthetic induction (if general anesthesia is to be used) or at a similar time before surgical incision (if local anesthesia is to be employed). This allows time for the injection site to be gently massaged and for the patient to exercise the relevant body part, when the anatomical location of the primary melanoma site makes this possible. Both of these maneuvers increase the likelihood that satisfactory passage of blue dye to the regional lymph node field will have occurred by the time of surgical exploration of that field. They are particularly important if, as frequently happens, the patient has become cold while being transferred from the ward to the operating suite, and while in a cool holding bay or anesthetic room awaiting surgery. Unless special precautions are taken, it is not uncommon for limb cutaneous temperatures of 32–33°C to be recorded when patients arrive in an operating theater. When local anesthesia is used, epinephrine (with lidocaine) is best avoided because of its potential effect on lymphatic flow.

If the preoperative lymphoscintigram has shown very slow movement of tracer from the primary melanoma site to the regional nodes [9,10], earlier injection of blue dye is desirable 10–20 min before anesthetic induction, with more prolonged exercise of the relevant body part. The temptation to more vigorously massage the injection site should be resisted because it is theoretically possible that this could redirect drainage of the dye in a nonphysiological way and could result in blue staining of nodes which are not true sentinel nodes draining the original melanoma site.

THE SURGICAL PROCEDURE

Planning the Skin Incision

The position, direction, and extent of the skin incision appropriate for sentinel lymphadenectomy is primarily determined by the mark or marks made on the overlying skin by the nuclear medicine physician at the time of preoperative lymphoscintigraphy. However, the position of the incision should also be such that complete excision of it would easily be possible as part of a full regional node dissection if the sentinel node was found to contain micrometastatic disease.

Exposing and Removing the Sentinel Nodes

Dissection must proceed cautiously, taking care not to damage any blue-stained lymphatics. When a blue lymphatic vessel is encountered, it should be traced until it reaches a lymph node, which should itself be at least partly blue stained if it is to be identified confidently as a sentinel node (Fig. 3). The number of sentinel nodes in a regional lymph node field will be known from the preoperative lymphoscintigram, as well as their approximate depth below the skin surface, making location of these nodes a relatively easy matter in most instances. It is nevertheless desirable to seek and trace blue-stained afferent lymphatics, as nodes can sometimes be elusive even when their approximate position is known and the degree to which they are themselves blue-stained may not be intense. Sometimes, a sentinel node will be only partly blue stained, in that part which is immediately adjacent to the point of entry of the afferent lymphatic bringing blue dye from the skin injection site. If this blue-stained area is on the undersurface so that it is not visible on that part of the node which has been exposed, its identity as a sentinel node may be overlooked unless a blue-stained afferent lymphatic is traced right to the node.

The objective must always be to remove sentinel nodes with as little interference to surrounding tissues as possible—particularly nonsentinel lymph nodes and their afferent lymphatics. This will not only minimize the risk of causing

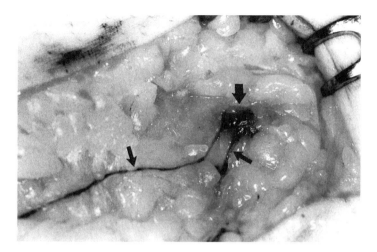

FIGURE 3   Blue-stained afferent lymphatics (thin arrows) entering a sentinel lymph node, which is itself blue stained (thick arrow).

lymphedema but will also help to ensure that if a sentinel node is determined to be positive and a full regional node dissection is therefore required, complete clearance of the sentinel lymphadenectomy site is possible without transgressing previously dissected and thus potentially contaminated areas.

When each sentinel node is found, it is removed, with care being taken to clip or ligate afferent and efferent lymphatics in order to minimize the risk of subsequent lymphocoele formation. Having ensured that hemostasis is complete, the wound is then closed, with use of a small drain if considered appropriate.

Frozen-Section Examination of Sentinel Nodes

During early experience with the sentinel lymphadenectomy technique, routine frozen-section examination of each sentinel node was performed in some centers [14,16], and immediate regional node dissection was undertaken if the sentinel node was reported to contain micrometastatic disease. However, even when experienced melanoma pathologists examined the frozen tissue sections, the results proved unreliable. There was also concern about the amount of tissue lost (and potentially containing the only deposits of micrometastatic disease) when trimming the tissue blocks for frozen-section examinations and cutting the tissue on the cryostat. In their initial clinical studies, Morton's group performed routine immediate immunohistochemistry on frozen tissue sections [14]. Although undoubtedly more accurate than standard frozen-section examination, this technique was very labor intensive, technically demanding, and time-consuming and is not a realistic proposition as part of a standard clinical protocol. For all the above reasons, frozen section is now not performed in most centers and it is generally considered preferable to await formal paraffin section histology and immunohistochemistry. If necessary, a full regional node clearance can then be undertaken as a separate procedure at a later date, after full discussion of the situation with the patient.

"In-Transit" Sentinel Nodes and Lymphatic Lakes

At the time of preoperative lymphoscintigraphy, a focus of intense isotope accumulation will occasionally develop on a lymphatic pathway leading from the skin injection site toward a regional lymph node field. Usually this is, by definition, a true sentinel node, even though it lies outside a recognized lymph node field, and it must be removed and examined if a sentinel lymphadenectomy procedure is to be performed. Occasionally, however, the focus of isotope uptake will simply be an area of lymphatic dilatation or a "lake" (Fig. 4). If there is a chain of such foci, it becomes much more likely that they are not nodes but lymphatic lakes. However, on rare occasions a chain of two, three, or even four sentinel nodes is present. Unless the area is surgically exposed, it is not feasible to differentiate between these two entities. This means that formal exploration of all such hot spots is required if missing a sentinel lymph node or nodes is to be avoided. In these cases, it makes sense to first explore the site furthest from the primary site because first exploring the proximal nodes carries the risk of disrupting channels to the more distant nodes (Fig. 5).

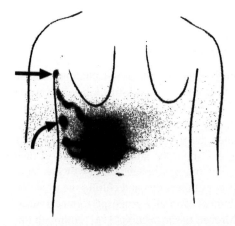

FIGURE 4   Focus of isotope uptake due to the presence of a lymphatic "lake" (curved arrow). On delayed scans, this focus had disappeared completely. There is a single sentinel node in the right axilla (straight arrow).

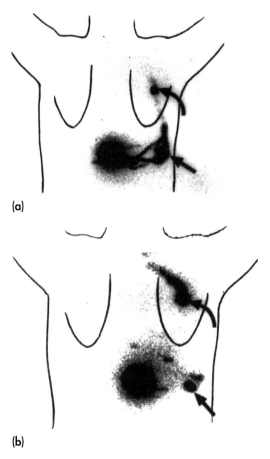

(a)

(b)

Figure 5 Interval lymph node outside a recognized lymph node field. Initial scan (a) shows channels passing to an interval node on the right back (straight arrow) and to a sentinel node in the right axilla (curved arrow). Delayed scan (b) also shows the interval node on the right back (straight arrow) plus the sentinel node in the right axilla (curved arrow). Both are sentinel nodes. Second-tier nodes in the right axilla are also visualized.

INTRAOPERATIVE USE OF A GAMMA PROBE

Although definite blue staining of a sentinel node with identification of at least one blue-stained afferent lymphatic channel entering the node currently remains the gold standard for assessment of whether a lymph node is or is not a true sentinel node, intraoperative use of a gamma detection probe can provide valuable confirmatory evidence.

A number of compact, lightweight gamma probes are now available which can be used intraoperatively to assist with the sentinel lymphadenectomy procedure. All these devices are fundamentally similar in design and function, and their relevant features are described in detail in Chapter 5. They comprise a hand-held probe containing a gamma detecting crystal connected to an easily portable control box (Fig. 6). The probe and the cable connecting it to the control box can be inserted into a sterile plastic sleeve for intraoperative use.

A gamma probe can be used for three distinctly separate purposes during a sentinel lymphadenectomy procedure: (1) to assist in locating each sentinel node, (2) to confirm that a node is "hot" both in vivo and after it has been removed, and (3) to check that there are no residual hot nodes in a lymph node field after removal of the presumed sentinel node or nodes.

Sentinel Node Location

Although the estimated position of each sentinel node will ideally have been marked on the overlying skin at the time of preoperative lymphoscintigraphy, it is useful to confirm its location with a gamma probe before making a skin incision. This is particularly valuable when the position of the patient on the operating table differs from the position they were in when the lymphoscintigram was obtained. The surgeon may occasionally decide, for example, to perform an axillary sentinel lymphadenectomy with the patient in a lateral position so that the subsequent wide excision of a primary melanoma site on the back can be performed

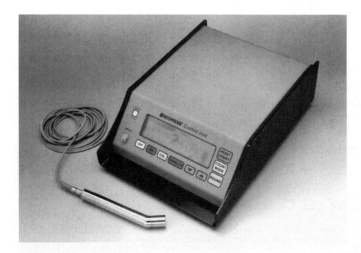

FIGURE 6   Hand-held gamma probe and control box (Neoprobe 1000, Neoprobe Corporation, Dublin, OH, U.S.A.).

without having to reposition and redrape the patient, whereas the preoperative lymphoscintigram was performed in routine fashion with the patient in the supine position, with the arm extended at a 90° angle to the body. Checking the position of the sentinel node with a gamma probe prior to skin incision can also be very useful in situations where anatomical considerations make it difficult for the nuclear medicine physician to mark the position of the sentinel node(s) accurately, for example, in the submandibular region or in the groin of a grossly obese patient with an overlying fatty apron. Having made the skin incision, if the sentinel node cannot be located readily by its blue dye staining, the tip of the gamma probe, clad in its sterile sheath, can be inserted into the wound and moved around, with adjustment of the angle of the probe to indicate the direction of the hot sentinel node. During this maneuver, care must be taken, however, to ensure that residual activity at the primary melanoma site does not provide misleading information (e.g., when the axilla is being explored and the primary melanoma site is on the upper back).

Confirming Sentinel Node Identity

Even 24 h after intradermal radionuclide injection at a primary melanoma site, the sentinel node invariably remains the hottest node in the draining lymph node field [5,18]. It is valuable to use the gamma probe to confirm the identity of any node suspected to be a sentinel node (Table 1; Fig. 7). The probe can be used for the purpose of confirmation both in vivo and after removal of the node. Sometimes the sentinel node is not obviously blue stained [11,12]. It is very rare, however, for a true sentinel node not to contain radioactive colloid, provided the intradermal isotope is injected at the primary melanoma site at least 1 or 2 h preparatively. If the isotope is injected immediately preoperatively, either alone or in combination with blue dye (as is the practice in some centers), the reliability of sentinel node confirmation with the gamma probe is diminished. Nevertheless,

TABLE 1 Gamma Probe Recordings for a Woman Aged 24 Years Undergoing Sentinel Node Biopsy

Site of nodes removed at operation	Blue staining?	Indicated by scintigraphy?	Node counts ex vivo (per 10 s)	Field count following removal of node(s) (per 10 s)	Ratio of node to lymphatic field count	Micro-metastases identified?
Left axilla (superficial)	Yes	Yes	43,598	7,391	5.9	Yes
Left axilla (deep)	Yes	Yes	28,105	7,391	3.8	Yes
Right axilla	Yes	Yes	10,604	2,563	4.1	No

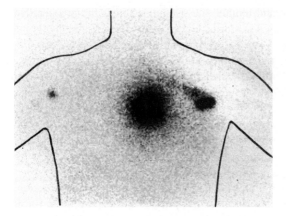

Figure 7   Preoperative lymphoscintigram (delayed scan) showing two sentinel nodes (partly superimposed in this view) in the left axilla and a single sentinel node in the right axilla. (Gamma probe counts for the sentinel nodes are listed in Table 1.) Excision–biopsy of a melanoma 1.5 mm in thickness on her left upper back had been performed 3 weeks earlier. Preoperative lymphoscintigraphy had revealed that there appeared to be two sentinel nodes in the left axilla lying one immediately deep to the other, and on delayed imaging, a single fainter sentinel node in the right axilla. All three sentinel nodes were identified without difficulty at the time of surgery and removed. Subsequent histological examination of the left axillary sentinel nodes revealed micrometastatic disease in both of them, and a full regional node dissection of the left axilla was therefore performed. No additional positive nodes were present.

the objectivity of the technique is still very useful. Detection of gamma radiation, measured in counts per second with a gamma probe, is completely objective, whereas confident detection of blue staining of a node can sometimes be difficult and operator dependent (and thus less reliable). The relatively less objective nature of lymphatic mapping and sentinel node identification with blue dye has led to suggestions that its use is unnecessary. However, it is readily demonstrable that second-tier nodes in the regional lymph node field (i.e., nodes which are not sentinel nodes) can become hot quite quickly after isotope injection [9,10,18]. Thus, any technique that relies on the gamma probe alone to identify sentinel nodes is likely to result in the removal of additional, nonsentinel nodes [18], defeating the main purpose of the sentinel lymphadenectomy procedure which is to be superselective and to avoid unnecessary disturbance of nonsentinel nodes and their afferent and efferent lymphatics.

Checking for Residual "Hot" Nodes

After removal of the presumed sentinel node or nodes, the residual count in the regional lymph node field can be checked with a gamma probe, and any residual hot areas can be explored. Usually, such hot spots are due to activity in second-tier nodes [19], which when exposed are not blue stained and do not have blue-stained afferent lymphatics draining directly from the primary melanoma site. The degree of residual activity in a node field must be assessed in relation to the activity present in the sentinel node(s) and is determined by the time elapsed since isotope injection at the primary melanoma site. Absolute levels of radio-activity are clearly meaningless. What is important is the ratio of counts in a given node to the counts in the remainder of the node field [12,20].

It has been suggested, for example, that to be identified as a sentinel node on the basis of gamma probe assessment the ratio of counts in sentinel and non-sentinel nodes should be over 3:1 in vivo and 10:1 ex vivo [20]. However, this is not a useful guide if attempts are made, in the true spirit of a selective ''sentinel node only'' biopsy policy, not to remove nonsentinel nodes. Others have suggested comparing sentinel node activity with ''background'' activity, but without specifying how background levels are to be determined. After analysis of the data from a large number of patients undergoing sentinel node biopsy, we have proposed that the ratio of sentinel node activity to residual activity in the node field after removal of the sentinel node should be over 3:1 [12]. In most cases, this ratio is greatly exceeded, but it appears to provide a useful lower level below which the likelihood of a node being a true sentinel node is very low. If, on checking a node field after removal of all presumed sentinel nodes, a node with activity of more than three times the activity elsewhere in the node field is found, it should thus be regarded as a possible sentinel node and removed for histological examination, even if it is not blue stained.

CONCLUSIONS

Although elegantly simple in concept, selective lymphadenectomy can be a technically complex and challenging procedure. Unless great care is taken to optimize the accuracy of sentinel node identification and the completeness of sentinel node removal, misleading information may be obtained. This could lead to inaccurate staging of the patient, resulting in inappropriate treatment and ultimately a worse prognosis. Use of all three currently available techniques—preoperative lympho-scintigraphy, perioperative blue dye mapping, and a gamma probe intraoperatively—will ensure that the greatest possible accuracy is achieved and that reliable information about sentinel lymph node status is obtained.

REFERENCES

1. JF Thompson. Sentinel node biopsy. How I do it. J Surg Oncol 66:270–272, 1997.
2. DL Morton, JF Thompson, R Essner, R Elashoff, SL Stern, OE Nieweg, DF Roses, CP Karakousis, N Mozzillo, D Reintgen, H Wang, EC Glass, AJ Cochran. Validation

of the accuracy in a multicenter trial of intraoperative lymphatic mapping and sentinel lymphadenectomy for early-stage melanoma. Ann Surg 230:453–465, 1999.

3. J Norman, CW Cruse, C Espinosa, C Cox, C Berman, R Clark, H Saba, K Wells D Reintgen. Redefinition of cutaneous lymphatic drainage with the use of lymphoscintigraphy for malignant melanoma. Am J Surg 162:432–437, 1991.

4. RF Uren, RB Howman-Giles, HM Shaw, JF Thompson, WH McCarthy. Lymphoscintigraphy in high risk melanoma of the trunk; predicting draining node groups, defining lymphatic channels and locating the sentinel node. J Nucl Med 34:1435–1440, 1993.

5. RF Uren, R Howman-Giles, JF Thompson, HM Shaw, MJ Quinn, CJ O'Brien, WH McCarthy. Lymphoscintigraphy to identify sentinel lymph nodes in patients with melanoma. Melanoma Res 4:395–399, 1994.

6. JF Thompson, RF Uren, HM Shaw, WH McCarthy, MJ Quinn, CJ O'Brien, R Howman-Giles. The location of sentinel lymph nodes in patients with cutaneous melanoma: new insights into lymphatic anatomy. J Am Coll Surg 189:195–204, 1999.

7. RF Uren, JF Thompson, RB Howman-Giles. Lymphatic drainage of the skin and breast: locating the sentinel nodes. Amsterdam: Harwood Academic Publishers, 1999.

8. SD Nathanson, L Nelson, KC Karvelis. Rates of flow of technetium 99m-labeled human serum albumin from peripheral injection sites to sentinel lymph nodes. Ann Surg Oncol 3:329–335, 1996.

9. RF Uren, RB Howman-Giles, JF Thompson. Variation in cutaneous lymphatic flow rates. Ann Surg Oncol 4:279–280, 1997.

10. RF Uren, RB Howman-Giles, JF Thompson, J Roberts, E Bernard. Variability of cutaneous lymphatic flow rates in melanoma patients. Melanoma Res 8:279–282, 1998.

11. R Pijpers, PJ Borgstein, M Sybren, OS Hoekstra, LH van Hattum, GJJ Teule. Sentinel node biopsy in melanoma patients: dynamic lymphoscintigraphy followed by intraoperative gamma probe and vital dye guidance. World J Surg 21:788–792, 1997.

12. JF Thompson, P Niewind, RF Uren, CMJ Bosch, R Howman-Giles, BC Vrouenraets. Single-dose isotope injection for both pre-operative lymphoscintigraphy and intraoperative sentinel lymph node identification in melanoma patients. Melanoma Res 6: 500–506, 1997.

13. JH Wong, LA Cagle, DL Morton. Lymphatic drainage of skin to a sentinel node in a feline model. Ann Surg 214:637–641, 1991.

14. DL Morton, DR Wen, JH Wong, JS Economou, LA Cagle, FK Storm, LJ Foshag, AJ Cochran. Technical details of intraoperative lymphatic mapping of early stage melanoma. Arch Surg 127:392–399, 1992.

15. D Reintgen, CW Cruse, K Wells, C Berman, N Fenske, F Glass, K Schroer, R Heller, M Ross, G Lyman, D Rapaport, HF Seigler, CM Balch. The orderly progression of melanoma nodal metastases. Ann Surg 220:759–767, 1994.

16. JF Thompson, WH McCarthy, CMJ Bosch, CJ O'Brien, MJ Quinn, S Paramaesvaran, K Crotty, SW McCarthy, RF Uren, R Howman-Giles. Sentinel lymph node status as an indicator of the presence of metastatic melanoma in regional lymph nodes. Melanoma Res 5:255–260, 1995.

17. CP Karakousis, AF Velez, JE Spellman, J Scarozza. The technique of sentinel node biopsy. Eur J Surg Oncol 22:271–275, 1996.

18. WH McCarthy, JF Thompson, RF Uren. Invited commentary on article by Krag DN, Meijer SJ, Weaver DL, Loggie BW, Harlow SP, Tanabe KK, Laughlin EH, Alex JC. Minimal access surgery for staging malignant melanoma. Arch Surg 130: 659–660, 1995.

19. RF Uren, RB Howman-Giles, JF Thompson. Demonstration of second tier lymph nodes during preoperative lymphoscintigraphy for melanoma: incidence varies with primary tumor site. Ann Surg Oncol 5:517–521, 1998.

20. JJ Albertini, CW Cruse, D Rapaport, K Wells, M Ross, R DeConti, CG Berman, K Jared, J Messina, G Lyman, F Glass, N Fensk, D Reintgen. Intraoperative radioloymphoscintigraphy improves sentinel lymph node identification for patients with melanoma. Ann Surg 223:211–224, 1996.

5

Comparison of the Physical Characteristics of Different Gamma Detection Devices

Sara H. Muller
The Netherlands Cancer Institute, Amsterdam, the Netherlands

Tatiana B. Sazonova-Tiourina and Albert Jan Arends
Catharina Hospital, Eindhoven, the Netherlands

INTRODUCTION

The purpose of this chapter is to outline the relevant physics of gamma ray detection probes. More extensive information can be found in other publications [1,2]. A gamma detection device for surgical use consists of two main parts: a hand-held sensor which contains the gamma-sensitive crystal with a preamplifier, and a reading unit. Both the sensor itself and the whole device are often referred to as a "probe." In this chapter, however, we use the word "probe" to indicate the sensor only. Because the radionuclide technetium-99m (^{99m}Tc) is almost exclusively used as a label for tracers in lymphatic mapping, discussion of the physical characteristics of the probe concerns the performance with ^{99m}Tc unless explicitly stated otherwise. Measurements on probes are often performed using a cobalt-57 (^{57}Co) source. Because the energy of the gamma photons emitted by ^{57}Co is only slightly lower than that of ^{99m}Tc (122 versus 140 keV), these measurements are, in general, representative for the performance with ^{99m}Tc. However, the transmission through shielding material must be measured using ^{99m}Tc because using ^{57}Co the correction factor will strongly depend on the thickness of the shielding.

TABLE 1 Probes and Crystals

Probe name	Detector type	Manufacturer
C-Trak	Scintillation	Care-Wise, U.S.A.
Neoprobe	CdZnTe	Neoprobe Corp, U.S.A.
RMD	CdTe	Radiation Monitoring Devices, U.S.A.
Gammed	CdTe, scintillation	Eurorad, France

CRYSTAL CHARACTERISTICS

Two basically different types of intraoperative probe are currently available: one based on a scintillation crystal and the other based on a semiconductor crystal. A scintillation detector consists of a scintillation crystal, a light guide, a photomultiplier tube, and electronics. Thallium-activated sodium iodide [NaI(Tl)] is the most widely used scintillation crystal in gamma cameras and is also used in this type of probe, although mostly cesium iodide (CsI) is used in probes. Semiconductor probes are more common. This type of detector consists of a semiconductor crystal, a preamplifier, and electronics. A cadmium–telluride (CdTe, or sometimes zinc-doped: CdZnTe) crystal is most commonly used in semiconductor probes.

Intrinsic detector efficiency (the ratio between the number of gamma photons entering the probe and the number detected) depends on crystal material, on the dimensions (area and thickness) of the crystal, and on the gamma energy. For CdTe, the intrinsic efficiency decreases with increasing gamma energy and will be 20–30% lower for ^{99m}Tc than for ^{57}Co when a 2-mm–thick crystal is used.

Energy resolution is the ability to discriminate between gamma photons with different energies. This depends not only on the crystal that is used in the probe but also on the thickness of the crystal. Semiconductor detectors generally have a better energy resolution than scintillation detectors. An overview of several available probes based on both types of crystals is given in Table 1. One should be aware of the fact that new devices enter the market rapidly and that characteristics may change.

PROBE CHARACTERISTICS

A gamma detection device consists of a probe detector, a preamplifier, and a housing with adequate metal screening around the detector for collimation and shielding.

The performance of a gamma detection probe can be described by the following physical characteristics:

- Sensitivity
- Spatial (or angular) resolution: collimation
- Shielding
- Energy discrimination (or energy resolution).

Sensitivity (the fraction of gamma photons emitted by the source that is detected by the probe) depends mainly on intrinsic detection efficiency (see the section on Crystal Characteristics, p. 88) and probe geometry. Spatial resolution and shielding are determined by the probe geometry. Therefore, sensitivity, spatial resolution, and shielding are not completely independent of each other, although they are often specified separately for a probe. Some probes are provided with add-on collimators or shields (Fig. 1), which enable the user to modify these properties. Because they are not independent, usually all three characteristics will change if an additional collimator is used (e.g., the spatial resolution and shielding will improve, but the sensitivity will decrease).

Energy resolution is useful for the discrimination between direct and scattered radiation, as described in a subsequent section.

In addition to these physical characteristics, the ergonomic properties of an instrument are relevant to its use by the surgeon: weight and shape of the probe, visual display and ease of operation, sound, and the hygienic aspects and safety. The weight will largely be determined by the amount of collimation and

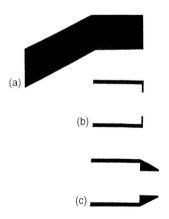

FIGURE 1 Cross-section through (a) the Neoprobe 19-mm sensor, (b) the add-on shield, and (c) the add-on cone collimator.

shielding. Excellent reliability and stability are a requirement for any surgical probe.

CHARACTERISTICS FOR SUCCESSFUL SENTINEL NODE DETECTION

The physical characteristics of the probe must be such that detection of radioactive lymph nodes is optimized. The following aspects are important:

- The uptake of radioactivity in lymph nodes is highly variable. Uptake in the sentinel node in melanoma patients varies between about 40 Bq* and 250 kBq with a median of 13 kBq (22 h after injection of 58 MBq ^{99m}Tc) [3].
- The depth of the sentinel node is variable. It may be just below the skin or more than 5 cm deep.
- The activity in the tissue surrounding the lymph nodes is very low, but ''background'' radiation can be considerable if a hot injection site is close to the sentinel node. In particular, this will be the case when the primary tumor in the breast is located in the upper outer quadrant, close to the axilla.

If the injection site is far from the node (or if it can be excised before localization of the sentinel node) and if the sentinel node has a high uptake and/ or is close to the surface, locating the sentinel node will be straightforward. Any probe will locate it. In practice, conditions are usually less favorable. Then, the characteristics of the probe will determine the probability of successful localization. Focusing on these less favorable circumstances, we will discuss the physical characteristics of the probe.

DETECTION OF NODES WITH A LOW UPTAKE: SENSITIVITY

Sensitivity is defined as the fraction of gamma photons emitted by the source that is detected by the probe. It is specified as the count rate per amount of activity (cps/Bq or cps/kBq). Sensitivity should be as high as possible. Sensitivity is a combination of intrinsic detector efficiency and geometric factors such as detector area and collimation. Differences in sensitivity between different types of probes may be considerable. We measured values between 1 and 43 cps/kBq for the probes in Table 1 at a distance of 1 cm from a source (Table 2, measured between

---

* 1 mCl = 37 MBq.

TABLE 2 Sensitivities Measured in Air for a [57]Co Source Using the Full Energy Spectrum, at a Distance of 1 cm and 5 cm (Measured Relative to the Tip of the Probe or Collimator)

Probe	Collimator	Sensitivity (cps/kBq)	
		at 1 cm	at 5 cm
C-Trak,[a] NaI	None	16	1.4
	With	8.4	1.3
Neoprobe, CdZnTe	None	43	3.5
	Shield	36	2.8
	Cone	10	1.5
RMD CdTe	None	1.2	0.08
Gammed CdTe	None	39	0.25
Gammed CsI	None	5.2	0.45

Note: Values for ^{99m}Tc will be lower, in particular for the probes with CdTe crystals.
[a] C-Trak also supplies a MiniProbe which has a low weight, but the sensitivity of this probe is about three times less than that of the standard probe.
Source: Ref. 4.

July 1996 and April 1997). Also given in Table 2 are the (reduced) sensitivities that were measured when additional collimators were used.

If a probe has no collimation at all, the crystal can be brought very close to the node. Increasing the distance between node and probe will mean that the sensitivity decreases with the square of the distance (double the distance: fourfold reduction of the sensitivity). A collimator may shield part of the crystal, which will reduce the sensitivity. In addition, the minimum distance between node and crystal will be larger (of the order of 1 cm depending on the length of the collimator; see Fig. 1). This means that the maximum sensitivity (with the probe as close as possible to the node) is considerably reduced by a collimator, but if the probe is far from the node, the collimated sensitivity will be relatively closer to the uncollimated value (compare the values for 1 cm and 5 cm in Table 2 for the same probes with and without the collimator). Closer than 1 cm to the source, the differences are even larger: At about 1 mm, the sensitivity of the Neoprobe 1000 with shield is about 175 cps/kBq, but with the cone collimator, it is only 35 cps/kBq. The sensitivity of the C-Trak probe without an additional collimator is about 40 cps/kBq. These data were measured using [57]Co. For the Neoprobe, the sensitivity for ^{99m}Tc is 20–30% lower.

Sensitivity may be of crucial importance during intraoperative use of the probe because the uptake of the tracer in the sentinel node may be very low or the node may be at a large distance from the probe. When the large amount of radioactivity at the injection site is nearby, the combination of collimation, scatter suppression, and sensitivity becomes important. This will be discussed in one of the next sections. Therefore, sensitivities of the probe in different configurations should be carefully evaluated. Manufacturers should specify the sensitivity in cps/kBq for a specified radionuclide in well-defined geometric configurations with the different collimators available.

NODE LOCALIZATION: SPATIAL RESOLUTION, SENSITIVITY AT A DISTANCE

Spatial resolution describes the ability of the probe to distinguish between two sources that are close together, or to locate the precise position of a source from a distance. The latter is important if we want to locate a sentinel node through the intact skin before the incision is made. Figure 2 shows the relative spatial resolution scanning in a straight line over a source with a closest distance of 26 mm with respect to the front of the probe or collimator for different probe configurations. If a probe is scanned at a fixed distance around the source (and

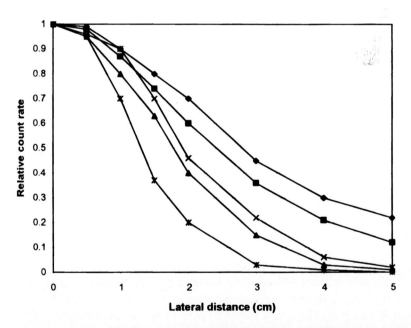

FIGURE 2   Relative spatial resolution for different probes and collimators at a distance of 26 mm in air. A ^{57}Co source was used. For each configuration, data are normalized to the value for a lateral distance of 0 cm. ●: Neoprobe, no collimator; ▲: Neoprobe, cone collimator; ■: Neoprobe shield; *: C-Trak probe, collimator; X: C-Trak probe, no collimator.

pointing at the source) the term "angular resolution" would be more appropriate. The spatial resolution of a probe at this distance can be improved considerably by the use of additional collimation. The C-Trak probe has a strong built-in collimation: Without additional collimation, the spatial resolution is comparable to that of Neoprobe with the add-on collimator. Scanning at larger distances reduces the spatial resolution, as is illustrated in Fig. 3 for collimated probes. In Fig. 4, it is shown that the collimator no longer improves spatial resolution at a depth of 5 cm in water: The spatial resolution with and without the collimator is nearly identical.

Adding a collimator to a probe also has disadvantages. As has been mentioned earlier, the effective area of the detector becomes smaller and the minimal distance to the detector is increased so that the maximum sensitivity decreases. Moreover, because the field of view is narrowed, searching for a node the location of which is not precisely known becomes more time-consuming. In general, it is important to use as little collimation as possible, unless it is certain that the

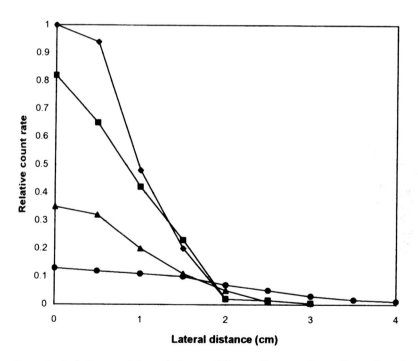

FIGURE 3 Relative spatial resolution at different distances for collimated probes. A ⁵⁷Co source was used. Values are normalized to the value for air at a distance of 1 cm. ◆: 1 cm air; ■: 1 cm water; ▲: 2 cm water; ●: 4 cm water.

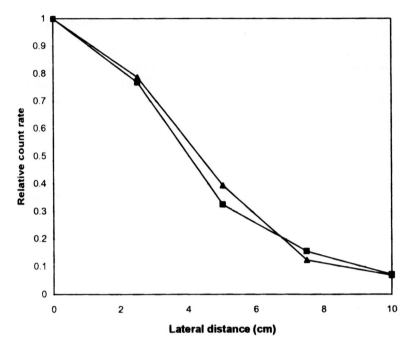

Figure 4   Relative spatial resolution at a depth of 5 cm in water for a probe with a shield (no collimation) and a collimator. A ^{57}Co source was used. For each configuration, data are normalized to the value for a lateral distance of 0 cm. ▲: collimator; ■: shield.

activity in the target is sufficient (e.g., in the case of a 1-day sentinel protocol). Probes that are supplied with different collimators enable the user to adapt the instrument to their own specific requirements and to the needs of the situation in individual patients.

DETECTION IN THE VICINITY OF AN INJECTION SITE: SHIELDING AND ENERGY DISCRIMINATION

Radiation from an injection site close to a node may be considerably stronger than that from the node. As long as the probe is not pointed in the direction of the injection site, its radiation may be blocked quite efficiently with side shielding. If necessary, an add-on shield or collimator can be used to improve side shielding. A 100–1000-fold reduction of the direct radiation can easily be obtained in this way, which is quite sufficient for the typical situation in which not more than 4 MBq is left at the injection site and the distance between injection site and node is at least a few centimeters.

However, blocking direct radiation is not sufficient. Radiation from the injection site also reaches the aperture of the probe via (multiple) scattering in the patient. Using the Neoprobe sensor and a ^{99m}Tc source at an off-axis distance of about 7 cm, we found that the scattered radiation is about one-tenth of the direct radiation that is measured if the sensor is pointed directly at the source.

Scattered radiation is diffuse. It enters the probe from different directions and cannot be eliminated by side shielding. However, it can be reduced by the use of collimation. Table 3 shows the amount of activity that must be present in a node so that the count rate from the node is twice that from an injection site of 2 MBq. Data are shown for the Neoprobe with a cone collimator and the Neoprobe with a shield, with injection sites at distances of 2.5, 5, and 7.5 cm. The injection site is positioned adjacent to the probe (at an angle of 90° relative to the node) so that direct radiation from the injection site is shielded. Two node positions have been chosen: a superficial node 5 mm from the probe and a deep node below 5 cm of tissue. The performance of the shielded and the collimated probe are identical in the case of the superficial node. For the deep node, the collimator performance is superior: It detects nodes that are twice as weak as nodes that can be detected with the shield. The injection site causes a high ''background'' count rate, so that the sensitivity of the probe does not limit detection.

An alternative method to suppress the counts from scattered radiation is to use the ability of the probe to discriminate between different energies. If the instrument is equipped with an energy threshold setting, the user can select the threshold below which radiation will be discarded, so that scattered radiation with its lower energy is not counted. However, for a lower threshold at which scattered radiation is nearly completely suppressed, the sensitivity will typically be reduced with about one-third of its full spectrum value, because radiation that is scattered inside the probe is also not counted.

Figure 5a shows the performance of the Neoprobe sensor with the additional shield as a function of lower threshold setting. The numbers along the

TABLE 3 Measurements for Nodes Close to Injection Site

Collimator	Distance probe–node	Distance to injection site			Unit
		2.5 cm	5 cm	7.5 cm	
Shield	5 mm	58	26	17	kBq ^{99m}Tc
Cone	5 mm	56	26	16	kBq ^{99m}Tc
Shield	5 cm tissue	2350	1030	660	kBq ^{99m}Tc
Cone	5 cm tissue	1250	600	360	kBq ^{99m}Tc

Note: The ^{99m}Tc activity in nodes, which is required to give twice the count rate from an injection site of 2 MBq ^{99m}Tc at distances of 2.5, 5, and 7.5 cm, is given. Data are given for a superficial node at 5 mm from the probe and for a deep node below 5 cm tissue. The data are calculated for a Neoprobe with a collimator and with a shield.

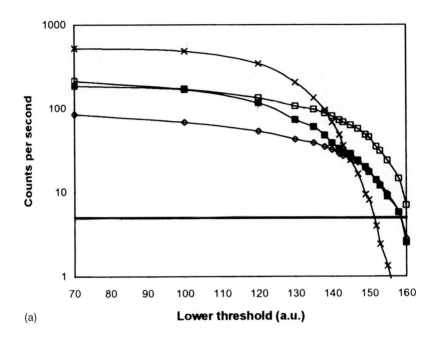

(a)

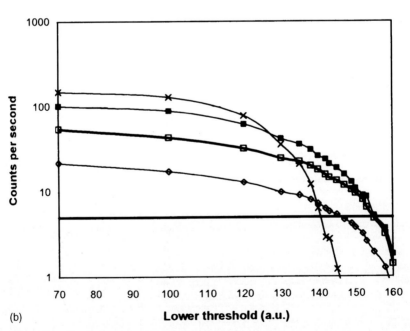

(b)

threshold axis are arbitrary units (and not keV). Both the count rate from a simulated injection site at a distance of 5 cm adjacent to the probe and the count rate from three simulated nodes (weak nodes of 2 and 5 kBq just in front of the probe and a strong node of 200 kBq at a depth of 5 cm in water) are shown. If the threshold is raised to a value above 140, the count rate of the node of 5 kBq is higher than that of the injection site. For a threshold of 150, all three nodes have count rates which are at least twice the count rate from the injection site. Figure 5b shows the same data for the probe with a collimator. In this case, raising the threshold to a value of about 140 is sufficient to find two nodes. For the third node, a threshold of 145 is required.

In Figs. 5a and 5b, a detection limit of about 5 cps is also indicated. The cone collimator reduces the sensitivity at short distances so that the count rate of the node of 2 kBq is barely above the detection limit if the threshold is raised sufficiently far to suppress scattered radiation from the injection site. Unless the probe has an extremely high sensitivity, only a shield is a better choice for shallow nodes. Use of the collimator is superior for a deep node. Raising the threshold is less efficient for deep nodes, because a larger proportion of the radiation from deep nodes is scattered and is no longer counted.

Actual nodes from melanoma patients contain 13 kBq on average, with a very wide range as mentioned earlier [3]. If an injection site is nearby, most shallow nodes will still be found with the correct technique. However, the identification of deep nodes will only be possible for nodes that have accumulated a substantial amount of the tracer.

WEIGHT, SIZE, AND SHAPE

Most surgeons prefer a thin, lightweight probe. Both collimation and shielding are required to improve sentinel node detection but are the major determinants of the weight of the probe. A thin probe necessarily has a small detector area and, consequently, a low sensitivity. A compromise must be found between these conflicting requirements.

The optimal shape of the probe will depend on personal preference. A probe with a 15° angled tip may be most versatile. Such a probe can easily be manipu-

---

FIGURE 5   Count rates as a function of lower threshold for an "injection site" of 2 MBq ^{99m}Tc at different distances from the probe and for three "nodes": two nodes of 2 and 5 kBq ^{99m}Tc close to the probe and one of 200 kBq ^{99m}Tc at a depth of 5 cm in water. (a) Neoprobe with a shield, (b) Neoprobe with cone collimator. X: injection at 5 cm, 2 MBq; □: node at 5 mm, 5 kBq; ◆: node at 5 mm, 2 kBq; ■: node depth 5 cm water, 200 kBq; solid horizontal line; detection limit 5 cps.

lated through a small incision in a fairly deep wound. A straight probe has the advantage that the sense of direction is better.

USER INTERFACE

The front panel of the control unit should have a clear layout and should be easy to read from a distance and under variable lighting conditions. Push buttons are easier to use than turning knobs.

Intraoperative probes are usually equipped with an audio signal, which indicates the detected count rate. Different types of audio signals exist. Exercising on a phantom (for instance, a source with a weak background) enables the surgeon to determine whether the audio signal is useful. With the new generation of probes, the sound pitch goes up with an increasing count rate. This has the advantage that the surgeon gets an impression of the count rate without having to take his eyes from the operative field.

The probe should be able not only to measure count rate continuously (counts per second) but also to collect counts during a longer time interval (at least up to 10 s). This feature will be used in the case of a very low target uptake and a non-negligible background. Because the standard deviation (SD) of nuclear count measurements is approximately proportional to the square root of number of counts, the error in very low count values is relatively high. With 10,000 counts, the SD is 100 (1%); with 100 counts, it is 10 (10%); and with 10 counts, the SD is 3 (30%). If the observed count value is 10, a chance of about 3% exists that the true count value is actually larger than 16! In such a case, discrimination between target and background is more reliable if the number of counts is increased by counting for a longer period. It would be useful if the probe gave an indication of the statistical reliability of the measurement.

HYGIENIC ASPECTS AND SAFETY

The instrument should be designed for use in the operating room and not for the laboratory. If possible, probe, cable, and collimators should be sterilizable or disposable, but this may be too expensive to be acceptable. The probe must also satisfy safety requirements for surgical equipment. Electrical safety must be considered in particular [5].

PROBE MAINTENANCE

Any probe selected for clinical use should have excellent reliability and stability. Quality control consists mainly of a check of the background value and the sensitivity of the probe. The shielding should be looked at as well. Although in our experience stability is not a problem, it is recommended that before each use, the background value and sensitivity are determined. A background count will also detect any contamination with radioactivity of the probe. It is necessary to check the sensitivity regularly, because a gradual decrease may be unnoticed. A ^{57}Co source is convenient to use for a check of the sensitivity, but the readings should be corrected for the half-life of 270 d. Initially the source should not be too strong to avoid dead-time effects, which would cause a reduced count rate. The maximum count rate of the probe (typicaly 10,000 counts per second) should not be exceeded. After 5 years, the count rate will then have decreased to 100 counts per second. In that case, the sensitivity can still be determined with an accuracy of 3% if a counting interval of 10 seconds is used, which is acceptable. Therefore, it is recommended to obtain a new ^{57}Co source at least every 5 years.

PROBE SELECTION

Before a probe is selected, it is important to analyze the specific requirements for which the probe will be used. An optimal solution does not exist, because improvement of one characteristic will mean deterioration of one or more of the other characteristics.

Because uptake in lymph nodes may be low, a high sensitivity is the primary requirement. Collimation will increase the precision of localization of nodes before an incision is made. The side shielding of the probe should be excellent when a hot injection site is nearby. Collimation is recommended in this situation and the threshold setting must be raised to such a level that scattered radiation from the injection site is eliminated. Depending on the estimated radioactivity uptake, depth of the node, and the position of the injection site, the shield or collimator to be used is chosen. Optimally, the surgeon might want to be able to switch between different probe configurations during the surgical procedure, starting with excellent spatial resolution and (if necessary) energy discrimination, then switching to a higher sensitivity if needed.

Summarizing, a probe is required with high sensitivity, a choice of add-on collimators, and the ability to suppress low-energy radiation at a level that can be specified by the user.

REFERENCES

1. M Thurston. Development of the gamma detecting probe for radioimmunoguided surgery. In: EW Martin, ed. Radioimmunoguided surgery (RIGS) in the detection and treatment of colorectal cancer. RG Landes Company, 1994, pp. 41–65.
2. JM Woolfenden, HB Barber. Radiation detector probes for tumor localization using tumor-seeking radioactive tracers. Am J Roentgenol 153:35–39, 1989.

3. BAE Kapteijn, OE Nieweg, SH Muller, IH Liem, CA Hoefnagel, EJTh Rutgers, BBR Kroon. Validation of gamma probe detection of the sentinel node in melanoma. J Nucl Med 38:362–366, 1997.
4. T Tiourina, B-J Arends, D Husmans, H Rutten, B Lemaire, SH Muller. Evaluation of surgical gamma probes for radioguided sentinel node localization. Eur J Nucl Med 25:1224–1231, 1998.
5. Medical Electrical Equipment. Part 1: General Requirements For safety. IEC publication 601.1. Geneva, Switzerland: International Electrotechnical Commission, 1988.

6

Results of Lymphatic Mapping in Melanoma

Richard Essner, Stacey Stern, Peter Bostick, and Donald L. Morton
John Wayne Cancer Institute at Saint John's Health Center, Santa Monica, California

> In respect of surgical treatment, two cardinal phenomena . . . call for emphatic notice and indicate corresponding principles of action. These are (a.) the usually insignificant dimensions of the primary lesion and (b.) its tendency to rapidly infect the nearest lymph glands.
> Herbert L. Snow, M.D., London, Lecture on melanotic cancerous disease, 1892

INTRODUCTION

The controversy regarding the surgical management of regional lymph nodes in early-stage melanoma began over 100 years ago. In 1892, Herbert L. Snow in his lecture ''Melanotic Cancerous Disease'' advocated wide excision and elective (prophylactic) lymph node dissection as a method to control lymphatic permeation of metastases [1]. His studies suggested a direct connection of the primary site with the regional lymph nodes and he concluded that treatment of melanoma should routinely include excision of the draining lymph nodes. Elective lymph node dissection for patients with early-stage melanoma has remained controversial since Dr. Snow first proposed this management approach. Although multiple retrospective studies suggest a survival benefit for patients treated with elective lymph node dissection as compared to those whose treatment is limited to the primary site alone, the therapeutic benefit of removing clinically normal lymph nodes has never been proved by randomized prospective studies [2–17]. Although elective lymph node dissection is considered a valuable staging procedure, its cost, morbidity, and overall low yield of tumor-containing nodes have led most surgeons to abandon this procedure as a routine part of patient care. Yet,

101

the tumor status of the regional lymph nodes has become exceedingly important for determining patient prognosis and directing the use of adjuvant therapy [18,19].

A number of alternative methods have been proposed for staging the regional lymph nodes. However, none of these other methods is as accurate as lymph node dissection. Clinical examination of the nodes and needle aspiration biopsy leads to an unacceptable rate of false negatives. Cutaneous lymphoscintigraphy can demonstrate the exact location of the draining regional nodes but cannot differentiate tumor-containing nodes from reactive or normal nodes [20,21]. Ultrasound, computed tomography (CT) scanning, and magnetic resonance imaging (MRI) can identify nodes exceeding 1 cm in size but are not specific for malignancy. Positron emission tomography (PET) is a promising staging technique but is expensive and the lower limit of detection of metastases is probably 5 mm [22,23].

In recent years, the ability to detect occult regional lymph node metastases has been improved by intraoperative lymphatic mapping and selective lymphadenectomy. This technique enables the surgeon to map the direct route of lymphatic spread from the primary lesion to the regional drainage basin and then to selectively excise the first lymph node(s) (sentinel node, first-tier node, first-echelon node). Because the sentinel node has been shown to be the most likely site of tumor cells in the regional drainage basin, focused pathological examination of the selective lymphadenectomy specimen is a useful method of ultrastaging the regional nodes. Selective lymphadenectomy can be performed with minimal morbidity and expense and has proved to be highly accurate and sensitive for detecting occult regional metastases in patients with early-stage melanoma.

In 1990, Morton and associates first proposed the technique of selective lymphadenectomy as a minimally invasive alternative to elective lymph node dissection in patients with clinically uninvolved regional lymph nodes [24,25]. They hypothesized that the dermal lymphatics provide a direct connection from the primary melanoma to the regional lymph node basin, where a sentinel node could be identified. The sentinel node should therefore be the first regional site of metastasis; if the sentinel nodes do not contain tumor cells from a primary melanoma, then it is probable that there is no regional lymph node involvement.

TECHNIQUE

Selective lymphadenectomy is preceded by preoperative cutaneous lymphoscintigraphy. In the United States, the most commonly employed agents are technetium-99m (^{99m}Tc)-labeled albumin colloid (Cis-US, Inc., Bedford, MA, U.S.A.), ^{99m}Tc sulfur colloid (Cis-US, Inc.), or ^{99m}Tc human serum albumin (HSA; Amersham Medi-physics, Arlington Heights, IL, U.S.A.) [21,26,27]. Approximately 18.5–30 MBq (0.5–0.8 mCi) of radiopharmaceutical is injected at the primary melanoma site. A scintillation camera is used to document the drainage pattern from the primary site via the dermal lymphatics to the regional nodes. The skin overlying the sentinel node is marked. Because there is some variation in the transit time among the various pharmaceuticals, the nuclear medicine physician performing the procedure must be careful to differentiate the sentinel node from second-tier (nonsentinel) nodes. In our experience, the sentinel node can be identified by 30 min (depending on the agent and the distance of the primary to the regional nodes), and usually by 4 h, the sentinel node can no longer be differentiated from the adjacent second-tier nodes [28]. We typically perform lymphoscintigraphy on the day of surgery to allow the radiopharmaceutical to be used for sentinel node identification. Lymphoscintigraphy is used to determine the regional lymph node basin at risk for metastases and is particularly helpful in sites

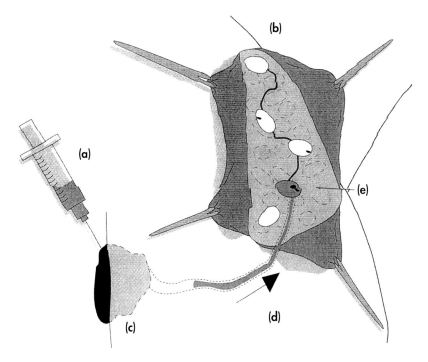

FIGURE 1   Schematic representation of intraoperative lymphatic mapping shows blue dye being injected into a primary melanoma. The dye moves along the lymphatic channel into the drainage basin. The first node(s) to turn blue—*not* necessarily the proximal node—is the sentinel node. This node is removed during selective lymphadenectomy and sent to the pathologist for analysis. (a) Blue dye injection; (b) other lymph nodes with or without metastases; (c) primary tumor; (d) regional lymph nodes; (e) sentinel node.

on the head and neck or torso, which may have ambiguous lymph drainage [21,26–28].

The patient is brought to the operating room on the same day as the lymphoscintigraphy. After induction of local or general anesthesia, 0.5–1.0 mL of isosulfan blue dye (Lymphazurin, Hirsch Industries, Inc., Richmond, VA, U.S.A.) is injected intradermally using a 25-gauge needle at the site of the primary melanoma (Fig. 1). If the primary lesion has already been excised, the injection is made on either side of the scar. An incision is made over the regional lymph node basin and oriented so that a complete lymphadenectomy can be performed if needed. The skin flap closest to the primary is dissected free of the underlying tissue and the subdermal lymphatics are observed as they and the sentinel node turn blue (Fig. 2). The blue dye typically takes from 5 to 20 min to reach the regional nodes and the transit time can usually be predicted by the distance of the primary from the dissected basin. The further the distance between the primary site and the regional lymph node basin, the greater the transit time. Injections are repeated every 20 min during the procedure. The sentinel node is excised and evaluated for the presence of metastasis (usually permanent section analysis). Complete lymph node dissection is performed at a later date if metastases are demonstrated.

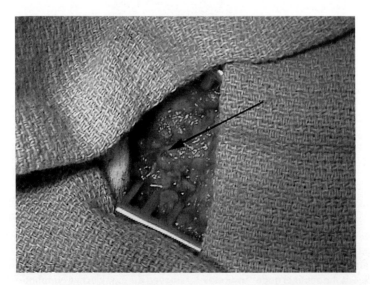

FIGURE 2 Demonstration of blue dye in a single axillary sentinel lymph node. A single blue-stained sentinel lymph node was identified 5 min after injection of blue dye around the primary tumor on the back.

RESULTS

In 1992, Morton and associates reported their initial experience with selective lymphadenectomy [24,25]. They were able to identify a blue-stained sentinel node in 194 (82%) of 237 regional lymphatic drainage basins (Table 1). All 223 patients underwent complete lymph node dissection regardless of the pathology of the sentinel node. Of these specimens, 40 (21%) contained metastases in at least one lymph node. In only 2 of 194 (1%) lymph node dissection specimens were nonsentinel nodes, the exclusive site of regional metastasis. These results are quite remarkable considering the fact that in most cases, preoperative lymphoscintigraphy was not used and the kinetics of the blue dye had not been well defined [29]. Yet, this early report demonstrates the strength of selective lymphadenectomy as a staging procedure.

Occult regional metastases were identified by both standard Hematoxylin & Eosin (H&E) staining and newer immunohistochemical techniques. Fifty-seven percent of nodal metastases were found using conventional techniques; the remainder were identified by immunohistochemical staining alone [24,25]. Using immunohistochemical staining techniques with an antiserum to S-100 protein, Cochran and associates had previously demonstrated that 29% of lymph nodes stained negative with H&E actually contained metastatic melanoma [30,31]. The 3338 lymph nodes excised in the selective lymphadenectomy patients were stained with the melanoma-specific murine monoclonal antibody NKI/C3 to confirm the presence of melanoma cells. They found few additional metastases with serial sectioning of the nodes as compared to just examining the bivalved faces. The role of additional sectioning of the sentinel nodes is unknown [32]. Whereas newer molecular biology techniques looking for specific gene sequences particu-

TABLE 1   Initial Experience with Selective Lymphadenectomy for Early-Stage Melanoma: Distribution of Metastases in Sentinel and Second-Tier Nodes

	N	%
Total lymphadenectomies	237	100
Lymphadenectomies with identified sentinel nodes	194	82
Lymphadenectomies with tumor in nodes	40	21
Lymphadenectomies with tumor in sentinel nodes	38	20
Lymphadenectomies with tumor in second-tier nodes (exclusively)	2	<1
Total lymph nodes	3338	100
Total sentinel nodes	259	8
Sentinel nodes with tumor	47	18
Total second-tier nodes	3079	92
Total second-tier nodes with tumor (exclusively)	2	<0.1

lar to melanoma may further enhance the sensitivity of detecting metastases in the sentinel node [33–35], their role in the routine management of melanoma is also unknown.

Selective lymphadenectomy is a relatively difficult procedure, but its learning curve is steep. During his initial 58 cases, Morton identified only 81% of blue-stained sentinel nodes. However, during the next 58 cases, his rate of sentinel node identification increased to 96%, and it now approaches 100%. The surgeon with the most experience with the procedure achieved an early success rate of 96%, whereas the surgeon with the least experience had the lowest level of success: 72% ($p < 0.01$). The gradual improvement in the rate of sentinel node detection is partially based on the increased experience with the technique. We have found that the blue-stained afferent lymphatics and nodes can be difficult to identify. Most surgeons have little experience dissecting lymphatic channels prior to ever performing a selective lymphadenectomy. We have found that patients who have undergone wide excision of the primary with margins of more than 1.5 cm or have had any procedure that disrupts the lymphatic drainage are not candidates for selective lymphadenectomy [24,25,36].

The routine use of preoperative lymphoscintigraphy in all cases has played a significant role in decreasing the incidence of missed sentinel nodes. Glass and associates from the John Wayne Cancer Institute [28] recently reviewed their experience with lymphoscintigraphy using three commonly employed radiopharmaceuticals: ^{99m}Tc-labeled albumin colloid, ^{99m}Tc sulfur colloid, and ^{99m}Tc-HSA. They compared the three agents for their utility to identify the afferent lymphatics and sentinel lymph nodes. Using early (up to 30 min) images, the three agents were equally effective for identifying the sentinel nodes. On average, two lymph nodes were identified in each basin. When they delayed their images up to 4 h after injection of the radiopharmaceutical, the average number of nodes visualized did not change significantly. There appeared to be a wide variation in the number of lymph nodes seen on lymphoscintigraphy from patient to patient: ^{99m}Tc-labeled albumin colloid (range: 1–7), ^{99m}Tc sulfur colloid (range: 1–14), and ^{99m}Tc-HSA (range: 0–9).

Yet more importantly, in more than half of the cases, we reviewed, more than one ''sentinel'' node was identified, often in basins or sites which would not be expected by strict anatomic definition [37]. Because the blue dye appears to travel along the same pathways as the radiopharmaceuticals, lymphoscintigraphy is critical for the accuracy of the selective lymphadenectomy procedure.

Morton's initial experience with selective lymphadenectomy also demonstrated the technical differences between dissection in the groin, neck, and axillary basins [24,25]. Sentinel nodes were easier to identify in the groin (89% accuracy) and increasingly more difficult in the neck (81% accuracy) and axilla (78% accuracy). In 1993, Morton's group reported their experience with selective lymphadenectomy for melanoma of the lower torso and extremities that drained to the groin basin [38]. One hundred twenty-eight patients had selective lymphadenectomy performed. Preoperative lymphoscintigraphy was used only for non-extremity primaries. Sentinel nodes were identified in 96% of the 51 patients who had complete groin dissections and in 98% of the next 77 patients having had a selective lymphadenectomy alone. In less than 1% of these patients, the sentinel node was free of disease while other (nonsentinel) nodes were involved. Even with this high rate of success with selective lymphadenectomy in this basin, we now employ preoperative lymphoscintigraphy in all cases. In 12% of selective lymphadenectomy procedures, lymphatic drainage was to two lymph node basins, including those rare primaries on the calf or foot that also drained to the popliteal region. In most cases, a single sentinel node was identified just inferior to the inguinal ligament. However, some of the sentinel nodes were located at the apex of the femoral triangle and occasionally two sentinel nodes were identified, usually on opposite sides of the femoral vein. Although lymphoscintigraphy may be considered unnecessary for some primaries on the lower extremities, the routine use of this procedure helps to identify the occasional aberrant lymph node in the groin or popliteal basins.

In 1993, Morton's group also reported their experience of selective lymphadenectomy for head and neck melanoma that drained to the cervical nodes [39]. All patients had preoperative cutaneous lymphoscintigraphy. At the time of surgery, blue dye alone was used to identify the sentinel nodes. The sentinel node was found in 71 of the 79 cervical drainage basins (90%). Most of the missed sentinel nodes were from the occipital, postauricular, or parotid basins, where the blue dye is difficult to identify. There were no regional recurrences in those patients with tumor-negative dissections during a mean follow-up of 27 months. Although preoperative lymphoscintigraphy was used in all cases, this early experience with selective lymphadenectomy demonstrated the intrinsic difficulty with the cervical basin. The lymphatic drainage from the head and neck is difficult to determine from the anatomical location of the primary [20]. As our own experience suggests, sentinel nodes in the midst of the parotid gland, deep in between the neck muscles or adjacent to the numerous facial veins, are difficult to identify. We have recently updated our experience with selective lymphadenectomy for early-stage melanoma of the head and neck employing both blue dye and radiopharmaceutical. Bostick and associates reported on 117 patients undergoing selective lymphadenectomy with either blue dye alone (94 cases) or in combination with a radiopharmaceutical (23 cases) for probe-directed selective lymphadenectomy [40]. The accuracy rate for blue-dye–directed selective lymphadenectomy was 92% (only slightly better than our earlier report) but improved to 96% with the combination of blue dye and radiopharmaceutical. The probe was helpful for identifying sentinel nodes in the difficult sites such as the postauricular, occipital, and parotid basins. Ten percent of patients had drainage to two basins. Eighty-nine percent of the patients avoided complete neck dissection after undergoing a tumor-negative selective lymphadenectomy. There have been no regional lymph node recurrences over a median follow-up of 46 months (range: 1–125 months) [40]. Our improved accuracy rate probably relates not only to our increased experience with selective lymphadenectomy for this basin but also to the use of the hand-held gamma probe. Although the probe helped improve the accuracy rate of selective lymphadenectomy, the background radioactivity in adjacent lymph nodes in the cervical basin can lead to the removal of excessive (second-tier) nodes.

In Morton's initial experience, the axilla was the most difficult of basins in which to identify the sentinel lymph node. The anatomy of the axilla prevents the nuclear medicine physician from marking the site of the sentinel node with the patient under the gamma camera, even with the patient positioned for surgery. With a hand-held gamma detection probe, this is considerably easier. We have also found that drainage patterns to the axilla vary greatly, especially from primaries on the chest and back.

In order to improve on the accuracy rate and diminish the learning curve for selective lymphadenectomy, we explored the technique of selective lymphadenectomy directed by a radiopharmaceutical and a gamma detection probe [41]. A gamma-probe–guided directed biopsy was first performed using the combination of blue isosulfan dye injected intraoperatively with 0.5–1.0 mL or 18.5 MBq (0.5 mCi) of ^{99m}Tc-HSA (Amersham) at the primary site. A hand-held gamma counter (Neoprobe 1000, Neoprobe Corp., Dublin, OH) was used to follow the radioactive tracer to the regional basin. Morton's group tested this approach initially in 30 melanoma patients. Thirty-four lymph node basins were identified by preoperative lymphoscintigraphy. At least one sentinel node was identified in each basin. The blue dye identified 36 sentinel nodes, and the gamma probe detected all 36 nodes plus an additional 6 nodes. Overall, blue-stained sentinel lymph nodes had a roughly twofold higher radioactive count rate than adjacent nonblue nodes, and up to an eightfold higher count rate than the lymph basin background. Although none of the sentinel nodes contained metastatic disease, this study demonstrated the utility of the hand-held gamma counter to help identify blue-stained sentinel nodes and the close concordance between the findings from blue dye and the radiopharmaceutical. One of the difficulties with the combined technique is the logistics of injecting a radiopharmaceutical in the operating room.

Bostick and associates recently reviewed the John Wayne Cancer Institute experience with gamma-probe-guided selective lymphadenectomy in 100 lymph node basins from 87 patients [42]. All patients underwent preoperative lymphoscintigraphy with one of the three radiopharmaceuticals commonly used in the United States. Selective lymphadenectomy was performed with either concurrent injection of blue dye and ^{99m}Tc-labeled human serum albumin or the ^{99m}Tc sulfur colloid injected up to 4 h prior to the operative procedure. One hundred thirty-six blue-stained and radioactive lymph nodes and eight additional non–blue-stained but "hot" nodes were removed in 98 lymph node basins (success rate 98%) (Table 2). A hand-held gamma probe was used to determine the radioactive counts over the blue nodes, adjacent nonblue nodes and an irrelevant background site. Ninety-two percent of the blue-stained lymph nodes had an in vivo count to background ratio of more than 2, and 87% had in vivo count ratios exceeding 3. Seventeen sentinel nodes from 15 basins contained metastases: 16 were located with blue dye and gamma probe and 1 was found with blue dye alone. None of the tumor-positive lymph nodes was identified with the gamma probe alone. Using the definition of a radioactive sentinel node as having an in vivo count ratio of more than 2 compared to the background, a success rate of 85% would be achieved. When the sentinel-node-to-background ratio was increased to a minimum of 3 to improve the specificity of the technique, the success rate decreased to 78% (Fig. 3). The concordance between the two techniques was not 100%. Not all blue-stained lymph nodes have an elevated count ratio and, conversely, not all nodes with an elevated count ratio are blue. In fact, when the in vivo count ratios for all the blue-stained lymph nodes were examined, a wide variation ranging from less than 1 to over 100 was noted. Similar results were observed when the ex vivo count ratio of the nodes was examined, suggesting that the

TABLE 2 **Results from Blue-Dye–Directed and from Radiopharmaceutical-Directed Selective Lymphadenectomy: Lymph Node Basins and Sentinel Lymph Nodes**

	N	%
Lymph node basins		
Total	100	
Sentinel node identified	98	
Sentinel node blue	93	
Sentinel node blue and radioactive (ratio ≥ 2)	83	
Sentinel node blue and radioactive (ratio ≥ 3)	77	
Sentinel node blue only (ratio <2)	10	
Sentinel node radioactive only (ratio ≥ 2)	5	
Sentinel node radioactive only (ratio ≥ 3)	5	
Sentinel nodes		
Total	144	100
Blue	136	94
Radioactive (ratio ≥ 2)	132	92
Radioactive (ratio ≥ 3)	125	87
Blue only (ratio <2)	12	8
Blue and radioactive (ratio ≥ 2)	124	86
Blue and radioactive (ratio ≥ 3)	117	81
Radioactive only (ratio ≥ 2)	8	6

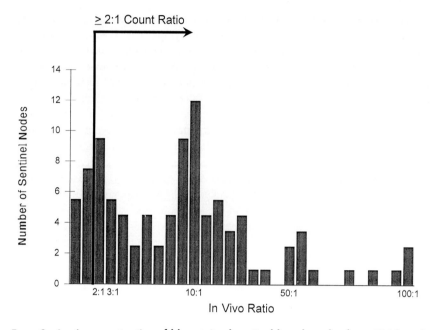

FIGURE 3   In vivo count ratios of blue-stained sentinel lymph nodes from 100 lymph basins. In vivo count ratios were calculated by determining the counts overlying the blue-stained sentinel nodes and comparing these counts to an irrelevant background site. Of sentinel nodes, 85% had an in vivo count ratio of more than 2 and 78% had a ratio exceeding 3.

radiopharmaceuticals alone can be misleading for sentinel node dissection. Both the radiopharmaceuticals were found to give similar count ratios for radio-lymphoscintigraphy and led to surgical excision of similar numbers of lymph nodes. At our center, we have little difficulty with performing lymphoscintigraphy and selective lymphadenectomy on the same day, but, logistically, this approach can be difficult. We are currently examining the use of ^{99m}Tc sulfur colloid administration for next-day selective lymphadenectomy.

One of the theoretical advantages of selective lymphadenectomy over conventional staging of the regional lymph nodes is the potential reduction in morbidity and cost compared to elective lymph node dissection. In 1997, Essner and associates reported their updated experience with selective lymphadenectomy for patients with melanoma of the torso and lower extremities that drained to the groin [43]. Fifty-two patients all underwent selective lymphadenectomy followed by complete groin dissection. Only a select portion of the patients underwent lymphoscintigraphy. A subsequent group of 114 consecutive patients all underwent lymphoscintigraphy followed by selective lymphadenectomy, with complete groin dissection only if the sentinel node contained metastasis. Three patients had bilateral drainage patterns. The average primary tumor thickness was 2.08 mm. The average number of lymph nodes removed for the 114 patients undergoing selective lymphadenectomy alone was 4.2 ± 6.5, and for those undergoing selective and complete node dissection, it was 13.0 ± 6.6 ($p < 0.05$). Seventy-three percent of patients having a selective lymphadenectomy alone had only one lymph node excised. The frequency of tumor positive dissections was similar in the two groups. Eighty percent of patients had one tumor-positive lymph node and additional tumor-positive lymph nodes were found in 20% of cases during completion lymph node dissection. We found no difference in survival between patients treated by either of the two approaches. Patients with tumor-negative dissections had a 5-year survival of $89.5 \pm 5\%$ following selective lymphadenectomy alone and $93 \pm 3\%$ after combined selective and complete node dissection. To determine the differences in costs of the two operative procedures, we compared both the length of in-patient stays and the total estimated hospital costs. Patients undergoing selective lymphadenectomy had an average hospital stay of less than 1 day. Patients treated by complete groin dissection had an average hospital stay of 6.05 days ($p = 0.01$) (Fig. 4). We included in our

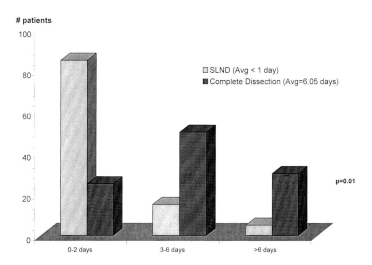

FIGURE 4   Length of hospital stay following selective lymphadenectomy (SLND) or complete groin dissection. Hospital stays were determined for patients treated by either selective lymphadenectomy or complete groin dissection. Most patients undergoing selective lymphadenectomy had less than 1 day of hospitalization. Patients with skin grafts usually required longer hospitalization.

calculation the hospital, nuclear medicine services, and pathology services (Table 3). Although the total costs will vary from institution to institution, our results represent the relative cost differences between these procedures at our community cancer center. When selective lymphadenectomy was performed under local anesthesia in our clinic, the cost was only $1,018. When the same procedure was performed through the out-patient operating room with participation of an anesthesiologist (either general or regional anesthesia), the costs increased to $7,150. Both superficial and deep groin dissections were even more expensive, as the costs increased substantially with patient admission to the hospital. The costs of the pathology evaluation were higher for selective-lymphadenectomy–treated patients only because of the routine use of immunohistochemical staining of the lymph nodes. Although this study focused on patients having selective lymphadenectomy of the groin basin, we would expect similar cost savings for patients having selective lymphadenectomy of the axillary or cervical basins. This study did not focus on the morbidity of the two operative procedures, but we expect that patients treated by the less extensive selective lymphadenectomy would have a lower risk of complications than those who also underwent the more radical dissection [44,45].

Because selective lymphadenectomy has virtually replaced elective lymph node dissection for staging the regional lymph nodes, we chose to compare the therapeutic value of selective lymphadenectomy to elective lymph node dissection. In 1998, Essner and associates performed a method pair statistical analysis to compare the outcome of 534 early-stage melanoma patients [46–48]. Half were treated by selective lymphadenectomy and the other half by elective lymph node dissection. Patients were matched from our computer-assisted database by age (54% over 50 years of age), gender (63% male), site of the primary (49% extremity, 36% on the trunk, and 15% on the head and neck), and thickness of the primary (7% <0.75 mm, 42% 0.75–1.5 mm, 43% 1.51–4.0 mm, and 8%

TABLE 3 Estimated Hospital Costs for Patients Undergoing Groin Dissections (U.S. Dollars)

	Hospital	Nuclear medicine	Pathology	Total
Out-patient clinic SLND[a]	833	54	131	1,018
Out-patient OR[b] SLND	6,965	54	131	7,150
In-patient OR superficial groin dissections	8,274	—	85	8,359
In-patient OR superficial and deep groin dissections	11,929	—	170	12,099

[a] SLND = selective lymph node dissection.
[b] OR = operating room.

>4 mm). Patients treated by selective lymphadenectomy only had a complete lymphadenectomy if the sentinel node contained metastasis. Overall, the incidence of lymph node metastases was not different between selective lymphadenectomy (15.7%) and elective lymph node dissection (12%) groups. Yet, the incidence of nodal metastases in patients with intermediate thickness primaries (1.51–4.0 mm) was significantly higher when treated by selective lymphadenectomy (23.7%) instead of elective lymph node dissection (12.2%) ($p = 0.025$). Although unexplained, this difference may relate to the improved staging accuracy of selective lymphadenectomy over elective lymph node dissection. Selective lymphadenectomy and elective lymph node dissection carried equivalent 5-year rates of disease-free survival (79 ± 3.3% and 84 ± 2.2%, respectively, $p = 0.25$) and overall survival (88 ± 3.0% and 86 ± 2.1%, respectively, $p = 0.98$).

Groups of 225 selective lymphadenectomy and 235 elective lymph node dissection patients had tumor-negative dissections. Overall 5-year survival was identical for the two treatments ($p = 0.37$). Twenty-six selective lymphadenectomy patients (11.5%) and 35 elective lymph node dissection patients (14.9%) have recurred over a median follow up of 45 and 169 months, respectively. Eleven of the recurrences after selective lymphadenectomy were confined to the dissected basin. We have since reexamined the original pathology of these sentinel nodes. In four (36%) cases, metastases were located in the sentinel node. The true surgical false-negative sentinel node rate is 3%. Among the 35 patients to have recurrences following elective lymph node dissection, five were in the dissected lymph node basin. The dissected basin recurrence rate (2%) was the same as in selective lymphadenectomy.

Fifteen of the 26 (58%) selective lymphadenectomy and 12 of the 35 (34%) elective lymph node dissection recurrences occurred within 2 years of lymph node dissection. We calculated the yearly probability of recurrence following the two techniques. Seven percent of selective lymphadenectomy patients recurred within 2 years compared to 5.1% of elective lymph node dissection patients. Although we have a relatively short follow-up for selective-lymphadenectomy–treated patients, these results demonstrate that selective lymphadenectomy and elective lymph node dissection are therapeutically equivalent procedures. We anticipate that longer follow-up of our selective-lymphadenectomy–treated patients will help to determine the true recurrence rates following a tumor-negative dissection [49].

DISCUSSION

Selective lymphadenectomy was devised as an alternative to either elective lymph node dissection or delayed therapeutic dissection for the management of the clinically negative lymph nodes in early-stage melanoma. The initial series from Morton and associates from the John Wayne Cancer Institute (Santa Monica, CA) demonstrated the feasibility of this technique [24,25,50]. Reintgen and associates from the Moffitt Cancer Center (Tampa, FL) were the first group to confirm the original series by Morton [51]. Forty-two patients underwent selective lymphadenectomy, all had undergone preoperative lymphoscintigraphy, with a blue-stained lymph node found in each basin (100% accuracy). In eight of the cases metastases were found in the sentinel lymph node, and in seven of the eight (88%), the sentinel lymph node was the exclusive site of disease. None of the remaining 34 patients had metastases either in sentinel or nonsentinel nodes. Their initial experience demonstrated the value of preoperative lymphoscintigraphy for localizing the site of the sentinel nodes. They also validated Morton's hypothesis that the sentinel node was reflective of the tumor status of the entire regional basin.

Thompson and his Sydney Melanoma Unit colleagues subsequently reported their initial experience with selective lymphadenectomy followed by complete regional node dissection [52]. A group of 118 patients underwent preoperative lymphoscintigraphy to identify the 120 basins at risk. At the time of surgery, blue-stained sentinel lymph nodes were located in 105 of the 120 basins (88%). In 18 of the 22 basins (82%) with metastatic disease, the sentinel node was the exclusive site of dissemination. Their rate of false-negative selective lymphadenectomy in the whole group of patients (1.9%) was similar to that reported in Morton's series. Thompson and colleagues confirmed the steep learning curve associated with this procedure. In the first half of their experience, sentinel nodes were found in 74% of the cases, and during the second half in 92%. A number of other investigators have also reported their experience with selective lymphadenectomy using blue dye alone (see Table 4) [24,25,51–55]. Most investigators had no prior experience with selective lymphadenectomy while achieving an accuracy rate of at least 90%. This relatively high rate of success is based on the

TABLE 4   Success Rate of Sentinel Node Identification
with Blue Dye Alone

Investigator [Ref.]	*N*	Accuracy rate (%)
Morton 1992 [24]	223	82
Morton 1993 [39]	72	90
Reintgen 1994 [51]	42	100
Thompson 1995 [52]	118	88
Karakousis 1996 [53]	55	93
Kapteijn 1997 [54]	110	84
Lingam 1997 [55]	35	100

more rapid learning of the technique through the experience gained by Morton and the other early pioneers of this procedure. The blue dye technique remains the gold standard for selective lymphadenectomy.

In order to improve the accuracy of selective lymphadenectomy and diminish the learning curve of this procedure, a number of investigators have attempted to use radiopharmaceuticals for probe-directed selective lymphadenectomy. Krag and associates were among the first groups to claim a high success rate for sentinel node identification with the use of a radiopharmaceutical alone [56]. Their 121 patients underwent selective lymphadenectomy, the majority with radiopharmaceutical alone. A sentinel node was defined as having at least 15 counts in 10 s and a count ratio three times the background. Ninety-eight percent of patients had a successful selective lymphadenectomy. Yet, the interval between injection of the radiopharmaceutical and surgery ranged from 15 min to 24 h. With this variation in technique, we suspect that the true sentinel node may have not always been properly identified. Other investigators have used an assortment of methods to define a radioactive sentinel lymph node (Table 5) [42,56–60]. Our own data suggest that the in vivo count ratios for blue-stained lymph nodes can vary almost 100-fold even when surgery was uniformly performed within 4 h after injection of the radiopharmaceutical [42]. Although the use of radiopharmaceutical and probe alone for selective lymphadenectomy would simplify the technique, our results with the filtered ^{99m}Tc sulfur colloid suggest that it is not ideal for this procedure. Although larger-sized particles such as the ^{99m}Tc sulfur colloid and the ^{99m}Tc albumin colloid would be expected to be trapped in the afferent lymphatics of the sentinel node, some of the particles are shunted through to adjacent lymph nodes. Similarly, our experience with ^{99m}Tc-HSA demonstrated that this agent passes quickly from the primary site to the sentinel node and to adjacent nonsentinel nodes. The ideal radiopharmaceutical for this procedure would be one that travels quickly from the primary site to the sentinel node and concentrates without leakage to adjacent lymph nodes. Until the kinetics of the radio-

TABLE 5 Definitions of Radioactive Sentinel Lymph Nodes

Investigators, Year [Ref.]	Definition
Krag 1995 [56]	15 counts/10 s and in vivo sentinel node to background ratio ≥ 3
Mudun 1996 [57]	300–3000 counts/10 s and in vivo sentinel node to background ratio ≥ 3
Albertini 1996 [58]	In vivo sentinel node to background ratio ≥ 2 or ex vivo sentinel node to nonsentinel node ratio ≥ 10
Pijpers 1995 [59]	Lymph node with highest counts
Bostick 1998 [42]	In vivo sentinel to background ratio ≥ 2

pharmaceuticals are better defined for selective lymphadenectomy or better agents are developed, we recommend that these agents not be employed alone for this purpose [61,62].

Most investigators now employ both blue dye and a radiopharmaceutical for selective lymphadenectomy. Preoperative lymphoscintigraphy is performed using one of the colloid agents on the same day as surgery. At the time of surgery, the hand-held gamma probe directs the surgeon to the site of the blue-stained sentinel node. Occasionally, the probe will lead the surgeon to an unexpected blue-stained lymph node (Fig. 5) [63–69]. We have found the concordance between the two techniques to be at least 80%. Although there is a variety of methods for defining a radioactive sentinel lymph node, a blue-stained lymph node with an afferent blue lymphatic coming from the direction of the primary lesion remains the gold standard for this procedure.

The technique of selective lymphadenectomy has been shown by a number of investigators to be a reliable indicator of the tumor status of the regional lymph nodes. Based on these studies, selective lymphadenectomy has become a popular alternative to conventional elective lymph node dissection and has become almost

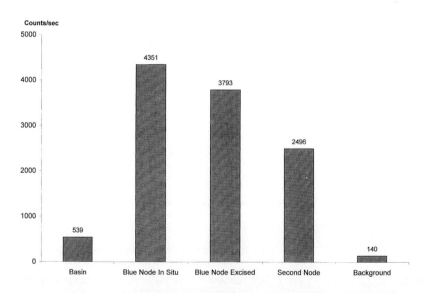

FIGURE 5 **In vivo count ratios demonstrating a second sentinel lymph node. A hand-held gamma probe was used to determine the radioactive counts of the blue-stained sentinel lymph node. High residual counts in the lymph node basin led the surgeon to continue exploration and ultimately to identify a second blue-stained sentinel lymph node.**

the standard procedure for staging regional lymph nodes. Yet, the successful performance of selective lymphadenectomy is dependent on the experience of the multidisciplinary team of surgeon, pathologist, and nuclear medicine physician. We recommend that each sentinel node team complete a learning phase of at least 15 cases (and perhaps up to 50) before selective lymphadenectomy becomes a routine procedure at any center [70]. Our studies clearly indicate that successful mapping of the sentinel nodes is directly related to the surgeon's experience. While progressing through the learning phase the surgeon must perform a complete lymph node dissection to monitor his own false-negative rate. Although the reported rates of missed sentinel nodes are extremely low, we have observed dissected basin recurrences as late as 5 years after negative selective lymphadenectomy. The true accuracy rate of this technique has yet to be determined for the casual user. Although this procedure has become increasingly popular, its therapeutic value is not yet proven [69].

Two major studies are underway examining the utility of selective lymphadenectomy. In 1994, Morton and colleagues at the John Wayne Cancer Institute initiated an international multicenter randomized prospective trial comparing wide excision and selective lymphadenectomy to wide excision alone in patients with clinically localized melanoma. Patients with intermediate (1–4 mm)-thickness melanoma who have not had a wide excision (>1.5-cm margins), skin graft or other procedures that would alter the lymphatic drainage are eligible [71]. Complete lymph node dissection is performed only in lymphatic drainage basins containing tumor-positive sentinel nodes. The purpose of this study is to determine the therapeutic benefit of selective lymphadenectomy and the true accuracy of the technique on a large scale. As of September 1999, 1300 of the anticipated 1600 patients had entered the study. The trial's organizers hope that selective lymphadenectomy will eventually replace conventional elective lymph node dissection or the wait-and-watch approach as the standard of management for patients with clinically localized melanoma [72–74].

A second randomized prospective trial examines the efficacy of selective lymphadenectomy as treatment for tumor-positive regional lymph nodes. The Sunbelt Melanoma Trial compares patients with one tumor-positive lymph node determined by conventional H&E or immunohistochemical techniques (followed by complete lymph node dissection) to observation or treatment with adjuvant interferon-alpha (Schering-Plough, Kenilworth, NJ, U.S.A.). A second group of patients who have a tumor-positive sentinel lymph node by reverse transcriptase–polymerase chain reaction (RT-PCR) alone are randomized to observation, complete lymph node dissection, or complete lymph node dissection and interferon-alpha. The organizers of this study anticipate that this trial should provide further insight into the therapeutic value of selective lymphadenectomy for patients with a single tumor-positive lymph node identified by either routine techniques or RT-PCR.

THE FUTURE

We anticipate that the selective lymphadenectomy procedure will continue to evolve as we gain more insight into the molecular biology of melanoma and the significance of micrometastatic disease. Although it is tempting for the oncology community to treat patients following tumor-negative and tumor-positive selective lymphadenectomy without complete lymph node dissections, we must not be too quick to change our management approaches without the results of the ongoing clinical trials [75].

ACKNOWLEDGMENTS

This work was supported in part by grant CA29605 from the National Cancer Institute and Haim Sabon Foundation, Los Angeles, CA.

REFERENCES

1. H Snow. Melanotic cancerous disease. Lancet 2:872, 1892.
2. DS Reintgen, EB Cox, KS McCarty Jr, RT Vollmer, HF Seigler. Efficacy of elective lymph node dissection in patients with intermediate thickness primary melanoma. Ann Surg 198:379–385, 1983.
3. WH McCarthy, HM Shaw, GW Milton. Efficacy of elective lymph node dissection in 2,347 patients with clinical stage I malignant melanoma. Surg Gynecol Obstet 161:575–580, 1985.
4. DL Morton, L Wanek, JA Nizze, RM Elashoff, JH Wong. Improved long-term survival after lymphadenectomy of melanoma metastatic to regional nodes: analysis of prognostic factors in 1134 patients from the John Wayne Cancer Institute. Ann Surg 214:491–501, 1991.
5. CM Balch, GW Milton, N Cascinelli, FH Sim. Elective lymph node dissection: pros and cons. In: CM Balch, AN Houghton, GW Milton, AJ Sober, S-J Soong, eds. Cutaneous Melanoma. 2nd ed. Philadelphia: JB Lippincott Company, 1992, pp. 45–366.
6. DR Roses, JA Provet, MN Harris, SL Gumport, N Dubin. Prognosis of patients with pathologic stage II cutaneous melanoma. Ann Surg 201:103–107, 1985.
7. CM Balch, S-J Soong, TM Murad, AL Ingalls, WA Maddox. A multifactorial analysis of melanoma III. Prognostic factors in melanoma patients with lymph node metastases (stage III). Ann Surg 193:377–388, 1981.
8. GW Milton, HM Shaw, WH McCarthy, L Pearson, CM Balch, SJ Soong. Prophylactic lymph node dissection in clinical stage I cutaneous melanoma: results of surgical treatment in 1,319 patients. Br J Surg 69:108–111, 1982.
9. MH Cohen, AS Ketcham, EL Felix, SH Li, MM Tomaszewski, J Costa, AS Rabson, RM Simon, SA Rosenberg. Prognostic factors in patients undergoing lymphadenectomy for malignant melanoma. Ann Surg 186:635–642, 1977.

10. C Callery AJ, Cochran, DJ Roe, W Rees, SD Nathanson, JK Benedetti, RM Elashoff, DL Morton. Factors prognostic in patients with malignant melanoma spread to the regional lymph nodes. Ann Surg 196:69–75, 1982.

11. CM Balch, S-J Soong, GW Milton, HM Shaw, VJ McGovern, TM Murad, WH McCarthy, WA Maddox. A comparison of prognostic factors and surgical results in 1,786 patients with localized (stage I) melanoma treated in Alabama, USA and New South Wales, Australia. Ann Surg 196:677–684, 1982.

12. U Veronesi, J Adamus, DC Bandiera, IO Brennhovd, E Caceres, N Cascinelli, F Claudic, RL Ikonopisov, VV Javorskj, S Kirov, A Kulakowski, J Lacoub, F Lejeune, Z Mechl, A Morabito, I Rode, S Sergeev, E van Slooten, K Szcygiel, NN Trapeznikov. Inefficacy of immediate node dissection in stage I melanoma of the limbs. N Engl J Med 297:627–630, 1977.

13. U Veronesi, J Adamus, DC Bandiera, IO Brennhoud, E Caceres, N Caseinelli, F Claudio, RL Ikonopisov, VV Javorski, S Kirov, A Kulakowski, J Lacour, F Lejeune, Z Mechl, A Morabito, I Rode, S Sergeev, E van Slooten, K Szcygiel, NN Trapeznikov, RI Wagner. Delayed regional lymph node dissection in stage I melanoma of the skin of the lower extremities. Cancer 49:2420–2430, 1982.

14. FH Sim, WF Taylor, DJ Pritchard, EH Soule. Lymphadenectomy in the management of stage I malignant melanoma: a prospective randomized study. Mayo Clin Proc 61:697–705, 1986.

15. CM Balch, MM Urist, CP Karakousis, TJ Smith, WJ Temple, K Drzewiecki, WR Jewell, AA Bartolucci, MC Mihm, R Barnhill, HJ Wanebo. Efficacy of 2-cm surgical margins for intermediate-thickness melanomas (1 to 4 mm). Results of a multi-institutional randomized surgical trial. Ann Surg 218:262–269, 1993.

16. CM Balch, SJ Soong, AA Bartolucci, MM Urist, CP Karakousis, TJ Smith, WJ Temple, MI Ross, WR Jewell, MC Mihm, RL Barnhill, HJ Wanebo. Efficacy of an elective regional lymph node dissection of 1 to 4 mm thick melanomas for patients 60 years of age and younger. Ann Surg 224:255–266, 1996.

17. R Rompel, C Garbe, P Buttner, K Teichelmann, J Petres. Elective lymph node dissection in primary malignant melanoma: a matched-pair analysis. Melanoma Res 5: 189–194, 1995.

18. JM Kirkwood, MH Strawderman, MS Ernstoff, TJ Smith, EC Borden, RH Blum. Interferon alfa-2b adjuvant therapy of high-risk resected cutaneous melanoma: the eastern cooperative group trial EST 1684. J Clin Oncol 14:7–17, 1996.

19. DL Morton, A Barth. Vaccine therapy for malignant melanoma. CA Cancer J Clin 46:225–244, 1996.

20. JP Shah, DH Kraus, S Dubner, S Sarkar. Patterns of regional lymph node metastases from cutaneous melanoma of the head and neck. Am J Surg 162:320–323, 1991.

21. HJ Wanebo, D Harpole, CD Teates. Radionuclide lymphoscintigraphy with technetium 99m antimony sulfide colloid to identify lymphatic drainage of cutaneous melanoma of ambiguous sites in the head and neck and trunk. Cancer 55:1403–1413, 1985.

22. AC Buzaid, L Tinoco, MI Ross, SS Legha, RS Benjamin. Role of computed tomography in the staging of patients with local-regional metastases of melanoma. J Clin Oncol 13:2104–2108, 1995.

23. DL Damian, MJ Fulham, E Thompson, JF Thompson. Positron emission tomography

in the detection and management of metastatic melanoma. Melanoma Res 6:325–329, 1996.

24. DL Morton, D-R Wen, JH Wong, JS Economou, LA Cagle, FK Storm, LJ Foshag, AJ Cochran. Technical details of intraoperative lymphatic mapping for early stage melanoma. Arch Surg 127:392–399, 1992.

25. AJ Cochran, DR Wen, DL Morton. Management of the regional lymph nodes in patients with cutaneous malignant melanoma. World J Surg 16:214–221, 1992.

26. DS Robinson, WF Sample, HJ Fee, C Holmes, DL Morton. Regional lymphatic drainage in primary malignant melanoma of the trunk determined by colloidal gold scanning. Surg Forum 28:147–148, 1977.

27. J Norman, CW Cruse, C Espinosa, C Cox, C Berman, R Clark, H Saba, K Wells D Reintgen. Redefinition of cutaneous lymphatic drainage with the use of lymphoscintigraphy for malignant melanoma. Am J Surg 162:432–437, 1991.

28. EC Glass, R Essner, DL Morton. Kinetics of three lymphoscintigraphic agents in patients with cutaneous melanoma. J Nucl Med 39:1185–1190, 1998.

29. JH Wong, LA Cagle, DL Morton. Lymphatic drainage of skin in a sentinel lymph node in a feline model. Ann Surg 214:637–641, 1991.

30. AJ Cochran, DR Wen, DL Morton. Occult tumor cells in the lymph nodes of patients with pathological stage I malignant melanoma: An immunohistochemical study. Am J Surg Pathol 12:612–618, 1988.

31. AJ Cochran, DR Wen, HR Herschman. Occult melanoma in lymph nodes detected by antiserum to S-100 protein. Int J Cancer 34:159–163, 1984.

32. R Heller, J Becker, J Wasselle, P Baekey, W Cruse, K Wells, C Cox, B King, DS Reintgen. Detection of submicroscopic lymph node metastases in patients with melanoma. Arch Surg 126:1455–1459, 1991.

33. X Wang, R Heller, N Van Voorhis, CW Cruse, F Glass, N Fenske, C Berman, J Leo-Messina, D Rapaport, K Wells, R DeConti, L Moscinski, C Stankard C Puleo, D Reintgen. Detection of submicroscopic lymph node metastases with polymerase chain reaction in patients with malignant melanoma. Ann Surg 220:768–774, 1994.

34. JS Goydos, TS Ravikumar, FJ Germino, A Yudd, E Bancila. Minimally invasive staging of patients with melanoma: Sentinel lymphadenectomy and detection of the melanoma-specific proteins MART-1 and tyrosinase by reverse transcriptase polymerase chain reaction. J Am Coll Surg 187:182–190, 1998.

35. DSB Hoon, Y Wang, PS Dale, AJ Conrad, P Schmid, D Garrison, C Kuo, LJ Foshag, AJ Nizze, DL Morton. Detection of occult melanoma cells in blood with a multiple-marker polymerase chain reaction assay. J Clin Oncol 13:2109–2116, 1995.

36. R Essner. The role of lymphoscintigraphy and sentinel node mapping in assessing patient risk in melanoma. Semin Oncol 24(1 Suppl 4):S8–S10, 1997.

37. MPC Sappey. Injection, preparation et conservation des vaisseaux lymphatic. Thesis, Rignoux Imprimeur de la Faculte de Medecine, Paris, 1843.

38. R Essner, DR Wen, AJ Cochran, DL Morton, KP Ramming. Lymphatic mapping and selective lymph node biopsy: an alternative to elective lymphadenectomy for early-stage melanomas of the trunk and lower extremities. Proc Am Soc Clin Oncol 12:391, 1993.

39. DL Morton, D-R Wen, LJ Foshag, R Essner, A Cochran. Intraoperative lymphatic

mapping and selective cervical lymphadenectomy for early-stage melanomas of the head and neck. J Clin Oncol 11:1751–1756, 1993.

40. P Bostick, R Essner, T Sarantou, M Kelley, E Glass, L Foshag, S Stern, D Morton. Intraoperative lymphatic mapping for early-stage melanoma of the head and neck. Am J Surg 174:536–539, 1997.

41. R Essner, L Foshag, DL Morton. Intraoperative radiolymphoscintigraphy: a useful adjunct to intraoperative lymphatic mapping and selective lymphadenectomy in patients with clinical stage I melanoma (abstr). Society of Surgical Oncology 47th Annual Meeting, Houston 1994, p. 104.

42. P Bostick R Essner, E Glass, M Kelley, T Sarantou, L Foshag, S Stern, DL Morton. Comparison of blue dye and probe-assisted intraoperative lymphatic mapping in melanoma to identify sentinel nodes in 100 lymphatic basins. Arch Surg 134:43–49, 1999.

43. R Essner, A Conforti, MC Kelley, L Wanek, DL Morton. Cost-conscious management of the inguinal nodes in early-stage melanoma (abstr). Melanoma Res 7:S29, 1997.

44. MM Urist, WA Maddox, JE Kennedy, CM Balch. Patient risk factors and surgical morbidity after regional lymphadenectomy in 204 melanoma patients. Cancer 51: 2152–2156, 1983.

45. CP Karakousis, MA Heiser, RH Moore. Lymphedema after groin dissection. Am J Surg 145:205–208, 1983.

46. R Essner, A Conforti, MC Kelley, L Wanek, S Stem, E Glass, DL Morton. Efficacy of selective lymphadenectomy as a therapeutic procedure for early-stage melanoma. Ann Surg Oncol 6(5):442–449, 1999.

47. N Mantel, JL Ciminera. Use of logrank scores in the analysis of the litter-matched data on time to tumour appearance. Cancer Res 39:4308–4315, 1979.

48. JE Michalek, D Mihalko. On the use of log-rank scores in the analysis of litter-matched data on time to tumor appearance. Stat Med 2:315–326, 1983.

49. JE Gershenwald, MI Colome, JE Lee, PF Mansfield, C Tseng, JJ Lee, CM Balch, MI Ross. Patterns of recurrence following a negative sentinel lymph node biopsy in 243 patients with stage I or II melanoma. J Clin Oncol 16:2253–2260, 1998.

50. DL Morton, DR Wen, AJ Cochran. Management of early-stage melanoma by intra-operative lymphatic mapping and selective lymphadenectomy. Surg Oncol Clin North Am 1:247–259, 1992.

51. D Reintgen, CW Cruse, K Wells, C Berman, N Fenske, F Glass, K Schroer, R Heller, M Ross, G Lyman, C Cox, D Rapaport, HF Seigler, CM Balch. The orderly progression of melanoma nodal metastases. Ann Surg 220:759–767, 1994.

52. J Thompson, WH McCarthy, CMJ Bosch, CJ O'Brien, MJ Quinn, S Paramaesvaran, K Crotty, SW McCarthy, RF Uren, R Howman-Giles. Sentinel lymph node status as an indicator of the presence of metastatic melanoma in regional lymph nodes. Melanoma Res 5:255–260, 1995.

53. CP Karakousis, AF Velez, JE Spellman Jr, J Scarozza. The technique of sentinel node biopsy. Eur J Surg Oncol 22:271–275, 1996.

54. BAE Kapteijn, OE Nieweg, IH Liem, WJ Mooi, AJM Balm, SH Muller, JL Peterse, RA Valdés Olmos, CA Hoefnagel, BBR Kroon. Localizing the sentinel node in

cutaneous melanoma: gamma probe detection versus blue dye. Ann Surg Oncol 4: 156–160, 1997.

55. MK Lingam, RM Mackie, AJ McKay. Intraoperative identification of sentinel lymph node in patients with malignant melanoma. Br J Cancer 75:1505–1508, 1997.

56. DN Krag, SJ Meijer, DL Weaver, BW Loggie, SP Harlow, KK Tanabe, EH Laughlin, JC Alex. Minimal-access surgery for staging of malignant melanoma. Arch Surg 130:954–957, 1995.

57. A Mudun, DR Murray, SC Herda, D Eshima, LA Shattuck, JP Vansant, AT Taylor, NP Alazraki. Early stage melanoma: lymphoscintigraphy, reproducibility of sentinel node detection, and effectiveness of the intraoperative gamma probe. Radiology 199: 171–175, 1996.

58. JJ Albertini, CW Cruse, D Rapaport, K Wells, M Ross, R DeConti, CG Berman, K Jared, J Messina, G Lyman, F Glass, N Fenski, DS Reintgen. Intraoperative radiolymphoscintigraphy improves sentinel lymph node identification for patients with melanoma. Ann Surg 223:217–224, 1996.

59. R Pijpers, GJ Collet, S Meijer, OS Hoekstra. The impact of dynamic lymphoscintigraphy and gamma probe guidance on sentinel node biopsy in melanoma. Eur J Nuc Med 22:1238–1241, 1995.

60. JF Thompson, P Niewind, RF Uren, CMJ Bosch, R Howman-Giles, BC Vrouenraets. Single-dose isotope injection for both preoperative lymphoscintigraphy and intraoperative sentinel lymph node identification in melanoma patients. Melanoma Res 7: 500–506, 1997.

61. SD Nathanson, M Avery, P Anaya, T Sarantou, FW Hetzel. Lymphatic diameters and radionuclide clearance in a murine melanoma model. Arch Surg 132:311–315, 1997.

62. JH Wong, K Terada, P Ko, MN Coel. Lack of effect of particle size on the identification of the sentinel node in cutaneous malignancies. Ann Surg Oncol 5:77–80, 1997.

63. H Van der Veen, OS Hoekstra, MA Cuesta, S Meijer. Gamma probe-guided sentinel node biopsy to select patients with melanoma for lymphadenectomy. Br J Surg 81: 1769–1770, 1994.

64. E Joseph, J Messina, FL Glass, CW Cruse, DP Rapaport, C Berman, DS Reintgen. Radioguided surgery for the ultrastaging of the patient with melanoma. Cancer J Sci Am 3:341–345, 1997.

65. BW Loggie, AA Hosseinian, NE Watson. Prospective evaluation of selective lymph node biopsy for cutaneous malignant melanoma (abstr). Southeastern Surgical Congress, 65th Annual Science Meeting and Postgraduate Course Program, Nashville, 1997.

66. SPL Leong, I Steinmetz, FA Habib, A McMillan, JZ Gans, RE Allen Jr, ET Morita, M El-Kadi, HD Epstein, M Kashani-Sabet, RW Sagebiel. Optimal selective sentinel lymph node dissection in primary malignant melanoma. Arch Surg 132:666–672, 1997.

67. G Miliotes, J Albertini, C Berman, R Heller, J Messina, F Glass, W Cruse, D Rapaport, C Puleo, N Fenske, C Petsoglou, R Deconti, G Lyman, D Reintgen. The tumor biology of melanoma nodal metastases. Am Surg 62:81–88, 1996.

68. D Reintgen, CM Balch, J Kirkwood, M Ross. Recent advances in the care of the patient with malignant melanoma. Ann Surg 225:1–14, 1997.

69. OE Nieweg, BAE Kapteijn, JF Thompson, BBR Kroon. Lymphatic mapping and selective lymphadenectomy for melanoma: not yet standard therapy. Eur J Surg Oncol 23:397–398, 1997.
70. DL Morton. Intraoperative lymphatic mapping and sentinel lymphadenectomy: community standard care or clinical investigation? Cancer J Sci Am 3:328–330, 1997.
71. PR Keleman, R Essner, LJ Foshag, DL Morton. Lymphatic mapping and sentinel lymphadenectomy after wide excision of primary melanoma. J Am Coll Surg 189: 247–252, 1999.
72. DL Morton, DG Davtyan, LA Wanek, LJ Foshag, AJ Cochran. Multivariate analysis of the relationship between survival and the microstage of primary melanoma by Clark level and Breslow thickness. Cancer 71:3737–3743, 1993.
73. CM Balch, TM Murad, SJ Soong, AL Ingalls, PC Richards, WA Maddox. Tumor thickness as a guide to surgical management of clinical stage I melanoma patients. Cancer 43:883–888, 1979.
74. CM Balch, S-J Soong, HM Shaw, MM Urist, WH McCarthy. An analysis of prognostic factors in 8500 patients with cutaneous melanoma. In: CM Balch, AN Houghton, GW Milton, AJ Sober, S-J Soong, eds. Cutaneous melanoma. 2nd ed. Philadelphia: JB Lippincott Company, 1992, pp. 165–187.
75. E Joseph, A Brobeil, F Glass, J Glass, J Messina, R DeConti, CW Cruse, DP Rapaport, C Berman, N Fenske, DS Reintgen. Results of complete lymph node dissection in 83 melanoma patients with positive sentinel nodes. Ann Surg Oncol 5:119–125, 1998.

7

Surgical Pathology of Dye-Directed Selective Lymph Node Dissection

Alistair J. Cochran and Duan-Ren Wen
University of California at Los Angeles, Los Angeles, California

Donald L. Morton
John Wayne Cancer Institute at Saint John's Health Center, Santa Monica, California

INTRODUCTION

The local management of patients with primary melanoma is not controversial. The primary tumor is excised with an adequate margin of surrounding normal skin. In contrast, there has been a long-standing debate as to whether and when the regional lymph nodes should be removed in patients with high-risk (deep, thick) primary melanomas. One school considers that nodes should be excised at the time that the primary is removed: elective or prophylactic lymphadenectomy [1–4]. In favor of this approach is the better survival of patients with melanoma confined to the primary site, relative to patients with regional nodal involvement and the fact that 20–30% of patients with clinically uninvolved nodes have melanoma in the excised nodes on examination by histology and immunohistochemistry [5]. Against this approach is the fact that if all individuals with high-risk melanoma are so treated, 70–80% of patients will be subjected to an unnecessary surgical operation that carries potential significant morbidity and mortality. The other school considers that lymphadenectomy should be performed only when patients develop clinical evidence of tumor in the nodes—therapeutic lymphadenectomy [6–10]. This avoids unnecessary operations, but delay of definitive therapy until a relatively advanced stage of disease may deprive these individuals of their best chance of cure.

We have long considered that a proportion of patients with high-risk primary melanoma will benefit from elective nodal dissection. These patients are likely to have limited nodal metastases and no or minimal systemic spread. Because in the past we could not identify this subset of individuals, this dictated lymphadenectomy for all patients with high-risk melanoma, imposing an unnecessary operation on many patients.

We have, therefore, developed techniques to identify those specific individuals likely to benefit from lymphadenectomy. The first priority was to be able to identify small numbers of tumor cells in tissues, including lymph nodes. This became straightforward with our development of S-100 protein as a marker for melanocytic tumors [11–16] and the development of antibodies to melanoma-associated epitopes, such as HMB-45 and NKI/C3 [17,18]. Using these markers, we demonstrated that conventional histology underestimates by 14% the number of tumor-containing lymph nodes in lymphadenectomy specimens from patients with clinically localized primary melanoma [5]. Conventional histology also underestimates tumor positivity by 30% in patients with ostensibly tumor-free nodes [19]. In patients with nodal tumor identifiable only by immunohistology, the number of nodes containing occult tumor cells was small (usually one or two) and the number of tumor cells present was low. Consideration of the anatomic orientation of these nodes carefully related to the location of the primary tumor (in a study examining the relative immune reactivity of nodes near to and remote from tumor) revealed that the nodes that contained occult tumor were those closest to the primary lesion site [20,21].

To develop an alternative approach to the management of high-risk primary melanoma, we needed to be able to identify in vivo the nodes most likely to contain tumor. Identification of the node group to which lymph drains from a particular site is possible using lymphoscintigraphy with technetium-99m (^{99m}Tc)-labeled albumin or dextran [22]. The identification of the individual nodes within that node group that are most likely to contain tumor is more difficult. In animals, a marker dye injected intradermally passed reliably from comparable areas of skin to a predictable regional lymph node [23].

Application of this approach to humans showed that we could identify blue coloration of the afferent lymphatics and one or more sentinel lymph nodes in a high proportion of patients (lymphatic mapping). From these initial steps, we developed the techniques of lymphatic mapping and selective lymph node dissection [24]. The sentinel node, identified by lymphatic mapping, is evaluated by histology and immunohistochemistry for the presence of metastatic melanoma. If the sentinel node contains tumor, a complete lymphadenectomy is undertaken. If melanoma is not identified, no further surgery is performed and the patient is observed.

This technique has generated intense interest in the surgical oncology community and there are increasingly frequent reports of its successful application.

A multicenter prospective randomized trial is in progress under the auspices of the U.S. National Cancer Institute, comparing selective lymph node dissection with a "watch and wait" approach after wide excision.

Surgical pathologists are increasingly called upon to evaluate tissues removed during this type of procedure. To assist those asked to provide such evaluations, this chapter describes our experience of the pathological aspects of selective lymph node dissection and summarizes our recommendations.

MATERIALS AND METHODS

The recommendations in this article are based on our experience of removing 1119 sentinel lymph nodes from 446 patients entered into the National Cancer Institute multicenter trial of sentinel lymph node dissection in progress under the direction of the John Wayne Cancer Institute.

For each patient, we determined the following: (1) the number of sentinel lymph nodes provided; (2) the number of sentinel lymph nodes identified as containing tumor on examination of Hematoxylin & Eosin (H&E)–stained slides; and (3) the number of sentinel lymph nodes identified as containing tumor in sections stained by immunoperoxidase techniques using antibodies to S-100 protein and HMB-45 antigen. Where we have information on lymph nodes removed during completion lymph node dissections (all pretrial patients and trial patients with tumor-containing sentinel lymph nodes), we recorded the number of nonsentinel lymph nodes that contained tumor.

Determination that a node is a first-tier node largely depends on information obtained by the surgeon who will rely on preoperative lymphoscintigraphy [22], blue coloration of afferent lymphatic and sentinel lymph node [24], and/or enhanced radioactivity of the lymph node detected by a hand-held gamma-ray counter [25]. At present, the pathologist's contribution to sentinel node identification is to examine submitted lymph nodes closely for the presence of blue coloration. In some instances, the whole lymph node may not be colored blue, color being localized to one-half of the node or to even more limited segments. Although sentinel nodes are preferentially the site of early metastases, tumor status cannot be used to confirm sentinel node status, as not all sentinel nodes contain tumor and some nonsentinel nodes contain tumor. Studies are in progress to develop approaches that will allow pathologists to confirm, independently, whether a node is truly "sentinel."

USE OF FROZEN SECTIONS

The sentinel lymph node technique was developed using intraoperative interpretation of frozen sections. Assessment of tumor status was based on evaluation of sections stained by H&E and sections stained by S-100 protein and HMB-45 using a rapid immunoperoxidase technique.

During the trial, we moved away from using frozen sections, believing that the "facing up" required during frozen-section preparation to obtain a full-face section may be wasteful of the tissue in which it is most probable that occult tumor cells will be present. Additionally, for technical reasons, interpretation of H&E-stained frozen sections and sections stained by the rapid immunohistology approach is always more difficult than interpretation of well-fixed "permanent" material. We strongly recommend that all interpretation of sentinel nodes is performed on well-fixed full-face sections cut as close to the midline of the lymph node as possible.

It is arguable that in an ideal situation each sentinel lymph node would be serially sectioned to extinction, but such an approach would be prohibitively expensive and is clearly impractical. Any reasonable recommendation will inevitably represent a compromise between the ideal and the practical. Our present recommendation is that the lymph node be cut into two exactly equal halves

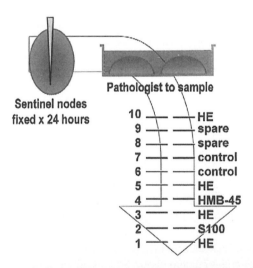

Figure 1 Technique of sentinel lymph node sampling. The node is cut into two exactly equal halves through the longest circumference. The two halves are placed cut face down in a cassette and fixed for 24 h and 10 "full-face" serial sections are cut from each block. Sections 1, 3, 5, and 10 are stained by H&E. Section 2 is stained for S-100 protein and section 4 for HMB-45. Sections 6 and 7 are used as negative controls. Sections 8–10 are available to repeat unsatisfactory preparations or for additional immunohistochemistry. If needed, additional groups of 10 sections are examined.

through the longest circumference of the node (Fig. 1). These two portions of the lymph node are placed face down in cassettes and fixed for at least 24 h. The technician is instructed to minimize "facing up" and to cut 10 serial sections as soon as a full-faced section can be obtained. Sections 1, 3, 5, and 10 are stained by H&E (Fig. 1), section 2 for S-100 protein, and section 4 for HMB-45. Section 6 and 7 are used for negative controls for the immunoperoxidase studies and sections 8 and 9 are available to repeat any of the studies that are technically unsatisfactory or for additional immunohistochemistry. If suspicious or anomalous appearances are seen within the first 10 sections, additional groups of 10 sections can be examined.

USE OF IMMUNOHISTOCHEMISTRY

It is absolutely essential that all lymph nodes be examined by immunohistology using antibodies to S-100 protein and HMB-45, unless the node contains overt tumor on gross inspection or review of H&E-stained slides. The antibody MART-1 (melanoma-associated antigen recognized by T lymphocytes) (Melan-A) can be substituted for HMB-45. Immunohistology will always increase the frequency of sentinel lymph nodes found to contain tumor. The proportion of sentinel nodes that require immunohistology to identify occult tumor decreases as pathologists gain experience in evaluating sentinel nodes. This is the pathologist's equivalent of the surgeon's learning curve [24].

S-100 protein is a highly robust marker for melanoma cells, staining virtually 100% of melanomas [14,16]. We look for epithelioid, oval, or spindle-shaped cells (usually located in the subcapsular sinus) that show S-100 protein positivity in both the cytoplasm and the nucleus (Figs. 2a–2c). There are other cells within the lymph nodes that contain S-100 protein. The dendritic leukocytes of the paracortex are the most prominent of these confounding cells. Identification of these cells is not difficult in reactive paracortices where they are polydendritic (Fig. 3a). Difficulty may be encountered in inactive lymph nodes where the dendritic leukocytes show either no or minimal dendrite formation (Fig. 3b). S-100 protein positivity may also be found in capsular nevi (Fig. 4b) [26] and in the Schwann cells of node-associated nerves (Fig. 5) [27].

HMB-45 is a more specific marker for melanoma cells but does not stain the cells of between 10% and 15% of melanomas. In contrast to S-100 protein, HMB-45-positive epitopes are confined to the cytoplasm. Nonetheless, antibodies to HMB-45 have the advantage that they do not stain dendritic leukocytes and either do not stain or stain weakly capsular nevocytes (Fig. 4c). The antibody MART-1 (Melan-A) may be used in a role similar to HMB-45, but it suffers from the same defect that a proportion of melanomas do not stain positively with this reagent.

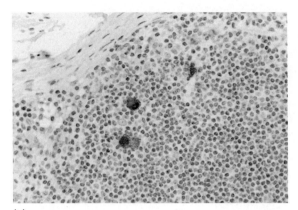

(a)

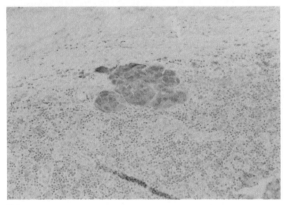

(b)

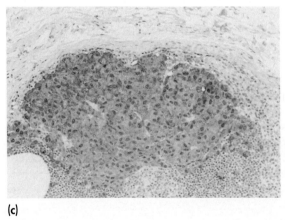

(c)

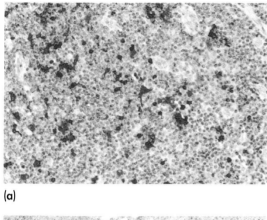

(a)

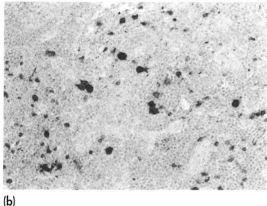

(b)

FIGURE 3 (a) Polydendritic S-100-protein-positive paracortical dendritic leukocytes in a reactive lymph node. Polyclonal antibody to S-100 protein. Original magnification ×240. (b) Nondendritic S-100-protein-positive paracortical dendritic leukocytes in a nonreactive sentinel lymph node. Polyclonal antibody to S-100 protein. Original magnification ×240.

FIGURE 2 (a) Single S-100-protein-positive melanoma cells in the subcapsular sinus of a sentinel node. Note that there is both cytoplasmic and nuclear staining. Polyclonal antibody to S-100 protein. Original magnification ×240. (b) Microfocus of S-100-protein-positive melanoma cells, predominantly in the subcapsular sinus. Polyclonal antibody to S-100 protein. Original magnification ×180. (c) Macrofocus of S-100-protein-positive melanoma cells in the subcapsular sinus and extending into the adjacent lymphoid tissue. Polyclonal antibody to S-100 protein. Original magnification ×180.

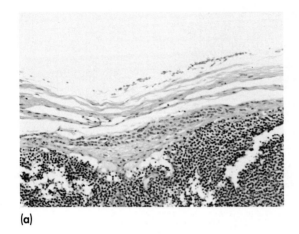

(a)

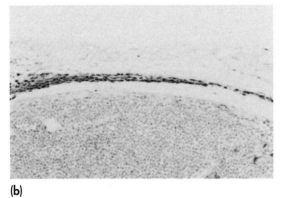

(b)

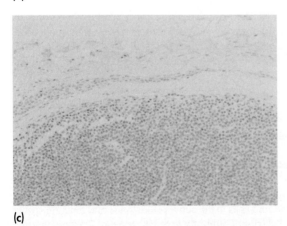

(c)

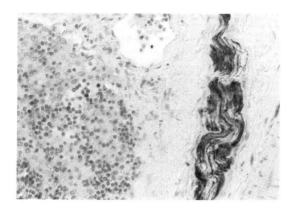

FIGURE 5   S-100-protein-positive perinodal nerve. Nerves that traverse the node and are cut transversely may present interpretative difficulty. Polyclonal antibody to S-100 protein. Original magnification ×240.

One potential source of error with HMB-45 is that in lymph nodes with trabecular calcification (mainly in nodes in the groin or iliac area), extracellular HMB-45 reactivity may be identified.

MANAGEMENT OF RADIOACTIVE NODES

The radionuclide used is generally ^{99m}Tc, which has a short penetration and a short half-life (6.2 h). The risk to operating-room personnel and pathologists from this radiation source is considered slight, but after bisection of the nodes, it is prudent to place them in formalin for 24 h after surgical excision. For a more detailed discussion of this matter, the reader is referred to the chapter on radiation protection in the sentinel node procedure (Chapter 13).

FIGURE 4   (a) Capsular nevus in a sentinel node. H&E staining. Original magnification ×180. (b) Capsular nevus in a sentinel node. Polyclonal antibody to S-100 protein. Original magnification ×180. (c) Capsular nevus in a sentinel node. Monoclonal antibody to HMB-45. Original magnification ×180. Note the capsular location of the lesion, the absence of cytologic atypia, and the immunophenotype, S-100 protein positive, HMB-45 negative. In contrast, occult melanoma is most often subcapsular and S-100-protein and HMB-45 positive.

RESULTS

In the initial studies, in which sentinel lymph node identification was followed by complete lymph node dissection, we evaluated 259 sentinel lymph nodes from 223 patients, an average of 1.2 sentinel lymph nodes per individual. Tumor was identified in 47 of these 259 sentinel lymph nodes (18%). Tumor cells were identified by H&E alone in 83.2% of patients with positive sentinel nodes and in the remaining 16.7% by immunohistology alone. The tumor cells occurred as single cells (Fig. 2a), small clumps of tumor cells (Fig. 2b), and as larger colonies (Fig. 2c). It is noteworthy that we found tumor in a nonsentinel node in the absence of tumor in the sentinel node in only two patients. These patients were treated very early in our evaluation of the technique. Because this situation has not been encountered since these early patients, we believe that the true sentinel lymph node was not correctly identified in these two patients. All patients in this group, regardless of the status of their sentinel lymph node, received a completion lymph node dissection. Tumor-containing nonsentinel nodes, associated with positive sentinel nodes, were identified in 33% of patients. Usually a single nonsentinel node was involved, rarely two or three. The amount of tumor in these nonsentinel nodes was small and presented as single cells or small microcolonies in the subcapsular sinus.

Subsequent patients were enrolled in the multicenter selective lymph node trial. These 446 patients represent the first series of patients entered into this trial, which will eventually comprise 1600 patients. In this group, 860 sentinel lymph nodes were removed from 512 lymph node basins and 99 sentinel nodes contained tumor (19% positive-analyzed by basin). Tumor was identified in 85 nodes by H&E histology (86%) and in the remaining 14 nodes by immunohistology alone (14%).

SOURCES OF ERROR IN INTERPRETING SENTINEL LYMPH NODES

Errors may be associated with S-100 protein staining. The major problem here is the interpretation of dendritic leukocytes or sinus macrophages. Dendritic leukocyte interpretation is especially difficult if the dendritic leukocytes are nondendritic, as is often the case in the immune-suppressed inactive sentinel nodes (Fig. 3b). With good quality immunohistochemical preparations, sinus macrophages do not stain for S-100 protein; however, if there is background staining, these may present interpretative difficulties. Capsular nevocytes (Figs. 4a–4c) occur in more than 20% of patients undergoing sentinel lymph node dissection and are made more visible by the use of immunohistochemistry. These cells are, in fact, confined to the capsule and trabeculae of the lymph node. They tend to be smaller and more cohesive than melanoma cells and while strongly S-100 protein positive (Fig. 4b) will either express no HMB-45 or HMB-45 at a relatively weak level (Fig. 4c). Nevocyte clusters are often arranged around capsular vessels. Another pitfall is the presence of neural tissue within the lymph node (Fig. 5). If the nerve has associated Schwann cells, these may stain relatively strongly, and if the nerve is cut transversely, an appearance suggestive of a cluster of S-100-protein-positive melanoma cells may result.

Errors may also be associated with HMB-45 staining. These are fewer than those encountered with S-100 protein, but some care is necessary. A minority of melanomas (10–15%) are made up of cells that do not express HMB-45. In hyalinized and calcified connective tissue within lymph nodes, especially lymph nodes from the groin and internal iliac area, extracellular HMB-45 positivity may be seen and care is necessary to avoid overcalling this appearance.

DISCUSSION

Sentinel lymph node technology has become very popular in the relatively short period of time since we first described the technique [24]. There is as yet no evidence that this approach is therapeutic. The technique certainly represents a considerable advance in the evaluation of the regional lymph nodes for prognosis assessment and may be useful in selecting patients for adjuvant therapy. Information of the therapeutic relevance of the approach must await the outcome of the multicenter trial, which is expected to be completed by the year 2003. Although the technique seems to be simple from both surgical and pathological standpoints, clearly there are pitfalls. The technique is also being used in a variety of other cancers, including breast cancer, colon cancer, and vulvar carcinoma. Although the broad lessons learned from our extensive experience with melanoma are likely applicable to other tumor systems, we urge caution and care in developing the techniques for each individual cancer system.

One proof of the effectiveness of the approach will be the frequency at which patients develop metastases in the ipsilateral regional nodes after removal of a reportedly negative lymph node. In our experience, this is infrequent. We have so far observed six patients in whom ipsilateral regional failure occurred despite an allegedly negative sentinel node. Detailed re-examination of the pathological material and clinical records of these individuals indicated that, in three patients, a tumor-positive sentinel lymph node had initially been incorrectly interpreted as negative. In two cases, tumor was not visible on the original H&E preparation and in neither case was immunohistochemistry performed. It is likely that if immunoperoxidase preparations had been available, a correct interpretation would have been made. In the remaining three patients, despite extensive sampling of the ''sentinel'' lymph node by H&E staining and immunohistochemistry, no evidence of tumor was identified. It is likely that in these patients the surgeons or nuclear medicine physicians did not correctly identify the sentinel nodes.

It is essential to identify with high certainty the sentinel lymph node. This remains primarily the responsibility of the surgeon. The process is rendered more accurate by a three-step procedure. The patient is subjected to lymphoscintigraphy prior to operation. This permits identification of the sentinel node, the site of which can be identified by a tattoo on the skin. Operating surgeons, in addition to injecting blue due in the area of the primary melanoma, often include a ^{99m}Tc-labeled radiopharmaceutical, which generates enhanced radioactivity in the sentinel node. Techniques are being developed to allow pathologists to confirm accurately the sentinel status of a submitted lymph node. Determination of the tumor status of the sentinel lymph node with complete accuracy is essential. This depends on careful sampling of the node and the routine use and accurate interpretation of immunohistochemistry. The technique that we recommend (Fig. 1) has served us well and is probably sufficient for the great majority of patients. In specific subsets of patients with unusually deep or thick melanoma, additional sampling may be necessary. Studies are in progress to evaluate that process.

There is much interest in the possibility that in evaluating nodes for the presence of tumor, molecular biological techniques may provide information additional to that provided by conventional pathology and immunohistochemistry. In considering these claims, it is necessary to recognize that conventional pathology and immunohistology identify approximately 20% of sentinel nodes as containing tumor, and that in patients treated by wide local excision alone, the regional failure rate is approximately 20%. Molecular biologists claim that by using reverse transcriptase–polymerase chain reaction (RT-PCR) technology they can identify signals for messenger RNA (mRNA), which may be associated with metastatic melanoma cells in a proportion of lymph nodes where H&E and immunohistochemistry are negative. This work was initially undertaken using primers for *m*-tyrosinase and it is widely accepted that cells other than metastatic melanoma cells contain mRNA for tyrosinase, including capsular nevocytes and Schwann cells in node-associated nerves. Studies in progress, in which multiple primers are being used, represent a scientifically more interesting situation. The need to evaluate the role and significance of molecular biology in the analysis of sentinel nodes is clear. Pathologists should, however, be careful to avoid providing sentinel lymph node tissue for scientific study in a manner that may compromise diagnosis. It is inappropriate to provide arbitrarily portions of a sentinel lymph node for research. We prefer to provide sections cut from the lymph node in a serial fashion and interspersed with sections stained by H&E and immunohistology. This approach has the additional advantage that it facilitates interpretation of the RT-PCR results.

Sentinel lymph node technology has much to offer melanoma patients in terms of staging and may have a therapeutic role. The technology will be investigated and exploited in many different tumor systems. Pathologists have a key role in evaluating the effectiveness of the approach. Careful attention to sampling and interpretation of the sentinel nodes is mandatory.

SUMMARY

We have evaluated 1119 sentinel lymph nodes from 669 patients with melanoma treated by selective lymph node dissection within an ongoing trial of the technique. Melanoma cells were identified in lymphadenectomy specimens from 126 patients (17.8%). Sixty-seven percent of specimens contained a single positive node, 25% had two positive nodes, and the remaining 12% had three. Tumor cells were identified singly or in small groups, usually in the peripheral sinus. A proportion of cases (approximately 14%) require immunohistochemistry to identify very small numbers of tumor cells. The proportion of lymph nodes identified as positive in H&E preparations increases with the pathologist's experience of the technique. The frequency of occult tumor cells directly correlates with increasing Clark level and Breslow thickness. Tumor cells are to be separated from capsular nevus cells, interdigitating dendritic leukocytes, macrophages, and intranodal neural tissues. With experience, the detection of small numbers of melanoma cells in nodes removed during selective lymphadenectomy is comparatively straightforward.

REFERENCES

1. HS Goldsmith, JP Shah, DH Kim. Prognostic significance of lymph node dissection in the treatment of malignant melanoma. Cancer 26:606–609, 1970.
2. CL Day, MC Mihm, RA Lew, MN Harris, AW Kopf, TB Fitzpatrick, TJ Harrist, FM Golomb, A Postel, P Hennesey, SL Gumport, JW Raker, RA Malt, AB Cosimi, WC Wood, DF Roses, F Gorstein, D Rigel, RJ Friedman, MM Mitzis, AJ Sober. Prognostic factors for patients with clinical Stage I melanoma of intermediate thickness (1.5–3.99 mm). Ann Surg 195:35–43, 1982.
3. CM Balch. The role of elective lymph node dissection in melanoma: Rationale, results and controversies. J Clin Oncol 6:163–172, 1988.
4. CM Balch, S-J Soong, AA Bartolucci, MM Urist, CP Karakousis, TJ Smith, WJ Temple, MI Ross, WR Jewell, MC Mihm Jr, R Barnhill, HJ Wanebo. Efficacy of an elective regional lymph node dissection of 1 to 4 mm thick melanomas for patients 60 years of age and younger. Ann Surg 224:255–266, 1996.
5. AJ Cochran, D-R Wen, DL Morton. Occult tumor cells in the lymph nodes of patients with pathological Stage I malignant melanoma: an immunohistological study. Am J Surg Pathol 12:612–618, 1988.
6. U Veronesi, J Adamus, DC Bandiera, IO Brennhovd, E Caceres, N Cascinelli, F Claudio, RL Ikonopisov, VV Javorskj, S Kirov, A Kulakowski, J Lacour, F Lejeune, Z Mechl, A Morabito, I Rode, S Sergeev, E Van Slooten, K Szczygiel, NN Trapezni-

kov, RI Wagner. Inefficacy of immediate node dissection in Stage I melanoma of the limbs. N Engl J Med 297:627–630, 1977.

7. U Veronesi, J Adamus, DC Bandiera, IO Brennhovd, E Caceres, N Cascinelli, F Claudio, RL, Ikonopisov, VV Javorski, S Kirov, A Kulakowski, F Lejeune, Z Mechl, A Morabito, I Rode, S Sergeev, E Van Slooten, NN Trapeznikov, RI Wagner. Delayed regional lymph node dissection in Stage I melanoma of the skin of the lower extremities. Cancer 49:2420–2430, 1982.

8. FH Sim, WF Taylor, JC Ivins, DJ Pritchard, EH Soule. A prospective, randomized study of the efficacy of routine elective lymphadenectomy in the management of melanoma. Cancer 41:948–956, 1978.

9. B Cady. ''Prophylactic'' lymph node dissection on melanoma: Does it help? J Clin Oncol 6:2–4, 1988.

10. AS Coats, CI Ingvar, K Peterson-Schaefer, HM Shaw, GW Milton, CJ O'Brien, JF Thompson, WH McCarthy. Elective lymph node dissection in patients with primary melanoma of the trunk and limbs treated at the Sydney Melanoma Unit from 1960 to 1991. Am Coll Surg 180:402–409, 1995.

11. BW Moore. Chemistry and biology of two proteins, S-100 and 14-3-2, specific to the nervous system. Biochem Biophys Res Commun 19:739–744, 1965.

12. R Gaynor, R Irie, DL Morton, HR Herschman. S-100 protein in cultured human malignant melanomas. Nature 286:400–401, 1980.

13. R Gaynor, HR Herschman, R Irie, PC Jones, DL Morton, AJ Cochran. S-100 protein: a marker for human malignant melanomas? Lancet 1:869–871, 1981.

14. AJ Cochran, D-R Wen, HR Herschman, RB Gaynor. Detection of S-100 protein as an aid to the identification of melanocytic tumors. Int J Cancer 30:295–297, 1982.

15. AJ Cochran, G Holland, D-R Wen, HR Herschman, WR Lee, BR Straatsma. Detection of S-100 protein in the diagnosis of primary and metastatic intraocular tumors. Invest Ophthalmol Vis Sci 24:1153–1155, 1983.

16. D-R Wen, RB Gaynor, AJ Cochran. S-100 protein: a marker for melanocytic tumors. Ann NY Acad Sci 420:261–266, 1983.

17. AM Gown, AM Vogel, D Heak, D Gough, MA McNutt. Monoclonal antibodies specific for melanocyte tumors distinguished subpopulations of melanocytes. Am J Pathol 123:195–203, 1986.

18. EC Hagen, C Vennegoor, RO Schlingemann, ER Van der Velde, DJ Ruiter. Correlation of histopathological characteristics with staining patterns in human malignant melanoma assessed by (monoclonal) antibodies reactive on paraffin sections. Histopathology 10:689–700, 1986.

19. AJ Cochran, D-R Wen, HR Herschman. Occult melanoma in lymph nodes detected by antiserum to S-100 protein. Int J Cancer 34:159–163, 1984.

20. AJ Cochran, E Pihl, D-R Wen, DSB Hoon, EL Korn. Zoned immune suppression of lymph nodes draining malignant melanoma: histologic and immunohistologic studies. J Natl Cancer Inst 78:399–405, 1987.

21. DSB Hoon, EL Korn, AJ Cochran. Variations in functional immunocompetence of human tumor-draining lymph nodes. Cancer Res 47:1740–1744, 1987.

22. DS Robinson, WF Sample, HJ Fee, C Holmes, DL Morton. Regional lymphatic

drainage in primary malignant melanoma of the trunk determined by colloidal gold scanning. Surg Forum 28:147–148, 1977.

23. JH Wong, LA Cagle, DL Morton. Lymphatic drainage of skin to a sentinel lymph node in a feline model. Ann Surg 214:637–641, 1991.

24. DL Morton, D-R Wen, JH Wong, JS Economou, LA Cagle, FK Storm, LJ Foshag, AJ Cochran. Technical details of intraoperative lymphatic mapping for early stage melanoma. Arch Surg 127:392–399, 1992.

25. SD Nathanson, P Anaya, KC Karvelis, L Eck, S Havstad. Sentinel lymph node uptake of two different technetium-labelled radiocolloids. Ann Surg Oncol 4:104–110, 1996.

26. KF Carson, D-R Wen, P-X Li, AM Lana, C Bailly, DL Morton, AJ Cochran. Nodal nevi and cutaneous melanomas. Am J Surg Pathol 20:834–840, 1996.

27. AJ Cochran, C Bailly, E Paul, F Remotti. Melanocytic Tumors: A Guide to Diagnosis. Philadelphia: Lippincott–Raven, 1997.

8

Molecular Staging of Malignant Melanoma

Douglas S. Reintgen
H. Lee Moffitt Cancer Center and Research Institute, University of South Florida, Tampa, Florida

Xiangning Wang, Weigno Li, and Steven Shiver
University of South Florida, Tampa, Florida

INTRODUCTION

A number of technological advancements have come together to allow more conservative surgery for the melanoma patient and, at the same time, provide a mechanism for more accurate staging. These advances involve the refinement of a nuclear medicine study, lymphoscintigraphy, to identify which basins are at risk for metastatic disease, the use of intraoperative lymphatic mapping, and sentinel lymph node biopsy to identify which node in the basin is most at risk for disease, and finally the development of more sensitive assays for detection of occult metastases. These assays are based on immunohistochemical staining and molecular biology techniques. The advances in the staging of the melanoma patient could not have happened without the advances intraoperatively, as it would be too time-consuming and too expensive to perform a technique like the reverse transcriptase–polymerase chain reaction (RT-PCR) on the 20–25 nodes from a complete regional node dissection. The fact that the lymphatic mapping techniques can identify the one or two sentinel lymph nodes that are most likely to contain the metastases makes the application of the more sensitive assays for occult metastases practical.

The staging of the melanoma patient is becoming more important with the recent publication of a multicenter, prospective, randomized trial that shows a benefit for the adjuvant treatment of T4 or Stage III melanoma patients with interferon-α [1]. Adjuvant therapy should be applied early when tumor burden

141

is minimal and in a selective fashion so that only those patients with a proven benefit are exposed to the toxicities and expense of the adjuvant therapies. The accurate staging of the melanoma patient will identify the subgroup of patients who have the most to benefit from interferon-α.

Focused on nodal status as the dominant prognostic factor for early-stage melanoma, investigators at the Moffitt Cancer Center initiated a line of research in an attempt to combine lymphatic mapping and more sensitive assays for occult metastases to better stage patients with this disease.

METASTATIC MELANOMA IN REGIONAL LYMPH NODES

Once patients develop metastatic melanoma in their regional nodes, prognostic factors based on the primary melanoma contribute very little to the prognostic model. For most solid tumors, including melanoma, the most powerful predictor of survival is the presence or absence of lymph node metastases. The presence of lymph node metastases decreases the 5-year survival of patients approximately 40% compared with those who have no evidence of nodal metastases. Much time, effort, and expense is placed on identifying prognostic factors based on the primary tumor, and not enough emphasis is given to identifying which patients really have signs of micrometastatic disease in their nodal basins. For instance, there are currently 26 prognostic factors (Table 1) for melanoma based on variables from the primary tumor. Yet, in multiple regression analysis performed on many collected populations in the literature, the lymph node status of the patient is the most powerful factor for predicting recurrence and survival. Primary tumor

TABLE 1 Twenty-six Prognostic Factors for Melanoma Based on the Primary Tumor

Tumor thickness	S phase
Ulceration	DR-1 expression
Clark level	DNA index
Histological type	Heat-shock protein expression
Cell type	HLA-DR staining
Primary site	p53 mutations
Regression	Cell adhesion molecule expression
Mitosis	Proteases expression
Lymphocytic infiltration	Migration-associated molecule expression
Vertical maturation grade	Angiogenesis-related factor expression
Blood vessel invasion	Oncogene expression
Lymphatic space invasion	Estrogen receptor expression
Ploidy	Cytokine; growth factor expression

Source: Ref. 2.

variables such as Breslow thickness, ulceration, primary site, and gender may add to the prognostic model, but only after nodal status is considered.

Routine histological examination of the regional lymph nodes, which typically involves making one or two sections of the central area of the node and staining with a standard Hematoxylin & Eosin (H&E) method, examines less than 1–5% of the submitted material and may miss micrometastatic disease (Fig. 1). The sensitivity of this examination is finding one abnormal melanoma cell in a background of 10,000 normal lymphocytes. If serial sectioning and immunohistochemical staining (Fig. 2) are added, the yield of positive dissections may double and the sensitivity becomes identifying one abnormal melanoma cell in a background of 100,000 normal lymphocytes. Serial sectioning and immunohistochemical staining techniques have been available for years, yet have not been incorporated into the everyday practice of the pathologist because of the time and expense involved.

New technology that enables the surgeon to map the cutaneous lymphatic flow from the primary tumor and identify the sentinel node (first-tier node, first-echelon node) in the regional basin could contribute to better nodal staging of the melanoma patient. This procedure, as initially proposed by Morton et al. [3,4],

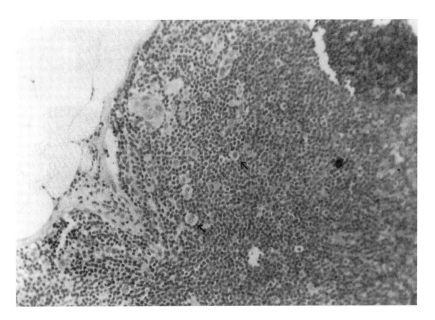

FIGURE 1   H&E photomicrograph of the sentinel lymph node in a patient with a 2.0-mm melanoma on the right arm. Metastatic melanoma can invade the sentinel node as single cells (arrows) and with low-volume disease.

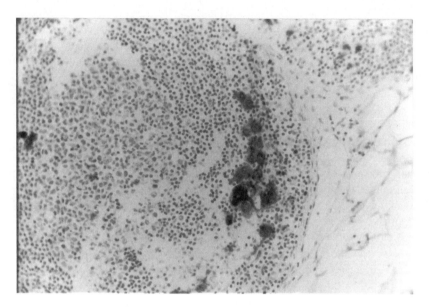

FIGURE 2   Immunohistochemistry staining with the melanoma specific S-100 stain. The metastatic cells will stain brown with the immunoperoxidase technique while the rest of the surrounding lymphocyte does not stain. The routine use of immunohistochemistry will increase the sensitivity of the examination for occult metastases. The figure also illustrates how metastatic melanoma can be a very low-volume disease.

has shown that the sentinel lymph node is the first site of metastatic disease, and if the sentinel lymph node is negative, then the remainder of the lymph nodes in the basin should also be negative [5,6]. Selective lymphadenectomy also allows for detailed examination of the sentinel node, because it is an examination of one or two nodes. This advance allows the pathologist to serial section the node and use immunohistochemistry to look for micrometastatic disease. Nevertheless, 25% of the histological node negative Stage I and II melanoma patients will recur and die of their disease within 5 years of diagnosis, suggesting that some of these patients have missed nodal micrometastases or these patients suffer from hematogenous metastases. A more sensitive method was needed to accurately identify the presence or absence of metastatic disease in the node.

ASSAYS FOR OCCULT METASTATIC MELANOMA: LYMPH NODE CULTURE

Investigators at the H. Lee Moffitt Cancer Center initially proposed a cell culture technique [7] in which the regional nodes were bisected, with half of the node sent to pathology and half of the node placed into tissue culture. Several patients with histologically negative nodes had melanoma cells grow in culture. Detailed characterization of these cells with immunohistochemical staining, monoclonal antibody staining, and electron microscopy confirmed that the growing cells were indeed melanoma cells. Thirty-one percent of the histologically node-negative population were upstaged to Stage III with the cell culture technique.

The clinical correlation between lymph node culture and disease-free survival was very good. Patients who were histologically node negative, but node positive by cell culture, had an increased recurrence rate compared with those patients with melanoma whose nodes were negative by both assays [8]. Widespread applicability was questioned with the lymph node culture technique because this would require hospitals to establish cell culture facilities and the results of the assay are not available for 4–6 weeks.

ASSAYS FOR OCCULT METASTASES: RT-PCR

A study was initiated to develop a highly sensitive method to detect micrometastases by examining lymph nodes for the presence of tyrosinase messenger RNA (mRNA) [9]. The assay is based on the biosynthetic pathway of melanin. It is known that tyrosine is converted to melanin in the melanocyte or melanoma cell. The key is that the first two steps of the synthesis are catalyzed by the enzyme tyrosinase. Tyrosinase is a mono-oxygenase that catalyzes the conversion of tyrosine to 3,4-dihydroxyphenylalanine (DOPA) and of DOPA to dopaquinone. Tyrosinase is one of the most specific markers of melanocytic differentiation. All cells of the body will have the gene for tyrosinase, but only cells that are actively producing pigment, such as melanoma cells or melanocytes, will express the mRNA for the tyrosinase gene. If this gene product is found in the lymph node preparation, in the peripheral blood, or in the bone marrow, then that finding is good evidence that metastatic melanoma cells are present in that compartment.

The test was modified and refined for lymph node work from an assay originally described by Smith and colleagues for peripheral blood using the combination of reverse transcription and two rounds of RT-PCR [10]. mRNA from the node is converted into a cDNA copy so that a stable product is obtained. The amplified samples were separated on a 2% agarose gel to examine for the presence of a 207-base pair (bp) fragment representing tyrosinase cDNA (Fig. 3). In a spiking experiment, one SK-Mel-28 melanoma cell in 1 million normal lymphocytes could be detected, indicating that the sensitivity of this method is two orders of magnitude greater than routine H&E examination.

In an initial study, sentinel nodes from 29 patients were analyzed by standard pathological staining and RT-PCR. Eleven of 29 lymph nodes samples (38%) from 29 patients with intermediate thickness melanoma were histologically positive. Nineteen of the 29 lymph node preparations (66%) were RT-PCR

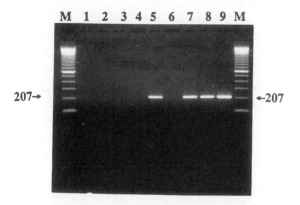

Figure 3   Gel of the tyrosinase RT-PCR assay with a positive signal being the 207-bp signal. Lane 9 is a melanoma control cell line that acts as the positive control. Lanes 2–4 are a breast cancer cell line, a colon cancer cell line, and normal lymph node, respectively, all of which are negative. Lanes 5–8 are from mRNA preparations of the sentinel nodes of three patients who were called histologically negative by the pathologist. In 75%, there is evidence of missed micrometastatic disease.

positive and these included all of the pathologically positive samples. Restriction enzyme analysis showed that the amplified 207-bp RT-PCR product was a part of the tyrosinase gene sequence. These data suggested that the RT-PCR method was an extremely sensitive, reproducible, and efficient technique for the identification of micrometastases in patients with melanoma [9].

CLINICAL CORRELATION OF THE RT-PCR ASSAY

New assays may be of academic interest only unless clinical correlation and reproducibility can be shown. There is indirect evidence of an association with clinically relevant disease in that the RT-PCR assay correlates with other known prognostic factors for primary melanoma. There is almost a linear relationship between increasing tumor thickness and decreasing survival. Figure 4 shows that as tumor thickness increases, the chance of finding RT-PCR positive cells in the sentinel lymph node also increases. In fact, the RT-PCR assay is probably a better predictor of the natural history of the disease for the intermediate thickness and thick melanoma population. For instance, patients with melanomas that are greater than 4.0 mm in thickness have a 10-year survival rate of 30%. If surgeons perform complete regional node dissections for patients with deep melanoma and give the pathologist 20–25 nodes to examine routinely, perhaps 30–40% will be found to have micrometastatic disease. However, 70% of patients with thick

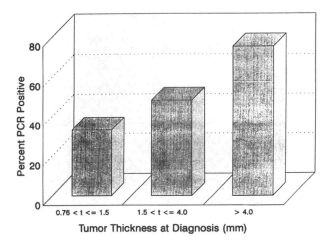

FIGURE 4   Tumor thickness versus nodal RT-PCR status showing that as tumor thickness increases, the chance of finding RT-PCR positive material in the sentinel nodes also increases.

melanomas are dead within 10 years of their diagnosis, suggesting that a complete lymph node dissection and a superficial histological examination may miss micrometastatic disease. The alternative explanation is that these patients have hematogenous spread of their melanoma to cause their death. Probably a combination of missed nodal metastases and hematogenous spread is responsible for this discrepancy between staging and survival. The RT-PCR assay may overpredict the natural history of patients with relatively thin melanomas between 0.76 and 1.5 mm in thickness. Only 15% of these patients have a recurrence and die of their disease within 10 years and yet the assay shows 33% of them to have RT-PCR material in their sentinel node. Perhaps tumor volume is low in these patients and confined to the sentinel node. These patients may be cured of their metastatic melanoma with the sentinel node biopsy. As is the case for increasing tumor thickness, ulcerated melanomas have a worse prognosis than tumors that do not have this poor prognostic factor. If a patient has an ulcerated melanoma, then there is a 70% chance of RT-PCR positive cells being present in the sentinel node (Fig. 5).

Sentinel nodes from melanoma patients have continued to be examined by RT-PCR. Table 2 shows the clinical correlation of this assay for the first 114 patients with melanomas greater than 1.0 mm who underwent lymphatic mapping and sentinel lymph node harvest. Their sentinel node was examined with the RT-PCR assay and a mean follow-up of 28 months after their definitive surgical therapy was obtained. This follow-up is a period of time in which 75% of all

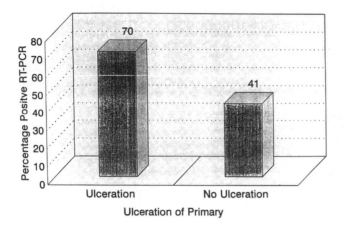

Figure 5 Ulceration versus RT-PCR sentinel lymph node status. Patients with ulcerated melanoma have a 70% chance of having RT-PCR positive material in the sentinel node.

the recurrences of melanoma should occur. Patients whose sentinel nodes were histologically positive and RT-PCR positive (20.2%) had a recurrence rate of 60.9%, whereas patients whose sentinel nodes were negative by both assays had a recurrence rate of 2.3%. The interesting group are 41.2% of patients whose sentinel node were histologically negative but RT-PCR positive. The patients in this category were upstaged with the RT-PCR assay and have an intermediate prognosis, with 12.8% of them recurring in the follow-up period [11].

Patients in group 1 in Table 2 are identified to be at an extremely low risk for recurrence and death. In fact, the one patient that recurred out of the 44 whose sentinel lymph node was both histologically negative and RT-PCR negative suffered a local recurrence, and one could argue that these cells never reach the regional basin to analyze. There have been no deaths in group 1 and these patients do not need further surgery (a complete lymph node dissection) or adjuvant ther-

Table 2 Clinical Correlation of the RT-PCR Sentinel Lymph Node Assay with Recurrence

Group	Sentinel node status	N (%)	Recurrence rate
1	Histo−/PCR−	44/114 (38.6%)	1/44 (2.3%)
2	Histo−/PCR+	47/114 (41.2%)	6/47 (12.8%)
3	Histo+/PCR+	23/114 (20.2%)	14/23 (60.9%)

apy. Group 3 patients have a guarded prognosis, with 61% of them recurring within 28 months. Patients in this group would be candidates for a complete lymph node dissection and adjuvant therapy. If the intermediate prognosis of the group 2 patients can be confirmed in an ongoing national multicenter trial (Sunbelt Melanoma Trial), then these patients may need further surgery or adjuvant therapy.

Figure 6 shows the disease-free survival curve of the three groups of patients stratified according to the status of their sentinel node. There were differences in disease-free survival in those patients whose sentinel node was histologically negative and RT-PCR positive versus those patients with melanoma whose sentinel node was negative with both assays. This difference is statistically significant with a *p*-value of 0.02 [11].

Univariate regression analysis that includes primary melanoma and clinical variables on these 114 patients shows that with each factor acting independently to predict disease-free survival, it is either the histology or the RT-PCR status of the sentinel node that best predicts recurrence (Table 3). In a multivariate regression analysis, an analysis that takes into account the interaction between variables, again it is either the histology or RT-PCR status of the sentinel lymph node that correlates best with disease-free survival (Table 4) [11]. Thus, once patients with melanoma develop nodal metastases, prognostic information from variables of the primary add little to how those patients will do after recurrence. It is really the fact that they have developed metastatic disease in their nodes that will influence their subsequent disease-free survival.

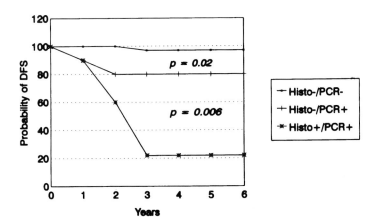

FIGURE 6 The disease-free survival of melanoma patients according to sentinel node status. Patients who are upstaged with the RT-PCR assay do significantly worse than patients whose sentinel node is histologically negative and RT-PCR negative.

TABLE 3   Univariate Regression Analysis of Disease-Free Survival Associated with Different Prognostic Factors

Variable	p-value
Thickness	0.09
Clark level	0.28
Ulceration	0.18
Primary site	0.25
Sex	0.30
Age	0.94
SLNPATH[a]	0.04
SLNPCR[b]	0.04

[a] The histology of the sentinel lymph node (SLN).
[b] The RT-PCR status of the SLN.

How do clinicians and pathologists find micrometastatic disease? In this series, 23 (20%) of the patients were found to have occult metastases. The standard examination of regional nodes throughout the world involved making one or two sections of the central part of the sentinel lymph node and an H&E stain and identified 17 of the 23 (73%) patients with metastatic disease. It was not until more sections and immunohistochemical staining with S-100 were performed that the remaining 27% of the patients with micrometastatic disease were identified (Table 5) [12]. Thus, the standard examination of the regional basin only identi-

TABLE 4   Multivariate Regression Analysis of Disease-Free Survival Associated with Different Prognostic Factors

Variable	p-value
Thickness	0.2
SLNPATH[a]	0.04
SLNPCR[b]	0.03

[a] The histology of the sentinel lymph node (SLN).
[b] The RT-PCR status of the SLN.

TABLE 5 Assays for Micrometastatic Disease in Sentinel Lymph Nodes

"Routine" histology Sentinel node +: 23/114 (20%)		Molecular assays Sentinel node +: 70/114 (61%)	
Technique	N (%)	Technique	N (%)
H&E	17/23 (73%)	H&E	17/70 (24%)
Serial sections	2/23 (9%)	Serial section and S-100	6/70 (9%)
S-100	4/23 (18%)	RT-PCR	47/70 (67%)

fies 73% of the patients with occult metastases. If one considers finding RT-PCR positive cellular material in the sentinel lymph node as being clinically relevant disease, then the routine pathological examination identifies a mere 24% of the patients with micrometastatic disease.

One possible source of a false-positive RT-PCR comes from the fact that 5% of the sentinel nodes in the Moffitt Cancer Center experience contain benign nevus cell rests [12]. These are relatively easy to identify, as they are almost uniformly located in the fibrous capsule or trabeculae of the node and their cytology is one of uniform small cells that have a benign appearance. For this reason, the entire node is not taken for the RT-PCR assay and only one-quarter to one-half of the node is analyzed. The remainder of the node is submitted to pathology, and if benign nevus cells are found with the sectioning, then a possible source of false-positive RT-PCR is identified.

RT-PCR ASSAY IN PERIPHERAL BLOOD

The development of new molecular biology techniques has provided a means by which molecular markers present at low copy numbers can be detected with a sensitivity higher than that of immunohistochemistry. In 1991, Smith et al. proposed for the first time that melanoma cells could be detected in the peripheral blood using RT-PCR to target any message from the tyrosinase gene [10]. Several other groups have pursued this lead, but the results have been extremely variable. The most striking discrepancies occur in patients with Stage IV melanoma, in which the incidence rates at finding RT-PCR-positive circulating cells varies from 0% to 100% [13,14].

In a series from Germany [13], 100% of the patients with Stage IV melanoma had RT-PCR evidence of circulating melanoma cells, whereas a report from Kunter showed that only 28% of the patients with Stage IV melanoma were marker positive [14]. In addition, in the latter series, a positive peripheral blood RT-PCR assay was associated with progression of disease. A more recent study from Barcelona studied 91 patients with all stages of melanoma [15]. There was a significant association between RT-PCR positivity in the peripheral blood and clinical stage. Circulating melanoma cells were detected in 36% of the patients with localized disease (Stages I and II), in 45% of the patients with regional nodal disease, and 94% of the patients with systemic metastases ($p < 0.001$). In Stage II and Stage III patients, the recurrence rate of patients who were RT-PCR positive in the peripheral blood was significantly higher than similar stage patients who were RT-PCR negative. In a multivariate analysis, RT-PCR positivity in the peripheral blood was an independent prognostic factor for recurrence ($p = 0.002$). Recently, another group reported their results with their version of the RT-PCR assay. One of 43 patients with primary melanoma (2.3%), none of 15 patients with Stage III melanoma, and 27.3% of patients with advanced disease were found to have circulating tumor cells [16].

How does one explain the discrepancies between the various laboratories? The causes are probably multifactorial, with the main difference being the different techniques used for processing the blood samples and the RT-PCR reaction. Recently, it has been shown that the use of a density gradient method to process the blood samples resulted in a higher detection rate of tyrosinase mRNA than extracting the RNA from whole blood [17]. It is also clear that the RT-PCR assay can be varied in sensitivity by the number of cycles, the type of gel development, and the temperatures and reagents used. Crossover contamination must be eliminated, but it is clear that one RT-PCR assay for tyrosinase from one laboratory may not be equivalent to another laboratory's assay.

Another reason given for the discrepancy between the assays and ultimate corelation with stage of disease and survival is that circulating melanoma cells may be present in the blood of patients in whom recurrent disease does not develop. Recently, it has been shown in an animal model that over 80% of the melanoma cells that enter the microcirculation will survive and extravasate, suggesting that most circulating cells have the potential to produce clinically relevant disease [18].

Other investigators have used a multiple-marker assay for occult metastases. Hoon and colleagues used an RT-PCR technique to detect occult circulating tumor cells in the blood of melanoma patients [19]. Four different markers were used to improve the sensitivity and specificity of the occult metastases assay. Preliminary studies of this multiple marker RT-PCR assay, which utilized the 4 melanoma markers, tyrosinase, MAGE-3 (*m*elanoma *A*nti*gen* 3), Muc-18 (*muc*in epithelial antigen 18), and p97, showed the presence of all 4 markers in 10 melanoma cell lines with none detected in the blood of 14 normal volunteers. The assay was used to detect circulating tumor cells in 74 melanoma patients of various clinical stage. The pattern of marker detection was as follows: tyrosinase (59%), MAGE-3 (9%), Muc-18 (66%), and p97 (65%). For all AJCC stages, the ability to detect circulating tumor cells was significantly higher ($p = 0.025$) in the 53 patients alive with disease than the 21 disease-free patients. For all patients alive with disease, as the clinical stage increased from I to IV, there was a corresponding increase in the ability of the assays to detect circulating melanoma cells. It was concluded that the detection of circulating occult tumor cells could provide a tumor marker for the early detection of metastatic or recurrent disease or evaluate the response to specific therapeutic modalities. Recently, clinical correlation was shown with this multiple-marker assay in that patients with up to two positive markers never recurred, whereas patients with three or four positive markers had a 1-year recurrence rate of 30%.

SUNBELT MELANOMA TRIAL

A recently started industry sponsored, multi-institutional trial attempts to confirm the clinical relevance of the RT-PCR assay. Patients with melanomas greater than or equal to 1.0 mm will undergo preoperative lymphoscintigraphy to identify all node basins at risk for disease and sentinel node biopsy of all basins identified by lymphoscintigraphy. If the patient's sentinel node is histologically negative and immunohistochemically negative (S-100 stain), then an RT-PCR assay for occult metastases will be performed on the sentinel node. Patients whose sentinel lymph node is histologically negative and RT-PCR negative will be observed. If the sentinel lymph node is histologically negative but RT-PCR positive, then patients will be randomized to either observation, complete lymph node dissection and observation, or lymph node dissection and adjuvant interferon-α-2b. This part of the trial will examine the clinical significance of a histologically negative but RT-PCR-positive sentinel node. In addition, the proper treatment for those patients upstaged with the RT-PCR assay will be investigated. The RT-PCR multiple marker assay will also be examined in the peripheral blood.

CONCLUSION

Intraoperative lymphatic mapping and sentinel node biopsy provide the mechanism to study the nodes most likely to contain tumor with a more detailed examination. Defined patterns of lymphatic drainage allow intraoperative determination of the first (sentinel) lymph node in the regional basin, and the absence of metastatic disease in the sentinel lymph node accurately reflects the absence of melanoma in the remaining regional nodes. Close collaboration among surgeons, nuclear medicine physicians, and pathologists is required to ensure optimal results.

Examination of serially sectioned sentinel nodes by H&E staining, immunohistochemical staining, and RT-PCR should reduce the number of patients with missed microscopic melanoma in their regional lymph nodes. Furthermore, the survival benefit recently reported in patients with melanoma metastatic to regional nodes prospectively randomized to receive high-dose interferon-α signals that patients should be aggressively examined for the presence of occult regional melanoma metastases in order to apply the adjuvant therapy in a selective fashion. One can make an argument that patients with a defined risk of melanoma metastases should have a nodal staging procedure. At the Moffitt Cancer Center, patients with melanomas greater than 0.75 mm undergo lymphatic mapping. Molecular staging of cancers is likely to become an important part of the everyday practice of the oncologist. ''Submicroscopic'' nodal disease will be identified and, combined with peripheral blood assays, will result in an ''ultrastaging'' of the melanoma patient. More sensitive assays for staging have been criticized in the past as just providing stage shifting without impacting on the survival of the patient. This ''Will Rodgers'' phenomenon implies that if a more accurate test is available for staging, patients may be upstaged and survival will increase across most stages with no overall impact on survival when the entire population with disease is considered. Stage migration or shifting occurs, without any overall effect on the survival of the entire melanoma population. This holds true as long as there are no effective adjuvant therapies for the patients at high risk of recurrence. With the emergence of interferon-α-2b as a standard for the adjuvant treatment of melanoma patients at an increased risk for recurrence, the mapping techniques that allow a more detailed examination of the sentinel lymph node will identify this patient population (Stage III) more accurately. These are the patients who have the most to benefit from this therapy. In this way, the therapy can be given in a selective fashion, exposing only those patients who have the most to benefit to the toxicities of the drug.

REFERENCES

1. JM Kirkwood, MH Strawderman, MS Ernstoff, TJ Smith, EC Borden, RH Blum. Adjuvant therapy of high-risk resected cutaneous melanoma: the Eastern Cooperative Oncology Group Trial EST 1684. J Clin Oncol 14:7–17, 1997.
2. DS Reintgen, J Albertini, C Berman, CW Cruse, N Fenske, F Glass, C Puleo, X Wang, K Wells, D Rapaport, R DeConti, J Messina, R Heller. Accurate nodal staging of malignant melanoma. Cancer Control: J Moffitt Cancer Center 2:405–414, 1995.
3. DL Morton, DR Wen, JH Wong, JS Economou, LA Cagel, KS Storm, LJ Foshag, AJ Cochran. Technical details of intraoperative lymphatic mapping for early stage melanoma. Arch Surg 127:392–399, 1992.
4. DL Morton, DR Wen, AJ Cochran. Management of early-stage melanoma by intraoperative lymphatic mapping and selective lymphadenectomy or ''watch and wait.'' Surg Oncol Clin North Am 1:247–259, 1992.
5. D Reintgen, CW Cruse, K Wells, C Berman, N Fenske, F Glass, K Schroer, R Heller, M Ross, G Lyman, C Cox, D Rappaport, HF Seigler, CM Balch. The orderly progression of melanoma nodal metastases. Ann Surg 220:759–767, 1994.
6. R Heller, J Becker, J Wassalle, P Beaky, CW Cruse, C Cox, B King, H Wood, DS Reintgen. Detection of occult lymph node metastases in malignant melanoma. Ann Plast Surg 28:74–77, 1992.

7. R Heller, J Becker, J Wasselle, P Beakey, W Cruse, K Wells, C Cox, B King, DS Reintgen. Detection of submicroscopic lymph node metastases in patients with malignant melanoma. Arch Surg 126:1455–1460, 1991.

8. R Heller, B King, P Beakey, W Cruse, D Reintgen. Identification of submicroscopic lymph node metastases in patients with malignant melanoma. Semin Surg Oncol 9: 285–289, 1992.

9. X Wang, R Heller, N VanVoorhis, CW Cruse, F Glass, N Fenske, C Berman, J Leo-Messina, D Rappaport, K Wells, R DeConti, L Moscinski, C Stankard, C Puleo, D Reintgen. Detection of submicroscopic metastases with polymerase chain reaction in patients with malignant melanoma. Ann Surg 220:768–774, 1994.

10. B Smith, P Selby, J Southgate, K Pittman, C Bradley, GE Blair. Detection of melanoma cells in the peripheral blood by means of reverse transcriptase and polymerase chain reaction. Lancet 338:1227–1229, 1991.

11. S Shivers, X Wang, W Li, D Rapaport, CW Cruse, R DeConti, F Glass, J Messina, C Berman, E Joseph, C Puleo, G Lyman, DS Reintgen. Molecular staging of malignant melanoma. JAMA 280:1410–1415, 1998.

12. J Messina, F Glass. Pathological exam of the sentinel lymph nodes. J Florida Med Assoc 84;153–156, 1997.

13. P Brossart, U Keilholz, M Willhauck, C Scheibenbogen, T Mohler, W Hunstein. Hematogenous spread of malignant melanoma cells in different stages of disease. J Invest Dermatol 101:887–889, 1993.

14. U Kunter, J Buer, M Probst, S Duensing, I Dallman, J Grosse, H Kirchner, EM Schluepen, M Volkenandt, A Ganser, J Alzpodien. Peripheral blood tyrosinase messenger RNA detection and survival in melanoma. J Natl Cancer Inst 88:590–594, 1996.

15. B Mellado, D Colomer, T Castel, M Munoz, E Carballo, M Galan, JM Mascaro, JLI Vives-Corrons, JJ Grau, J Estape. Detection of circulating neoplastic cells by reverse-transcriptase polymerase chain reaction in malignant melanoma: association with clinical stage and prognosis. J Clin Oncol 14:2091–2097, 1996.

16. R Glaser, K Rass, S Seiter, A Hauschild, E Christopers, W Tilgen. Detection of circulating melanoma cells by specific amplification of tyrosinase complementary DNA is not a reliable tumor marker in melanoma patients: a clinical two-center study. J Clin Oncol 15:2818–2825, 1997.

17. FA Jung, AC Buzaid, MI Ross, JV Woods, JJ Lee, M Albitar, EA Grimm. Evaluation of tyrosinase mRNA as a tumor marker in the blood of melanoma patients. J Clin Oncol 15:2826–2831, 1997.

18. S Koop, IC MacDonald, K Luzzi, EE Schmidt, VL Morris, M Grattan, R Khokha, AF Chambers, AC Groom. Fate of melanoma cells entering the microcirculation: over 80% survive and extravasate. Cancer Res 55:2520–2523, 1995.

19. DS Hoon, Y Wang, PS Dale, AJ Conrad, P Schmid, D Garrison, C Kuo, LJ Foshag, AJ Nizze, DL Morton. Detection of occult melanoma cells in blood with a multiple marker polymerase chain reaction assay. J Clin Oncol 13:2109–2116, 1995.

9

Breast Lymphoscintigraphy

Claudia G. Berman
University of South Florida, Tampa, Florida

INTRODUCTION

The predominant early application of radiocolloids in the imaging of lymph node basins in patients with breast carcinoma resulted from the difficulties entailed in contrast lymphography of the axillary and internal mammary nodes [1,2]. In analogy to lymphography, injection of the radiopharmaceutical would be made into the rectus muscle or the finger webbing and an abnormality was defined as diminished or absent visualization of either the internal mammary or axillary nodal group [3]. Typically, the study group included a diverse population of patients and treatments and, most important, the clinical implications and applicability of the technique remained uncertain. Limited, more recent work, utilizing this anatomic lymphoscintigraphic approach, has demonstrated poor reliability for identifying low-volume metastatic disease in internal mammary nodes [4].

LYMPHOSCINTIGRAPHY

Hultborn and colleagues were among the first to employ a physiologic strategy for radiocolloid imaging of lymph nodes draining breasts with malignant disease [5]. Their technique involved preoperative injection of the breast parenchyma with postoperative ex vivo imaging of the radical or extended radical mastectomy specimen. The gamma camera image directed the pathologist's dissection of the operative specimen. They also utilized a gamma probe for localization within indistinctly visualized specimens. Their 1954 report remarkably presaged the present-day thinking driving the development of lymphoscintigraphic sentinel node staging of breast carcinoma. They recognized a typical pattern of visualization of some but not all axillary nodes, and concluded, "This probably indicates a segmental arrangement of the lymph drainage from the breast to the axilla . . ." or, in our jargon, a sentinel node.

Krag and colleagues were the first to describe the rationale and use of radiocolloid for sentinel node localization in early-stage breast carcinoma [6]. Their technique was adapted from their prior use of a hand-held gamma probe for sentinel node radiolocalization in patients with melanoma [7,8]. Twenty-two consecutive women with biopsy-proved breast carcinoma underwent radiolocalized sentinel lymphadenectomy prior to full axillary dissection. Treatment of the primary lesion was accomplished by either mastectomy or partial mastectomy with planned postoperative radiation therapy. Three of the 22 women had clinically positive (palpable) axillary nodes.

The technique consisted of the injection of 15 MBq (0.4 mCi) technetium-99m (^{99m}Tc) sulfur colloid in a volume of 0.5 mL saline into the normal breast tissue adjacent to the lesion or biopsy cavity. Five 0.1-mL injections were made from 1 to 9 h prior to surgery in a 180° arc facing the axilla. Prior to incision, a gamma detector was passed over the axilla. An underlying sentinel node was presumed present when 30 counts in 10 s were detected at the skin surface. Sentinel nodes were found in 18 of the 22 patients. The sentinel node contained metastatic tumor in all seven patients ultimately found, on pathologic examination, to have metastatic axillary lymphadenopathy. In three patients, it was the only site of metastatic disease. Notably, they were unable to identify any sentinel node in 18% of their patients. The investigators did not include an imaging component in the study, commenting on the unsuccessful historical experience.

The same group has more recently reported an updated experience with 50 patients, maintaining their 100% sensitivity and specificity [9]. They have increased their injectate volume to 3 mL and raised a concern about diffusion of injectate obscuring hand-held gamma probe localization of a sentinel node adjacent to the primary lesion. This would, in particular, be a concern in extreme upper outer quadrant lesions.

What is most probably the first modern experience using a radiocolloid to visualize the physiologic lymphatic drainage of the breast was published by Vendrell-Torne and associates [10]. They mapped drainage from injections in the four quadrants of the breast as well as the subareolar region utilizing colloidal gold-198. No attempt to visualize the first draining focus was made. They clearly established the presence of unexpected, sometimes multiple, pathways of drainage to axillary, internal mammary and supraclavicular sites in a significant minority of normal subjects.

Uren and colleagues were the first to report the use of radiocolloid injection of the primary lesion site to image the pathways of lymphatic drainage in patients with breast cancer [11]. They used ^{99m}Tc-labeled antimony trisulfide (^{99m}Tc–

Sb$_2$S$_3$) with a 3–12-nm particle size. Injections of 0.1–0.2 mL were placed at the four clock quadrants using a tuberculin syringe and a 25-gauge needle. The depth of injection (and precise position of the tumor) was determined in each case by high-resolution ultrasound. Activity varied from 2.5 to 7.0 MBq (0.07–0.19 mCi) for each injection. All studies were performed prior to excision of the tumor. The tumor and adjacent injection sites were subsequently excised within

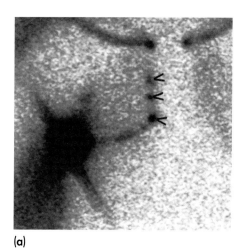

(a)

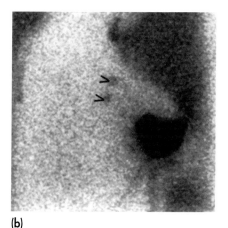

(b)

FIGURE 1　(a) Anterior view of right chest of a patient with a lower outer-quadrant lesion draining across midline of the breast to the internal mammary nodes. (b) Right lateral view depicting drainage to the ipsilateral axilla. The arrowheads mark the first-tier lymph nodes.

1 week. Imaging was performed immediately after injection and at 2.5 h in all patients. In patients with no nodal visualization, a repeat scan was obtained at 4 h. Images were obtained in an anterior view of the chest and axilla in all patients. A lateral or oblique view was added to assess the depth of axillary sentinel nodes. All scans were obtained with a large-field-of-view digital camera with a low-energy, high-resolution collimator. Immediate scanning was performed to identify lymph channels draining the tumor. Delayed scanning was performed to locate persistent uptake in nodes. The sentinel node was considered to be the first node to take up the colloid on the immediate scan or the node with the most activity on the delayed scan.

The ipsilateral axilla was a drainage site in 29 of the 34 patients (85%) and the only drainage site in 18 of them (53%). However, the unpredictability of drainage patterns previously described by Vendrell-Torne was confirmed. Approximately one-third of lateralized tumors demonstrated drainage to the ipsilateral axilla and/or internal mammary chain (Figs. 1a and 1b), whereas 20% of upper-quadrant lesions drained to supraclavicular or infraclavicular nodes (Fig. 2). Immediate scans were able to identify lymph channels in only 7 of the 34 patients (21%). This was a potential drawback only in patients with internal mammary node drainage because multiple nodal uptake candidates for sentinel node designation were characteristically present, on delayed scans, in the internal mammary but not the axillary or periclavicular basins. In three patients, no migra-

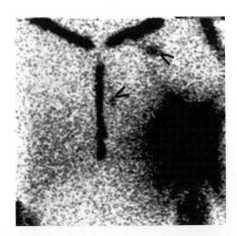

FIGURE 2   Anterior chest view showing left breast lesion draining directly into an infraclavicular lymph node as well as to an internal mammary lymph node. Arrowheads mark lymph nodes. Sternum and clavicles are delineated with a radioactive marker.

tion of tracer from the injection site was seen. In one of these, gross chest wall and axillary tumor masses were present.

DISCUSSION

Our experience at the H. Lee Moffitt Cancer Center and Research Institute at the University of South Florida dates from 1994 when we first undertook lymphatic mapping of the breast, prompted like others by our prior experience in melanoma [12]. Our technique for lymphoscintigraphy requires no specialized equipment. We use a standard gamma camera and a high-resolution collimator. The 140-keV energy level is windowed at a 10% level, as this is the ^{99m}Tc energy peak.

Historically, investigators have preferred ^{99m}Tc–antimony trisulfide for lymphoscintigraphic studies because its particle size of 3–30 nm is optimal for transit through lymphatics and localization in nodes without phagocytosis. This radiocolloid is no longer available in the United States, although it is still widely used elsewhere in the world. Hung and associates have produced acceptable lymphoscintigraphic images with the ^{99m}Tc sulfur colloid filtered to a maximum particle size of 100 nm. In practice, nearly all of its filtered activity was distributed in the 15–50-nm range [13]. Our radiopharmaceutical is the ^{99m}Tc sulfur colloid filtered to 200 nm maximum particle size. Our filtration technique uses a 0.2-μm (200-nm) filter and we have found this preparation satisfactory with best results obtained when used fresh. We use a dose of 17.5 MBq (0.45 mCi) unless the lesion is high in the axillary tail, in which case the dose is reduced to 9.25 MBq (0.25 mCi). For a discussion on the radiation safety aspects, the reader is referred to Chapter 13.

In the Nuclear Medicine Department, patients with palpable tumors are injected with six injections around the periphery of the tumor at the depth of the mass. Patients with nonpalpable tumors first undergo mammographic or ultrasound needle localization. If imaged by ultrasound, six equal aliquots are injected with ultrasound guidance around the tumor. If imaged by mammography, the same procedure is followed except the six injections are made equidistant to the localization wire. In small-breasted patients or patients with superficial tumors, it is often possible to perform the injections without compression of the breast tissue. In large-breasted patients or in patients with centrally located lesions, it may be necessary to perform the injections while the breast remains under compression to assure accurate depth.

A third group of patients is studied after lumpectomy or excisional biopsy has been performed. Most have seromas that are palpable and injections are performed as if the seroma were the tumor, so that the injection is into the breast parenchyma around the biopsy cavity. If the seroma is not readily palpable, ultrasound is used, and, in almost all cases, will identify a small residual seroma or area of architectural distortion within the breast so that the injectate can be instilled at the correct location. The physician making the injections must be able to distinguish the tumor seroma or scar from induration or scar related to the skin incision, which is often placed remote from the tumor to satisfy cosmetic concerns.

All injections are made through a tuberculin syringe. Care must be taken not to inject into the tumor or seroma cavity, as this impedes lymphatic flow. We have found injection through the localization needle to be undesirable as the needle acts as a wick causing much of the dose to migrate to the skin surface. This not only reduces the dose available for imaging but produces confounding contamination on the skin surface.

We have obtained good results using 2 mL total diluent. The ideal volume of injectate is unknown. On one hand, a larger volume should improve uptake within the lymphatic system. On the other hand, larger volumes may diffuse into the axilla, confounding imaging and detection. We are currently performing a randomized study comparing results of injected volumes of 2 mL versus 6 mL.

The patient is imaged immediately after injection, positioned supine under the gamma camera in the anterior oblique lateral projection. Unlike imaging in melanoma, it is very unusual to see afferent lymphatics (Fig. 3). As the regions of interest are the axilla, the clavicular region, and the internal mammary nodes, various maneuvers are attempted to remove breast activity from the camera's field of view. The injection site in the breast can be shielded with lead, but this may produce a penumbra effect which can camouflage lymph nodes. The breast

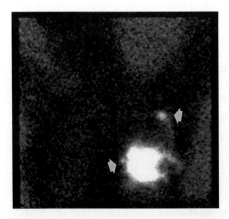

Figure 3 Left anterior oblique view of the chest. An afferent lymphatic is seen draining into a sentinel lymph node in the axilla. Drainage into an internal mammary lymph node is also present. White arrows denote the sentinel nodes.

can sometimes be taped out of the field of view. Alternately, the patient may be imaged sitting or standing so that gravity will act to position the breast. Small-breasted women or women with lesions near the chest wall or axilla often present a challenge and it may not be possible to separate the injection site from the regional lymphatic groups.

Low-density count images are acquired over 10 min. The lymph nodes are localized using a persistence scope and by triangulation, using changes in the patient's position. A small mark with an indelible pen or tattoo is placed on the skin overlying the lymph node. Alternatively, the ''hot'' node in the axilla can be marked with a hand-held gamma probe in the nuclear medicine suite. Sentinel lymph nodes are found with immediate imaging in approximately 50% of cases. Delayed imaging will be necessary in the remainder of cases. In our practice, the optimal time for delayed imaging as well as for surgery with use of a hand-held gamma probe is 4–6 h following injection.

THE FUTURE

There are two levels of questions pertinent to radiocolloid identification of sentinel lymph nodes in patients with breast cancer. The first relates to technical issues such as the optimum particle size, volume of injectate, and scanning interval. These issues are all currently under investigation at ours and other institutions. The second level pertains to the possible implications of this technique for clinical practice. What, for instance, is the significance of a positive supraclavicular sentinel node? Do these patients have Stage II disease in previously undissected areas (node positive, at high risk for metastasis and likely to benefit from adjuvant systemic treatment) or distant metastatic disease, as defined by the UICC/AJCC staging system? In either circumstance, do they represent a clinically unique subset who might benefit from a specialized treatment approach? What is the significance of a periclavicular or internal mammary sentinel node as to the need for performing any axillary surgical procedure and what types of surgical approaches should be used in these settings? Are there some women with invasive breast cancer, with perhaps inner-quadrant tumors who do not drain to the axilla and therefore do not need any axillary procedure? These and similar clinical questions are only beginning to be asked and, no doubt, will receive extensive attention in the future.

CONCLUSIONS

At the present time, the standard of care for definitive staging of clinically early-stage invasive breast cancer is axillary node dissection. Because of the morbidity of this procedure, sentinel lymphadenectomy has been suggested as a means of identifying patients without lymphatic metastases, allowing them to forego the more morbid axillary dissection. Sentinel nodes have been identified using both vital stains and radiocolloid injection, with the highest success achieved by the combination of the two techniques. The role of preoperative lymphoscintigraphy is uncertain at this stage, but we recommend that it be considered at the initiation of a breast carcinoma sentinel node radiocolloid localization program as a further aid to localization.

It is apparent that if an axillary sentinel node can be imaged, surgeons will have no difficulty identifying the node intraoperatively because the sentinel node is emitting a significant number of counts. The real potential of lymphoscintigraphy in breast cancer may be to identify a subpopulation of women who do not drain to the axilla and may not need any axillary procedure. In addition, this preoperative test may identify women whose tumors drain into the internal mammary nodes, and these nodes can then be included in the radiation ports if this modality is used with breast conservation.

REFERENCES

1. E Ohtake, H Toyama, M Iio, M Noguchi, S Kawaguchi, H Murata, K Chiba, H Yamada. The application of the bilateral collimator to parasternal lymphoscintigraphy: a new method to measure the depth of the lymph node. Nucl Med Commun 1:102–106, 1980.
2. GN Ege. Lymphoscintigraphy—techniques and applications in the management of breast cancer. Semin Nucl Med 13:26–34, 1983.
3. RG McLean, GN Ege. Prognostic value of axillary lymphoscintigraphy in breast carcinoma patients. J Nucl Med 27:1116–1124, 1986.
4. M Noguchi, T Michigishi, K Nakajima, N Koyasaki, T Taniya, N Ohta, I Miyazaki. The diagnosis of internal mammary node metastases of breast cancer. Int Surg 78: 171–175, 1993.
5. KA Hultborn, LG Larsson, I Ragnhult. The lymph drainage from the breast to the axillary and parasternal lymph nodes, studied with the aid of colloidal Au-198. Acta Radiol 43:52–64, 1954.
6. DN Krag, DL Weaver, JC Alex, JT Fairbank. Surgical resection and radiolocalization of the sentinel lymph node in breast cancer using a gamma probe. Surg Oncol 2:336–340, 1993.
7. JC Alex, DN Krag. Gamma-probe–guided localization of lymph nodes. Surg Oncol 2:137–143, 1993.
8. LC Alex, DL Weaver, JT Fairbank, DN Krag. Gamma probe–guided lymph node localization in malignant melanoma. Surg Oncol 2:303–308, 1993.
9. DN Krag. Gamma-probe–guided resection of axillary sentinel nodes (abstr). Society of Surgical Oncology. 48th Annual Meeting, Boston, 1995.
10. E Vendrell-Torne, J Setoain-Quinquer, FM Domenech-Torne. Study of normal lymphatic drainage using radioactive isotopes. J Nucl Med 13:801–805, 1972.
11. RF Uren, RB Howman-Giles, JF Thompson, D Malouf, G Ramsey-Stewart, FW

Niesche, SB Renwick. Mammary lymphoscintigraphy in breast cancer. J Nucl Med 36:1775–1780, 1995.

12. JJ Albertini, GH Lyman, C Cox, T Yeatman, L Balducci, N Ku, S Shivers, C Berman, K Wells, D Rapaport, A Shons, J Horton, H Greenberg, S Nicosia, R Clark, A Cantor, D Reintgen. Lymphatic mapping and sentinel node biopsy in the patient with breast cancer. JAMA 176:1818–1822, 1996.

13. JC Hung, GA Wiseman, HW Wahner, BP Mullan, TR Taggart, WL Dunn. Filtered technetium-99m-sulfur colloid evaluated for lymphoscintigraphy. J Nucl Med 36:1895–1901, 1995.

10

Lymphatic Mapping in Breast Cancer

Nora M. Hansen and Armando E. Giuliano
Joyce Eisenberg-Keefer Breast Center and John Wayne Cancer Institute at Saint John's Health Center, Santa Monica, California

INTRODUCTION

Axillary lymph node dissection has been an integral component in the surgical management of invasive breast cancer for many years. For most of this century, axillary dissection was thought to be both prognostic and therapeutic and was considered an important component of surgical cure. En bloc resection of the axillary lymph nodes was the standard of surgical therapy [1]. In the 1970s, Fisher suggested that breast cancer is a systemic disease at presentation, implying that small tumors may represent an early manifestation of a disease process that is already metastatic [2]. Therefore, nodal involvement becomes not an orderly contiguous extension as described by Halsted but rather a marker of distant disease. Fisher proposed that regional lymph node metastases are of biologic importance and an indicator of a poor tumor–host relationship. Axillary nodal metastasis remains the best and most important prognostic marker and remains the single strongest predictor of survival in women with breast cancer [3,4]. As a result of this, the National Institute of Health (NIH) Consensus Conference of 1991 recommended a Berg Level I and II axillary node dissection for patients with early-stage invasive breast cancer [5]. This will provide accurate information regarding the axillary nodal status and is associated with a low rate of axillary recurrence.

Although axillary node dissection has a low false-negative rate, it does result in significant morbidity. Permanent lymphedema has been reported in 15–30% of patients undergoing axillary dissection and the frequency, and severity of this complication increases with the extent of axillary surgery and the addition of radiation therapy [6–8]. Other complications such as wound infection, seroma, arm weakness, decreased shoulder range of motion, and neurologic changes can occur. These sequelae are a major source of emotional distress and functional impairment for women with breast cancer and they significantly increase the monetary cost of the procedure [6,11]. Unfortunately, there is no accurate alternative to histologic assessment of the axillary nodes. Clinical evaluation has been associated with a high false-negative rate ranging from 29–38% and a false-positive rate of 10–50%. Radiological evaluation using mammography, ultrasound, computed tomography (CT) scan, magnetic resonance imaging (MRI), and nuclear medicine evaluation using lymphoscintigraphy, positron emission tomography (PET), and radiolabeled monoclonal antibody scanning may detect axillary nodal metastases, but these techniques lack the sensitivity and specificity that are needed for clinical decision-making [12–16].

Over the last few years the need for axillary dissection for women with invasive breast cancer has been questioned. This is in part due to the increasing use of mammography and the detection of smaller tumors, which has led to a decreased incidence of nodal metastases in this subset of women. Adjuvant therapeutic decisions once based on the nodal status are no longer limited to patients with node-positive breast cancer and are now often dependent on the characteristics of the primary tumor [17,18]. Increased public awareness of the long-term sequelae of axillary dissection and the lack of evidence to support a survival advantage of axillary dissection have also contributed to this trend toward elimination of this procedure.

Perhaps the most exciting new development in the surgical management of invasive breast cancer is the emergence of sentinel lymphadenectomy and its potential to provide accurate prognostic information for the patient with breast cancer without the sequelae of an axillary dissection.

This chapter will review the history of breast sentinel lymphadenectomy, the various techniques used to identify the sentinel node, the histopathological workup of the sentinel node, the strengths and weaknesses of this technique, and its future goals.

HISTORY

Haagensen first introduced the concept of lymphatic mapping for breast cancer [19]. He did not coin the term ''sentinel node'' but rather used a blue dye to map the lymphatic drainage pattern in his patients with breast cancer. The concept of intraoperative lymphatic mapping and sentinel lymph node biopsy was popularized by Morton and colleagues in patients with melanoma [20]. This technique has since been validated by other independent investigators [21,22]. The sentinel node (first-tier node, first-echelon node) was identified using a vital blue dye and represented the first lymph node that drained a specific melanoma. This concept was subsequently applied to patients with breast cancer. Because a majority of women do not have axillary metastases at the time of diagnosis, this technique has the potential to eliminate a full axillary dissection in most patients.

INTRAOPERATIVE LYMPHATIC MAPPING USING A RADIOLABELED COLLOID

Krag et al. published the first pilot study of sentinel lymphadenectomy in patients with invasive breast cancer [23]. In this study, an unfiltered technetium-99m (^{99m}Tc)-labeled colloid was injected 1–9 h prior to surgery and was used to map the lymphatic tract and identify the sentinel node. The sentinel node was identified in 82% of a group of 22 patients using a hand-held gamma-ray counter. The sentinel node proved 100% predictive of the axillary status. This implies that if this node is free of disease, the remainder of the axillary nodes are also free of disease. Krag and co-workers updated their results in 248 cases [24]. The sentinel node was identified in 95.5% of patients with a false-negative rate of 6.5%. This led to the initiation of a multicenter trial to evaluate the success of intraoperative lymphatic mapping and sentinel lymphadenectomy using a radiolabeled colloid. The results of this trial have recently been reported and show a false-negative sentinel lymph node biopsy rate of 11.4% in a multicenter trial involving 12 institutions [25].

INTRAOPERATIVE LYMPHATIC MAPPING USING VITAL BLUE DYE

In 1994, Giuliano and co-workers published their initial work of intraoperative lymphatic mapping with a vital blue dye [26]. A 1% isosulfan blue dye solution (Lymphazurin, Hirsh Industries, Inc., Richmond, VA, U.S.A.) was used to identify the sentinel node in this study of 172 patients (174 lymph node basins). The sentinel node was identified in 66% of patients overall, but the identification rate improved as the investigator became familiar with the nuances of the technique. The 59% rate of sentinel node detection in the first 87 cases increased to 72% in the next 87 cases and the detection rate reached 78% by the last 50 cases in this series. The technique was modeled after the melanoma model, a cutaneous tumor, but had to be adapted to breast cancer, which is a parenchymal tumor. This led to significant changes in the technique. In this study, there were five false-negative cases reported in which the pathology of the sentinel node did not accurately predict the status of the axilla. All false negatives occurred in the first 87 cases. This was a critical problem with the technique because a false-negative result could potentially lead to the undertreatment of a node-positive patient. These five cases were reanalyzed and it was discovered that in three of the five cases, axillary fat was misidentified as the sentinel node. This prompted the use of intraoperative frozen section to confirm the presence of nodal tissue. A fourth patient was found to have occult metastasis when the pathology was reevaluated with immunohistochemical stains using anticytokeratin antibodies. With our current histopathological workup, involvement of the sentinel node would have been identified. Only one of the five patients examined had a ''true'' false-negative sentinel node improving the accuracy rate from 96% to 99%.

The initial modest identification rate of 66% is, in retrospect, interpreted as the ''learning curve.'' Although we do feel that experience is needed before mastering this technique, many of the problems during this learning curve are now avoided due to improvements in the technique itself as well as better patient selection. The volume of dye injected, the site of injection, the timing of the axillary incision, the histopathological workup of the sentinel node and the addition of massage to the injection site all aided in improving the probability of identifying the sentinel node. Using this mature technique in a subsequent study, the sentinel node was identified in 93% of patients and was 100% predictive of the nodal status [27]. Based on the results of this study, we abandoned completion axillary lymph node dissection in 1995 in patients whose sentinel nodes were tumor-free.

COMBINED TECHNIQUE

Albertini and co-workers combined both the blue dye and the radiopharmaceutical in an effort to improve the detection rate and reduce the ''learning curve'' [28]. This approach combines a filtered sulfur colloid with 1% isosulfan blue dye. The sentinel node was identified in 93% of 62 patients and proved 100% predictive of the axillary lymph node status. Cox et al. updated their experience and reported the results of 466 consecutive patients [29]. A sentinel node was successfully identified in 94.4% of patients with only a single false-negative case.

OTHER STUDIES

Other investigators have reported their success with sentinel node biopsy. The various studies of its applicability as a staging tool in breast cancer patients are summarized in Table 1. Veronesi et al. reported probe-directed mapping with a subdermal injection of a ^{99m}Tc-labeled human serum albumin colloid in 163 consecutive breast cancer patients who subsequently underwent completion axillary node dissection [30]. The sentinel node was identified in 98.2% of patients; however, there was a 5% false-negative rate. Guenther et al. in a large California-based health maintenance organization (HMO) had a 71% identification rate using blue dye alone in a cohort of 145 patients [31]. Although this identification rate is low, the predictive value of the sentinel node, when identified, was 97%.

TABLE 1 Summary of Sentinel Lymphadenectomy Publications

Study year [Ref.]	N	Mapping technique	Identification rate (%)	False-negative rate (%)
Krag et al. 1993 [23]	22	[99m]Tc colloid	82	0
Giuliano et al. 1994 [26]	174	Dye	66	11
Albertini et al. 1996 [28]	62	[99m]Tc colloid + dye	92	0
Pijpers et al. 1997 [33]	37	[99m]Tc colloid	92	0
Veronesi et al. 1997 [30]	163	[99m]Tc colloid	98	5
Giuliano et al. 1997 [27]	107	Dye	94	0
Guenther et al. 1997 [31]	145	Dye	71	10
Dale and Williams 1998 [32]	21	Dye	66	0
Borgstein et al. 1998 [34]	130	[99m]Tc colloid	94	2
Barnwell et al. 1998 [38]	42	[99m]Tc colloid + dye	90	0
O'Hea et al. 1998 [39]	59	[99m]Tc colloid + dye	93	13
Miner et al. 1998 [35]	42	[99m]Tc colloid	98	14
Offodile et al. 1998 [36]	41	[99m]Tc colloid	98	0
Cox et al. 1998 [29]	466	[99m]Tc colloid + dye	94	[a]
Koller et al. 1998 [40]	98	Dye	98	17
Crossin et al. 1998 [37]	50	[99m]Tc colloid	84	13
Krag et al. 1998 [25]	443	[99m]Tc colloid	93	11

Note: N = number of patients; false-negative rate = fraction of patients with tumor-free sentinel node(s) in group of patients with tumor-positive axilla.

[a] Majority of patients with tumor-negative sentinel node did not undergo completion of axillary node dissection.

Similarly, Dale and Williams published their results using blue dye alone in 21 patients. The sentinel node was identified in only 66% of cases but was 100% predictive of the axillary tumor status [32]. Pijpers et al. reported the use of peritumoral injection of ^{99m}Tc-labeled colloidal albumin in 37 patients [33]. They reported a 92% success rate and the sentinel node was 100% predictive of the axillary status. Borgstein et al. used the same tracer in patients with a T1 or T2 tumor [34]. There was a 94% identification rate and a 2% false-negative rate. Miner et al. applied the use of ultrasound to aid in the peritumoral injection of an unfiltered ^{99m}Tc sulfur colloid [35]. The sentinel node was identified in 98% of patients with a predictive value of 98%. Offodile et al. used ^{99m}Tc-labeled dextran as the radioactive tracer in 41 patients with an identification rate of 98% and an accuracy rate of 100% [36]. Crossin et al. utilized a peritumoral injection of the ^{99m}Tc sulfur colloid and found the sentinel node in 84% of cases with an accuracy rate of 98% [37]. Barnwell et al. reported a 90% identification rate and 100% accuracy rate using the combined technique [38]. The group at Memorial Sloan Kettering Cancer Center was successful in identifying the sentinel node in 93% of cases, but the tumor status of the axilla was accurately reflected in only 95% [39]. Koller et al. recently reported their results using either a methylene blue or patent blue dye [40]. A sentinel node was successfully identified in 98% of patients and was 97% accurate. It is clear from these studies using a variety of techniques that the success rate of identifying the sentinel node is greater than 90%. More importantly, the accuracy of the sentinel node in predicting the nodal status of the axilla was consistently over 95%. The average number of sentinel nodes excised in all of these studies ranged from 1 to 2.9 and was similar irrespective of the use of a vital dye, a radioactive tracer, or a combination. Sentinel lymphadenectomy can be successfully performed in a variety of centers both in academic and private settings.

TECHNIQUES

Intraoperative Lymphatic Mapping Using Vital Blue Dye

After the induction of general or local anesthesia with intravenous sedation, 3–5 mL of 1% isosulfan blue dye is injected into the breast parenchyma surrounding a primary breast tumor or into the wall of the cavity after an excisional biopsy [26,31,32]. If the lesion is nonpalpable, a mammographic or ultrasound localization procedure will be necessary. The timing of the axillary incision and the amount of dye injected depend on the location of the tumor (Table 2). Once the dye is injected, the area is massaged for several minutes to augment the action of the lymphatic pump and promote passage of the blue dye to the sentinel node. A transverse incision is made at the inferior aspect of the hair-bearing region of the axilla. The axillary space is entered and blunt dissection is performed to identify a blue-stained lymphatic channel, which is commonly located just below the

TABLE 2   Recommendations for Volume of Blue Dye and Time from Injection to Incision

Location of primary tumor	Volume of dye (mL)	Time to incision (min)
Upper outer quadrant	3–4	4–5
Upper inner quadrant	4–5	5–6
Lower outer quadrant	5	5
Lower inner quadrant	5	7

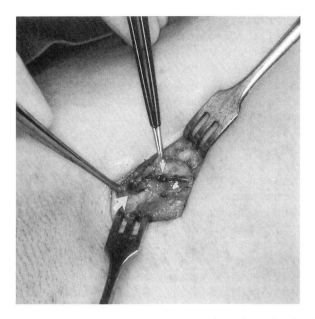

Figure 1 Sentinel node (large arrow) in the right axilla identified by dissecting a blue lymphatic duct (small arrow).

axillary fascia. The blue lymphatic channel is then dissected both proximally and distally until a blue-stained lymph node is identified (Fig. 1). Abduction of the arm above the patient's head will facilitate identification of the blue node. The sentinel node is then excised and sent for pathological evaluation.

At the John Wayne Cancer Institute, we perform a frozen-section examination, but other institutions rely only on evaluation of permanent sections. A completion level I and II axillary dissection should be performed when the sentinel node is found to contain metastatic cells or if the sentinel node is not identified.

Intraoperative Lymphatic Mapping Using a Radioactive Tracer

There are several different radioactive tracers that can be used to identify the sentinel node. In the United States, the most commonly used agents are the ^{99m}Tc-labeled sulfur colloid [23,35,37], the ^{99m}Tc albumin colloid [30,33,34], or ^{99m}Tc dextran [36]. These agents are injected 1–24 h prior to operation. Some investigators use filtered agents, which have a faster transit time; others prefer unfiltered agents. The timing of the injection depends on the type of radioactive colloid used. Prior to operation, 9–37 MBq (0.25–1.0 mCi) of the radiopharmaceutical is injected into the breast parenchyma surrounding a primary tumor or biopsy cavity. A lymphoscintigram may be performed to mark the location of the sentinel node prior to surgery. This is of value in medial hemisphere lesions, where it is important to document axillary drainage. Rarely, a medial hemisphere lesion may drain only to lymph nodes in the internal mammary chain, thereby decreasing the success rate of identifying an axillary sentinel node. Intraoperatively, a gamma probe is used to map the lymphatic drainage pattern. A background count is established by measuring the radioactive count over a neutral site. The skin is incised over the area of greatest activity. Blunt dissection is carefully performed until the gamma probe signal intensifies and a lymph node is found. Once the sentinel node is identified and removed, the axillary basin should be scanned for residual radioactivity. An attempt should be made to find a second sentinel node if the count rate is still increased. If the primary lesion is in the upper outer quadrant, the sentinel node may be difficult to identify due to the ''shine through'' from the injection site. The segmental mastectomy may be performed prior to searching the sentinel node to avert this problem.

The definition of a ''hot'' node varies among investigators and may be dependent on the type of radioactive colloid used. Krag et al. define the sentinel node as any node with radioactivity levels three times that of background and at least 15 counts per 10 s [23]. Veronesi et al. define the sentinel node as the node with the highest radioactivity counts [30], whereas Albertini et al. define the sentinel node as the node with at least 10 times the radioactivity of neighboring nonsentinel nodes [28]. Unfortunately, the various definitions used to define the sentinel node make it difficult to standardize the technique.

Intraoperative Lymphatic Mapping Using Both a Radioactive Tracer and a Vital Blue Dye

This approach utilizes both the blue dye technique and the radioactive tracer. The radioactive colloid is injected preoperatively, whereas the blue dye is injected in the operating room several minutes prior to the axillary incision. This technique may be the best technique for the beginner because it provides the surgeon with two modalities to identify the sentinel node.

HISTOPATHOLOGICAL ANALYSIS

The histopathological examination of the sentinel node is a critical component to the success of the procedure. Frozen section or touch prep cytology may be performed to confirm the presence of lymphoid tissue and to identify the presence of metastases. Frozen-section analysis can be difficult, particularly in invasive lobular cancers. False-negative results from 7% to 23% have been documented [41–43]. Permanent section hematoxylin & eosin (H&E) staining is imperative to confirm the results of frozen-section analysis. The addition of immunohisto-chemistry using antibodies to low- and intermediate-molecular-weight cytokera-tin (MAK-6, Ciba-Corning, Alameda, CA, U.S.A.) has improved the detection of micrometastases.

In a study by Giuliano and co-workers, 162 patients who underwent a senti-nel lymphadenectomy followed by a completion axillary node dissection (sentinel node group) were compared to 134 patients who underwent axillary node dissec-tion alone (axillary dissection group) [44]. All sentinel nodes were evaluated with standard H&E staining and immunohistochemistry; the other axillary nodes were evaluated by H&E alone. The sentinel node biopsy group had a 42% incidence of nodal metastases and the axillary dissection group had only a 28% incidence of nodal metastases ($p < 0.03$). The difference was primarily due to an increase in the detection rate of micrometastases. Micrometastasis (defined as a tumor deposit smaller than 2 mm) was detected in 38.2% of the sentinel node biopsy group compared to 10.3% of the axillary dissection group. Immunohistochemistry staining identified 11 of the 26 micrometastases in the sentinel node group after H&E stains were negative. The addition of immunohistochemistry to the histopathologic evaluation of the sentinel node upstaged an additional 16% of patients. By allowing a more focused histopathological analysis of the sentinel node, patients undergoing sentinel lymphadenectomy had improved axillary staging.

Turner and co-workers applied immunohistochemistry to all nonsentinel nodes in a cohort of patients who had undergone a sentinel lymphadenectomy followed by a completion axillary node dissection [45]. The purpose of this study was to determine if the enhanced detection of metastatic tumor in the sentinel node reflected a more intensive histopathological workup of the sentinel node as compared to nonsentinel nodes. A total of 1087 nonsentinel nodes were examined at two levels using immunohistochemistry and only one nonsentinel node was found to contain a micrometastasis. Therefore, if the sentinel node is negative on H&E and immunohistochemical staining, the probability of nonsentinel node involvement is less than 0.1%.

ROLE OF SENTINEL LYMPHADENECTOMY IN DUCTAL CARCINOMA *IN SITU*

The number of patients diagnosed with ductal carcinoma *in situ* (DCIS) has in-creased dramatically over the last 20 years with the increased use of screening mammography. The treatment of DCIS has ranged from mastectomy to segmen-tal resection. The role of axillary dissection has not been addressed in DCIS. The prognostic importance of axillary nodal metastases has focused on invasive can-cer and, therefore, there has been no consensus as to the optimal management of the regional nodes in patients with noninvasive breast cancer.

Axillary nodal metastases have been documented in patients with DCIS. The American College of Surgeons Study reported a 1–4% incidence of nodal metastases [46]. In spite of this low rate of nodal metastases, data from the National Cancer Data Base in 1991 indicated that 58.5% of patients with DCIS underwent an axillary dissection [47]. Several investigators have used the lymphatic mapping technology to identify the sentinel node in patients with DCIS. Zavotsky and co-workers at the John Wayne Cancer Institute evaluated a subset of DCIS patients with evidence of microinvasion. Two patients (14.3%) had tumor-involved sentinel nodes. In both cases, the sentinel node was the only tumor involved node. Cox and co-workers reported a 4.6% incidence of nodal metastases in their cohort of 87 patients with DCIS [29].

Ductal carcinoma *in situ* has been classified into histological subtypes that correlate with biologic behavior. *In situ* comedo carcinoma carries a greater long-term risk for infiltrating cancer and is more likely to become invasive. Although the incidence of nodal metastases is low, sentinel lymphadenectomy appears to be a good alternative to axillary node dissection, particularly in comedo lesions. The use of systemic treatment has not been advocated in patients with DCIS in general. However, patients with nodal metastases would require adjuvant therapy, making sentinel lymphadenectomy an important diagnostic tool for these individuals.

CLINICAL SIGNIFICANCE OF OCCULT METASTASES

Although the clinical significance of micrometastases in lymph nodes has not been validated in a prospective study, there have been several retrospective studies which have addressed this important question. It is well known that lymph node status is the most important prognostic factor for patients with breast cancer. Despite this observation, 15–20% of node-negative women develop a recurrence within 10 years. It is not clear whether or not the presence of occult dissemination may be a predictor of relapse. To date, the natural history of micrometastases is unknown and the published literature is contradictory. Earlier studies using serial sectioning and H&E staining reported no significant difference in survival between patients with uninvolved nodes and those with occult metastases. However, axillary micrometastases were associated with decreased survival in certain subgroups, including those with T1 tumors or tumors larger than 1.3 mm in diameter.

The Ludwig Breast Cancer Study group reevaluated 921 breast cancer patients whose original pathological workup did not identify axillary metastases [48]. The axillary nodes were sectioned at six different levels and examined with H&E stains. The incidence of nodal metastases increased by 9%. Patients with micrometastases had lower rates of 5-year disease-free survival (58%) and overall survival (74%) compared to those with truly negative nodes (79% and 88%, respectively). These differences were found to be statistically significant.

De Mascarel et al. used immunohistochemistry to identify micrometastases in 23% of their study population [49]. In patients with invasive ductal cancer, immunohistochemistry-detected dissemination was the most significant factor associated with recurrence and had a significant impact on overall survival. Trojani demonstrated a 14% increase in micrometastases with the addition of immunohistochemistry which correlated with a lower survival [50]. Hainsworth et al. in a similar study concluded that the presence of occult metastases increased the 5-year recurrence rate from 16% to 32% [51].

Other investigators have reported conflicting results [52–55]. Pickren et al. evaluated 199 breast cancer patients and found a 22% increase in micrometastases with the addition of serial sectioning, but this increase did not have an impact on overall survival [52]. Friedman et al. evaluated 1153 patients, and although there was an increase in the number of micrometastases, the relative risk of distant metastases was identical in the two groups [56].

The addition of immunohistochemistry to the entire axillary specimen is impractical due to both time and financial constraints. However, the addition of immunohistochemistry to the sentinel node alone may improve the detection of tumor spread and the natural history of micrometastases may eventually be elucidated. The American College of Surgeons' Oncology Group will be conducting a prospective study to evaluate the clinical significance of immunohistochemistry-detected dissemination.

CONCLUSION

Intraoperative lymphatic mapping and sentinel lymphadenectomy is an innovative technique to accurately stage patients with breast cancer with minimal morbidity. Although there have been no published reports of sentinel lymphadenectomy alone, one can anticipate that the complication rate will be lower when compared to a standard axillary node dissection. This may be particularly relevant to the majority of patients who are node negative at initial diagnosis. This group of patients would be at risk for the morbidity of an axillary node dissection without any known benefit from the procedure. Because the incidence of nodal metastases is related to tumor size, several investigators have suggested abandoning axillary node dissection in patients with T1a (up to and including 0.5 cm) or T1b (0.5–1.0 cm) lesions [57,58]. Nodal involvement, however, has been documented in 15–25% of such patients and 3–28% of patients with T1a tumors [59,60].

Because adjuvant therapy is generally reserved for patients with tumors larger than 1 cm regardless of nodal involvement or tumors of any size with nodal involvement, it is important to determine the nodal status particularly in patients with tumors less than 1 cm in size [17]. Sentinel lymphadenectomy is especially important in this subset of patients.

A recent review of 256 patients with T1 breast cancers at the John Wayne Cancer Institute documented nodal metastases with routine H&E staining in 10% of T1a tumors, 12% of T1b tumors, and 27% of T1c (1–2 cm) tumors. In a subset of T1 patients who underwent sentinel lymphadenectomy, the incidence of nodal metastases increased to 15% for both T1a and T1b lesions with the addition of immunohistochemistry [61]. The overall incidence of axillary metastases may need to be reevaluated because the addition of immunohistochemistry and a focused histopathological workup increases the detection of axillary metastases. Patients with a historically low risk of axillary metastases may be found to have a higher rate of positivity with the addition of lymphatic mapping. It will be interesting to see if the improved axillary staging with the addition of the sentinel node affects survival. A prospective trial will be necessary to answer this question and is the second goal of the American College of Surgeons trial.

Several investigators have found that the sentinel node is often the only lymph node to contain metastastic tumor cells. In our previous study of 107 consecutive patients, 67% of those with sentinel node involvement had no other tumor-positive nodes in the axillary basin [27]. Albertini published similar results [28], whereas Veronesi found that only 38% of his patients had no other nodal involvement [30]. Although there is no accurate means of predicting which patients will have axillary metastases limited to the sentinel node, the size of the primary tumor and the size of the sentinel node metastases may predict the likelihood of nonsentinel node metastases. Patients with T1 tumors and immunohistochemistry-detected sentinel node metastases had no additional metastastic lymph nodes identified [62]. Therefore, not all patients—even with sentinel node metastases—may need completion axillary node dissection. At this time, a completion axillary node dissection is advised for all sentinel-node-positive patients. However, if axillary dissemination is only a prognostic marker and has no effect on survival, the need for axillary dissection will have to be reevaluated. A prospective randomized trial will be necessary to answer this important question.

Sentinel lymph node biopsy should be considered an experimental technique. Although the accuracy of the technique has recently been validated in a multicenter trial, the procedure has not been validated for community use. This approach is still under investigation and any plan to immediately abandon axillary dissection without documenting the ability to successfully and accurately identify the sentinel node should be discouraged. The premature use of this technique has the potential to result in missed positive axillary nodes that may take months or years to become clinically evident. Although several investigators have published promising results, there are still many questions that must be answered before sentinel node biopsy can replace axillary dissection. Should preoperative lymphoscintigraphy be used? What is the best surgical technique? How should internal mammary sentinel nodes be managed? What is the role for the reverse transcriptase–polymerase chain reaction (RT-PCR) in the evaluation of sentinel nodes?

As with any new technique, it is imperative that each surgeon documents his or her ability to accurately identify the sentinel node by performing a subsequent completion axillary dissection. Quality control is paramount for successful application of this technique and involves not only surgeons but also the other specialists involved. Successful application of sentinel lymphadenectomy in clinical practice requires a coordinated effort among the surgeon, the nuclear medicine physician, the radiologist, and the pathologist to assure high quality and accurate staging.

It is clear that not all patients are candidates for this procedure. Patients with a large tumor or a large biopsy cavity may have a higher false-negative rate after sentinel node biopsy. Patients with prior axillary surgery may not be candidates due to disruptance of the axillary lymphatics. Multicentric disease is a contraindication due to the inability to determine which focus should be injected. The effects of pregnancy, lactation, or preoperative chemotherapy on this procedure are unknown and further investigation is needed to determine if these patients are candidates for this procedure.

Sentinel lymphadenectomy is perhaps the most exciting advancement in the surgical management of patients with early breast cancer because the advent of breast-conserving procedures. It provides the surgeon with a minimally invasive technique to accurately assess the axillary nodal status and limit morbidity in those patients who do not require a completion dissection. It is imperative that the procedure be done accurately and safely. Centers should avoid offering sentinel lymphadenectomy alone until they have formally trained surgeons and nuclear medicine physicians in place who are comfortable with the technique and have documented their success. The true test of sentinel lymphadenectomy in patients with breast cancer will only be available after a sufficient amount of time has elapsed in those patients undergoing sentinel lymphadenectomy alone. Axillary metastases are considered a poor prognostic marker, and, to date, there has not been a consensus regarding the effect of their surgical removal on overall survival. The sentinel node procedure offers the ability to further evaluate the effect of axillary metastases on both local recurrence and ultimately survival. A prospective randomized trial may help to answer some of these questions.

ACKNOWLEDGMENTS

This work was supported in part by funding from the Ben B. and Joyce E. Eisenberg Foundation, Los Angeles, California and the Fashion Footwear Association of New York.

REFERENCES

1. WS Halsted. The results of radical operation for the cure of carcinoma of the breast. Ann Surg 46:1–6, 1907.
2. B Fisher. The surgical dilemma in the primary therapy of invasive breast cancer: A critical appraisal. Curr Prob Surg 1–5, October 1970.
3. CD Haagensen. Treatment of curable carcinoma of the breast. Int J Radiat Oncol Biol Phys 2:975–980, 1977.
4. G Bonadonna. Karofsky Memorial Lecture: Conceptual and practical advances in the management of breast cancer. J Clin Oncol 7:1380–1397, 1989.
5. National Institutes of Health. NIH consensus conference on the treatment of early-stage breast cancer. JAMA 265:391–395, 1991.
6. MW Kissin, G Querci della Rovere, D Easton, G Westbury. Risk of lymphoedema following the treatment of breast cancer. Br J Surg 73:580–584, 1986.
7. D Larson, M Weinstein, I Goldberg, B Silver, A Recht, B Cady, W Silen, JR Harris. Edema of the arm as a function of the extent of axillary surgery in patients with stage I–II carcinoma of the breast treated with primary radiotherapy. Int J Radiat Oncol Biol Phys 12:1575–1582, 1986.
8. RD Penzer, MP Patterson, LR Hill. Arm edema in patients treated conservatively for breast cancer: Relationship to patient age and axillary node dissection technique. Int J Radiol Oncol Biol Phys 12:2079–2083, 1986.
9. D Ivens, AL Hoe, TJ Podd, CR Hamilton, I Taylor, GT Royle. Assessment of arm morbidity from complete axillary dissection. Br J Cancer 66:136–138, 1992.
10. MB Tobin, HJ Lacey, L Meyer, PS Mortimer. The psychological morbidity of breast cancer-related arm swelling: Psychological morbidity of lymphoedema. Cancer 72:3248–3252, 1993.
11. CJ Vecht, HJ Van de Brand, OJM Wajer. Post-axillary dissection pain in breast cancer due to a lesion of the intercostobrachial nerve. Pain 38:171–176, 1989.
12. B Fisher, N Wolmark, M Bauer, C Redmond, M Gebhardt. The accuracy of clinical nodal staging and of limited axillary dissection as a determinant of histologic nodal status in carcinoma of the breast. Surg Gynecol Obstet 152:765–772, 1981.
13. M Noguchi, N Ohta, M Thomas, H Kitagawa, M Earashi, I Miyazaki, Y Mizukami. Clinical and biological prediction of axillary and internal mammary lymph node metastases in breast cancer. Surg Oncol 2:51–58, 1993.
14. R De Freitas, Jr, MV Costa, SV Schneider. Accuracy of ultrasound and clinical examination in the diagnosis of axillary lymph node metastases in breast cancer. Eur J Surg Oncol 17:240–244, 1991.
15. AB Ball, R Waters, S Fish, JM Thomas. Radical axillary dissection in the staging and treatment of breast cancer. Ann R Coll Surg Engl 74:126–129, 1992.
16. OE Nieweg, EE Kim, WH Wong, WF Broussard, SE Singletary, GN Hortobagyi, RS Tilbury. Positron emission tomography with fluorine-18-deoxyglucose in the detection and staging of breast cancer. Cancer 71:3920–3925, 1993.
17. Early Breast Cancer Trialists' Collaborative Group. Systemic treatment of early breast cancer by hormonal, cytotoxic, or immune therapy [Part I]. Lancet 339:1–15, 1992.
18. Early Breast Cancer Trialists' Collaborative Group. Systemic treatment of early

breast cancer by hormonal, cytotoxic, or immune therapy [Part II]. Lancet 339:71–85, 1992.

19. CD Haagensen. Lymphatics of the breast. In: CD Haagensen, CR Feind, FP Herter, CA Slanetz, JA Weinberg, eds. The Lymphatics in Cancer. Philadelphia: WB Saunders, 1972, pp. 300–398.

20. DL Morton, DR Wen, JH Wong, JS Economou, LA Cagle, FK Storm, LJ Foshag, AJ Cochran. Technical details of intraoperative lymphatic mapping for early stage melanoma. Arch Surg 127:392–399, 1992.

21. D Reintgen, CW Cruse, K Wells, C Berman, N Fenske, F Glass, K Schroer, R Heller, M Ross, G Lyman, C Cox, D Rappaport, HF Seigler, CM Balch. The orderly progression of melanoma nodal metastases. Ann Surg 220:759–767, 1994.

22. JF Thompson, WH McCarthy, CM Bosch, CJ O'Brien, MJ Quinn, S Paramaesvaran, K Crotty, SW McCarthy, RF Uren, R Howman-Giles. Sentinel lymph node status as an indicator of the presence of metastatic melanoma in regional lymph nodes. Melanoma Res 5:255–260, 1995.

23. DN Krag, DL Weaver, JC Alex, JT Fairbank. Surgical resection and radiolocalization of the sentinel lymph node in breast cancer using a gamma probe. Surg Oncol 2:335–339, 1993.

24. D Krag, S Harlow, D Weaver, T Ashikaga. Technique of sentinel node resection in melanoma and breast cancer: Probe-guided surgery and lymphatic mapping. Eur J Surg Oncol 24:89–93, 1998.

25. D Krag, D Weaver, T Ashikaga, F Moffat, VS Klimberg, C Shriver, S Feldman, R Kusminsky, M Gadd, J Kuhn, S Harlow, P Beitsch. The sentinel node in breast cancer. A multicenter validation study. N Engl J Med 339:941–946, 1998.

26. AE Giuliano, DM Kirgan, JM Guenther, DL Morton. Lymphatic mapping and sentinel lymphadenectomy for breast cancer. Ann Surg 220:391–401, 1994.

27. AE Giuliano, RC Jones, M Brennan, R Statman. Sentinel lymphadenectomy in breast cancer. J Clin Oncol 15:2345–2350, 1997.

28. JJ Albertini, GH Lyman, C Cox, T Yeatman, L Balducci, N Ku, S Shivers, C Berman, K Wells, D Rapaport, A Shons, J Horton, H Greenberg, S Nicosia, R Clark, A Cantor, DS Reintgen. Lymphatic mapping and sentinel node biopsy and lymphatic mapping of patients with breast cancer. JAMA 276:1818–1822, 1996.

29. CE Cox, S Pendas, JM Cox, E Joseph, AR Shons, T Yeatman, NN Ku, GH Lyman, C Berman, F Haddad, DS Reintgen. Guidelines for sentinel node biopsy and lymphatic mapping of patients with breast cancer. Ann Surg 227:645–653, 1998.

30. U Veronesi, G Paganelli, V Galimberti, G Viale, S Zurrida, M Bedoni, A Costa, C de Cicco, JG Geraghty, A Luini, V Sacchini, P Veronesi. Sentinel-node biopsy to avoid axillary dissection in breast cancer with clinically negative lymph-nodes. Lancet 349:1864–1867, 1997.

31. JM Guenther, M Krishnamoorthy, LR Tan. Sentinel lymphadenectomy for breast cancer in a community managed care setting. Cancer J Sci Am 3:336–340, 1997.

32. PS Dale, JT Williams IV. Axillary staging utilizing selective sentinel lymphadenectomy for patients with invasive breast carcinoma. Am Surg 64:28–32, 1998.

33. R Pijpers, S Meijer, OS Hoekstra, GJ Collet, EF Comans, RP Boom, PJ van Diest, GJ Teule. Impact of lymphoscintigraphy on sentinel node identification with technetium-99m-colloidal albumin in breast cancer. J Nucl Med 38:366–368, 1997.

34. PJ Borgstein, R Pijpers, EF Comans, PJ van Diest, RP Boom, S Meijer. Sentinel lymph node biopsy in breast cancer: guidelines and pitfalls of lymphoscintigraphy and gamma probe detection. J Am Coll Surg 186:275–283, 1998.

35. TJ Miner, CD Shriver, DP Jaques, ME Maniscalco-Theberge, DN Krag. Ultrasonographically guided injection improves localization of the radiolabeled sentinel lymph node in breast cancer. Ann Surg Oncol 5:315–321, 1998.

36. R Offodile, C Hoh, SH Barsky, SD Nelson, R Elashoff, FR Eilber, JS Economou, M Nguyen. Minimally invasive breast carcinoma staging using lymphatic mapping with radiolabeled dextran. Cancer 82:1704–1708, 1998.

37. JA Crossin, AC Hohnson, PB Stewart, WW Turner Jr. Gamma-probe-guided resection of the sentinel lymph node in breast cancer. Am Surg 64:666–669, 1998.

38. JM Barnwell, MA Arredondo, D Kollmorgen, JF Gibbs, D Lamonica, W Carson, P Zhang, J Winston, SB Edge. Sentinel node biopsy in breast cancer. Ann Surg Oncol 5:126–130, 1998.

39. BJ O'Hea, AD Hill, AM El-Shinrbiny, SD Yeh, PP Rosen, DG Coit, PI Borgen, HS Cody III. Sentinel lymph node biopsy in breast cancer: Initial experience at Memorial Sloan-Kettering Cancer Center. J Am Coll Surg 186:423–427, 1998.

40. M Koller, D Barsuk, D Zippel, S Engelberg, G Ben-Ari, MZ Papa. Sentinel lymph node involvement—a predictor for axillary node status with breast cancer—has the time come? Eur J Surg Oncol 24:166–168, 1998.

41. CJ Fisher, S Boyle, M Burke, AB Price. Intraoperative assessment of nodal status in the selection of patients with breast cancer for axillary clearance. Br J Surg 80:457–458, 1993.

42. DJ Hadjiminas, M Burke. Intraoperative assessment of nodal status in the selection of patients with breast cancer for axillary clearance. Br J Surg 81:1615–1616, 1994.

43. M Noguchi, M Minami, M Eachachi, T Taniya, I Miyazaki, Y Mizukami, A Nonomura. Intraoperative histologic assessment of surgical margins and lymph node metastases in breast conserving surgery. J Surg Oncol 60:185–190, 1995.

44. AE Giuliano, PS Dale, RR Turner, DL Morton, SW Evans, DL Krasne. Improved axillary staging of breast cancer with sentinel lymphadenectomy. Ann Surg 222:394–401, 1995.

45. RR Turner, DW Ollila, DL Krasne, AE Giuliano. Histopathological validation of the sentinel lymph node hypothesis for breast carcinoma. Ann Surg 226:271–278, 1997.

46. D Rosner, RN Bedwassi, J Vana, HW Baker, GP Murphy. Noninvasive breast carcinoma: Results of a national survey by the American College of Surgeons. Ann Surg 192:139–147, 1980.

47. National Cancer Database. 1991.

48. International (Ludwig) Breast Cancer Study Group. Prognostic importance of occult axillary lymph node micrometastases from breast cancer. Lancet 335:1565–1568, 1990.

49. I De Mascarel, F Bonichon, JM Coindre, M Trojani. Prognostic significance of breast cancer axillary lymph node micrometastases assessed by two special techniques; reevaluation with longer follow-up. Br J Cancer 66:523–527, 1992.

50. M Trojani, I De Mascarel, F Bonichon, JM Coindre, G Delsol. Micrometastases to

axillary lymph nodes from carcinoma of breast: detection of immunohistochemistry and prognostic significance. Br J Cancer 55:303–306, 1987.

51. PJ Hainsworth, JJ Tjandra, RG Stillwell, D Machet, MA Henderson, GC Rennie, IF McKenzie, RC Bennett. Detection and significance of occult metastases in node-negative breast cancer. Br J Surg 80:459–463, 1993.

52. JW Pickren. The significance of occult metastases; a study of breast cancer. Cancer 14:1266–1271, 1961.

53. ER Fisher, S Swamidoss, CH Lee, H Rockette, C Redmond, B Fisher. Detection and significance of occult axillary node metastases in patients with invasive breast cancer. Cancer 42:2025–2031, 1978.

54. PP Rosen, PE Saigo, DW Braun, E Weathers, AA Fracchia, DW Kinne. Axillary micro- and macrometastases in breast cancer: Prognostic significance of tumor size. Ann Surg 194:585–591, 1981.

55. EJ Wilkinson, LL Hause, RG Hoffman, JF Kuzma, DJ Rothwell, WL Donegan, LJ Clowry, UA Almagro, H Choi, AA Rimm. Occult axillary lymph node metastases in invasive breast carcinoma: characteristics of the primary tumor and significance of the metastases. Pathol Annu 17(Pt 2):67–91, 1982.

56. S Friedman, F Bertin, H Mouriesse, A Benchabat, J Genin, D Sarrazin, G Contesso. Importance of tumor cells in axillary node sinus margins (''clandestine'' metastases) discovered by serial sectioning in breast carcinoma. Acta Oncol 27:483–487, 1988.

57. B Cady. The need to reexamine axillary lymph node dissection in invasive breast cancer. Cancer 73:505–508, 1994.

58. MG Silverstein, ED Gierson, JR Waisman, GM Senofsky, WJ Colburn, P Gamagami. Axillary lymph node dissection for T1a breast carcinomas. Is it indicated? Cancer 73:664–667, 1994.

59. RE Wilson, WL Donegan, C Mettlin, N Natarajan, CR Smart, GP Murphy. The 1982 National survey of carcinoma of the breast in the United States by the American College of Surgeons. Surg Gynecol Obstet 159:309–318, 1984.

60. CL Carter, C Allen, DE Henson. Relation of tumor size, lymph node status and survival in 24,740 breast cancer cases. Cancer 63:181–187, 1989.

61. DW Ollila, MB Brennan, AE Giuliano. Therapeutic effect of sentinel lymphadenectomy in T1 breast cancer. Arch Surg 133:647–651, 1998.

62. KU Chu, A Bilchik, MB Brennan. Do all patients with sentinel node metastases from breast carcinoma need complete axillary node dissection? Presented in plenary session, Society of Surgical Oncology, 51st Annual Meeting, San Diego, 1998.

11

Lymphatic Mapping and Sentinel Lymphadenectomy in Carcinoma of the Vulva

Joanne A. de Hullu, Do A. Piers, Heimen Schraffordt Koops, Jan G. Aalders, and Ate G. J. van der Zee
Groningen University Hospital, Groningen, the Netherlands

INTRODUCTION

The value of lymphatic mapping and identification of the sentinel lymph node is currently being investigated in a variety of malignancies. This chapter deals with the possible role that lymphatic mapping may play in vulvar cancer. In order to set the stage, epidemiology, clinical features, staging, prognosis, and treatment of vulvar cancer are briefly summarized. This provides the clinical background information necessary to understand why further development of techniques to identify the sentinel node (or first-tier node, or first-echelon node) in vulvar cancer is warranted. Subsequently, the literature on lymphatic mapping and sentinel lymphadenectomy in vulvar cancer is reviewed. Possible methods for implementation of this novel diagnostic technique in clinical practice will be discussed.

ABOUT THE DISEASE

Vulvar cancer accounts for 3–4% of all female malignancies. The incidence rises from one per 100,000 at age 40 to 20 per 100,000 after age 80 [1]. In the Netherlands, 235 new patients with vulvar cancer were diagnosed in 1994 [2]. The incidence of vulvar cancer has remained stable in recent decades [3]. A rise in absolute numbers of vulvar cancer is expected because of the proportional increase in the average age of the population. The mean age at presentation is

185

about 70 years. Figure 1 shows the age distribution of new patients at Groningen University Hospital from 1979 to 1997. The most prominent presenting symptom of vulvar cancer is localized pruritus. Other common symptoms are a vulvar mass, bleeding, pain, discharge, or urinary tract symptoms [4,5]. Vulvar itching is often noted many years before malignant changes are documented and is often investigated only after trials of various medical regimens have been unsuccessful. In more than 50% of patients, there is a (patient's and doctor's) delay of more than a year before the diagnosis is established [4,6].

About 90% of vulvar cancers are of the squamous cell type. Melanoma, Paget's disease, adenocarcinoma, basal cell carcinoma, and sarcoma are much less common [1,2,5,7]. Most squamous cell cancers of the vulva present on the labia majora, but the labia minora, clitoris, and perineum also may be primary sites [8]. About 5% of vulvar cancers are multifocal [3]. This chapter particularly deals with squamous cell cancer of the vulva.

Vulvar cancer may spread by three routes. Spread by direct extension is infrequent. Initial spread usually occurs to the inguinofemoral lymph nodes. Dissemination via the bloodstream to other sites occurs late in the course of the disease and is rare in the absence of lymph node metastases [3]. Table 1 shows the staging system for vulvar cancer. Seventy percent of the patients are Stage I or II and have an excellent prognosis, with 5-year survivals of 98% and 85%, respectively [5,10]. The most important prognostic factor is the inguinofemoral

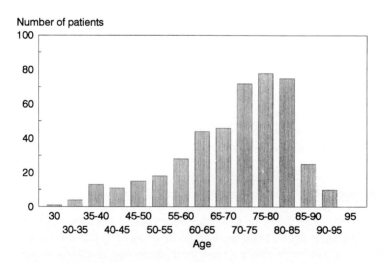

FIGURE 1   Age distribution of 440 patients with vulvar cancer at the Groningen University Hospital.

TABLE 1   Staging System for Vulvar Cancer of The International Federation of Gynecology and Obstetrics (FIGO)

Stage I	Lesions 2 cm or less in size confined to the vulva or perineum; no nodal metastasis
[Stage IA	Lesions 2 cm or less in size confined to the vulva or perineum and with stromal invasion no greater than 1.0 mm[a]; no nodal metastasis]
Stage II	Tumor confined to the vulva and/or perineum or more than 2 cm in the greatest dimension; no nodal metastasis
Stage III	Tumor of any size with (i) adjacent spread of the lower urethra and/or the vagina or anus and/or (ii) unilateral regional lymph node metastasis
Stage IVA	Tumor invades any of the following: upper urethra, bladder mucosa, rectal mucosa, pelvic bone, and/or bilateral regional node metastasis
Stage IVB	Any distant metastasis including pelvic lymph nodes

[a] The depth of invasion is defined as the measurement of the tumor from the epithelial–stromal junction of the adjacent most superficial dermal papilla to the deepest point of invasion.
Source: Ref. 9.

lymph node status. The 5-year survival rate for patients with uninvolved lymph nodes is approximately 90%, but this decreases to about 50% for patients whose nodes contain metastatic disease [3]. The number of diseased inguinofemoral lymph nodes is the most important single prognostic factor. Five-year survival decreases from 75% in patients with one or two metastatic lymph nodes to 24% when five or six lymph nodes are involved [10]. For Stages III and IV, 5-year survival rates are 40% and 13%, respectively [5].

TREATMENT

Surgery is first choice in the treatment of vulvar cancer. In the early part of this century, treatment mainly consisted of local excision and 5-year survival was a mere 20%. Overall survival figures rose to more than 60% when Taussig and Way introduced radical vulvectomy with *en bloc* bilateral inguinofemoral and pelvic lymphadenectomy to replace simple local excision [11,12]. Due to this dramatic improvement of prognosis, this radical surgical approach became the standard treatment for almost all patients with vulvar cancer. Over the past 15 years, however, the surgery has become more conservative. Significant advances have been made by the elimination of routine pelvic lymphadenectomy, introduction of radical local excision instead of radical vulvectomy, and unilateral or bilateral inguinofemoral lymphadenectomy via separate incisions in selected cases. In general, it appears that individualization of treatment results in high efficacy with less morbidity [3].

Postoperative adjuvant radiotherapy to the inguinofemoral and pelvic lymph nodes is indicated when more than one involved inguinofemoral lymph node is found or when tumor growth extends beyond the capsule of a lymph node [13,14]. Radiotherapy can also be part of alternative primary therapy in patients with midline tumors in order to preserve important anatomical structures like the clitoris, the urethra, and the anal sphincter [15,16]. In advanced disease, radiotherapy (in combination with chemotherapy and/or surgery) may be used as primary treatment [3]. The indications for chemotherapy are limited. A number of compounds are available as radiosensitizers and can be used in conjunction with radiotherapy, especially in advanced vulvar cancer [3].

COMPLICATIONS OF SURGICAL THERAPY

Radical vulvectomy with *en bloc* inguinofemoral lymph node dissection is remarkably well tolerated in spite of the extent of the surgery and the advanced age of the majority of the patients. The postoperative mortality rate is approximately 2%, usually as a result of pulmonary embolism or myocardial infarction [3,17]. Although overall survival figures are excellent with radical surgery, the short- and long-term morbidity associated with this procedure is substantial. Complications are related either to the radical vulvectomy or to the lymphadenectomy. Wound healing is often disturbed. Postoperative wound breakdown and infection occur with a frequency of up to 85%, often prolonging hospitalization [4]. Other early postoperative complications include urinary tract infection, seroma, phlebitis, deep venous thrombosis, and hemorrhage. Psychosexual disturbance is a major long-term problem, especially in young patients [18,19]. Edema of the lower extremities is an important late complication related to the lymphadenectomy. This unfortunate sequela is seen in up to 69% of patients, varying from minimal to moderate edema [4]. Fortunately, most patients respond favorably to elastic support. Urinary stress incontinence, hernia, prolapse, fistula, introital stenosis, and rectal dysfunction are less common late complications [3]. The excellent survival rate with—unfortunately—impressive postoperative morbidity have resulted in a search for less radical but equally effective surgery.

VULVECTOMY

Recent publications offer a still growing body of evidence that especially smaller primary vulvar tumors can be managed with hemivulvectomy or radical local excision instead of radical vulvectomy. An important factor to take into account when determining the management of the vulvar lesion is the condition of the remainder of the vulva. The presence of multifocal invasive lesions or widespread *in situ* neoplasia may preclude management by radical local excision [3]. Radical local excision implies a wide and deep excision of the primary tumor with surgical-free margins of at least 1 cm. The frequency of local recurrence is estimated to be 7% after local excision and 6% after radical vulvectomy for primary tumors less than 2 cm in size [20]. A tumor-involved margin is the most powerful predictor of local recurrence. A margin of less than 0.8 cm is associated with 50% chance of recurrence, whereas a 1-cm tumor-free margin results in a high rate of local control [21]. Tumors less than 2 cm in size can be treated with a local excision as long as surgical margins of 1 cm are obtained, resulting in lower morbidity but with a prognosis that is comparable with radical vulvectomy [22]. Close proximity to the anus may preclude adequate surgical margins in perineal lesions. Surgery in combination with radiotherapy should be considered in such cases. In conclusion, radical local excision appears to be a safe surgical alternative to radical vulvectomy in selected patients with an otherwise normal-appearing vulva.

LYMPHADENECTOMY

Thirty percent of all patients with vulvar cancer have inguinofemoral metastases and 20% of these patients will have pelvic metastases too [8,23]. For many decades, the generally accepted treatment has been to perform bilateral inguinofemoral lymphadenectomy in patients with vulvar cancer with a depth of invasion of more than 1 mm, even when the inguinofemoral nodes are not enlarged. The rationale for this approach is the assumption that the prognosis is better after elective inguinofemoral lymphadenectomy compared with surveillance of the groins. However, no randomized trials have addressed the issue of elective versus delayed inguinofemoral lymphadenectomy in patients with vulvar cancer and clinically normal nodes. Such a trial is unlikely to be performed in the future, as prospects are very poor for patients with vulvar cancer that recur in an initially untreated groin [24]. A trial comparing elective inguinofemoral lymphadenectomy versus elective radiotherapy of the groins was stopped prematurely because of an increased recurrence rate and a worse outcome for patients in the radiotherapy arm of the trial [25]. The substantial morbidity that ensues from lymph node dissection and the fact that the nodes are frequently free of disease justify the search for a more conservative approach. In this respect, the controversies surrounding the management of nonpalpable lymph nodes in carcinoma of the vulva resemble the situation in squamous cell cancer of the penis [26,27].

In vulvar cancer, it is generally accepted that inguinofemoral lymphadenectomy should be omitted only in patients with a tumor invading less than 1 mm (Stage Ia). Until now, only three cases of Stage Ia have been reported with inguinofemoral lymph node metastasis [28–30]. The existence of a more favorable ''microinvasive'' type of vulvar cancer was suggested in 1970, analogous to microinvasive cervical cancer [6,31]. The risk of lymph node metastasis in these vulvar cancers with a depth of invasion of less than 1 mm was estimated to be very low, which led to the advice to abandon routine inguinofemoral lymphadenectomy in these patients [6,32,33]. Further experience showed that the risk of inguinofemoral lymph node metastases is too high to omit lymphadenectomy in tumors that invade to a depth greater than 1 mm. Tumors with depths of invasion of 1–3 mm and 3–5 mm result in inguinofemoral lymph node metastases in 10% and 25%, respectively [3].

Pelvic lymph nodes are rarely, if ever, involved in the absence of metastatic vulvar cancer in the inguinofemoral nodes [8,23,34]. A randomized trial has been carried out to compare pelvic lymphadenectomy with pelvic radiotherapy in patients with inguinofemoral lymph node metastases after radical vulvectomy and bilateral inguinofemoral lymphadenectomy [35]. Survival proved to be better in the patients who received postoperative radiotherapy. Based on the low incidence of metastatic pelvic lymph nodes in patients with negative inguinofemoral nodes, routine pelvic lymphadenectomy should no longer be performed, whereas postoperative radiotherapy is indicated if more than one inguinofemoral lymph node metastasis is found [8,23,34,35].

The rationale for inguinofemoral lymphadenectomy via separate incisions instead of *en bloc* is that dissemination to the inguinofemoral lymph nodes does not occur in continuity but by embolization [36]. Preservation of a ''skin bridge'' results in a lower frequency of postoperative wound breakdown and less risk of lymphedema of the legs. Hacker and co-workers found no difference in survival between radical vulvectomy with *en bloc* inguinofemoral lymphadenectomy when compared with surgery via separate incisions, whereas the morbidity was less in the latter patient group [37]. Despite this decreased morbidity, seroma and lymphadema are still frequently observed [37]. Tumor recurrence in the skin bridge has been reported [38,39].

Unilateral inguinofemoral lymphadenectomy in lateral tumors with a medial margin of more than 1 cm from the midline is justified, because contralateral metastases are rarely present in the absence of ipsilateral inguinofemoral metastases [3,40]. However, contralateral lymphadenectomy should be performed in combination with postoperative radiotherapy when ipsilateral inguinofemoral nodes are involved. Isolated contralateral metastases have been found in only one study [41].

RATIONALE FOR SENTINEL LYMPH NODE BIOPSY IN VULVAR CANCER PATIENTS

Several of the characteristics of vulvar cancer as described earlier suggest the need for less invasive diagnostic techniques for evaluation of clinically uninvolved inguinofemoral lymph nodes. The majority of patients with vulvar cancer present with early-stage disease and have a low frequency of nodal involvement.

However, most clinicians are reluctant to abandon elective inguinofemoral lymphadenectomy and to follow a ''wait and watch'' policy because of the dismal prognosis in patients with a groin recurrence. Elective inguinofemoral lymphade-nectomy is associated with significant short-term and long-term morbidities. He-matogenous metastases are rare.

At present, no reliable noninvasive techniques for the detection of inguino-femoral lymph node metastases are available. Physical examination of the groins is inaccurate in 25% of cases [4]. The percentage of error in clinical appraisal increases progressively with the stage of disease: from 18% for Stage I to 44% for Stage IV [4]. Little information exists on the value of imaging techniques such as magnetic resonance imaging and computerized tomography. The results of the use of ultrasound and positron emission tomography are disappointing [42,43]. All these reasons provide a rationale for lymphatic mapping with sentinel lymphadenectomy in patients with vulvar cancer.

STUDIES ON LYMPHATIC MAPPING AND SENTINEL LYMPHADENECTOMY IN PATIENTS WITH VULVAR CANCER

DiSaia in 1979 was the first to postulate that the superficial groin nodes may serve as sentinel lymph nodes for more deeply situated nodes in patients with vulvar cancer [18]. Patients with clinically normal nodes underwent intraopera-tive mapping through a modified incision. No complete lymphadenectomy was performed if frozen-section analysis of the superficial lymph nodes did not show metastasis. However, in later studies of early vulvar cancer, femoral node metas-tasis was reported after biopsy of tumor-free superficial inguinofemoral nodes [44].

In 1983, Iversen and Aas presented a scintigraphy study of lymph drainage of the vulva in patients with cervical cancer scheduled for radical surgery [45]. The conclusions of this study were as follows: in all patients, the vulvar lymph flow passes to the inguinofemoral and pelvic lymph nodes; clitoris and perineum have bilateral drainage; the main lymphatic pathway is ipsilateral after injection in the labium, but nearly 70% also have some contralateral lymph drainage; and no direct pathways to pelvic nodes exist with bypassing of the inguinofemoral nodes. A subsequent pilot study was undertaken in vulvar cancer patients to corre-late patterns of lymphatic drainage with clinical and histopathological findings of the inguinofemoral lymph nodes [46]. However, radioactive tracer uptake pat-terns in the inguinofemoral lymph nodes were not predictive for the presence or absence of metastases.

In 1994, Levenback and co-workers published the first feasibility study of sentinel node biopsy using isosulfan blue in nine patients with vulvar cancer [47]. No technique-related complications were observed and the sentinel lymph node status was indicative of the lymph basin status in all patients. Extension of the study to 21 patients showed that the sentinel lymph node technique with isosulfan blue was a safe and simple technique and that it allowed identification of the sentinel node in 66% of the dissected groins [48]. In 1997, DeCesare and co-workers reported a pilot study on intraoperative gamma-ray detection for identification of the sentinel node [49]. After induction of general anesthesia, a technetium-99m (^{99m}Tc)-labeled nanocolloid (Nanocoll®, Sorin Radiofarmaci S.r.l., Saluggia, Italy) was injected around the tumor. A hand-held gamma detection probe (Neoprobe 1000®, Neoprobe Corporation, Dublin, OH) was used for identification of the first-tier node. This technique correctly indicated the nodal status in all four cases with metastatic inguinofemoral dissemination and in all 16 groins without disease. The ^{99m}Tc-labeled colloid had to be injected at least 1 h before the procedure in order to allow the background radiation in the groin to decrease sufficiently for the sentinel lymph node to be identified.

At our institution, a feasibility study involving 11 patients was performed to determine whether the sentinel node could be identified using a combination of a preoperatively administered ^{99m}Tc-labeled nanocolloid and intraoperatively administered patent blue dye (Blue Patenté V, Guerbet, Aulney-Sous-Bois, France) [50]. Lymphoscintigraphy was performed on the day before the operation, with a peritumoral injection of a ^{99m}Tc nanocolloid. The first-appearing persistent focal accumulation was designated as the sentinel lymph node. The location of this sentinel lymph node was marked on the overlying skin. The subsequent day, patent blue dye was injected intradermally around the primary tumor, approximately 10 min prior to the surgical resection. A hand-held gamma detection probe was used during the operation to localize the sentinel lymph node. After removing the sentinel lymph node(s), complete inguinofemoral lymphadenectomy was performed and these lymph nodes were sent for histopathological examination separately. In 10 evaluable patients, preoperative administration of the ^{99m}Tc nanocolloid was well tolerated. One patient refused further participation just before the injection of the radioactive tracer because of anxiety about pain. All 18 sentinel lymph nodes were identified with the probe. Ten of the 18 nodes were stained blue or had a blue-stained lymphatic duct leading up to them (56%). The inguinofemoral lymph nodes were free of disease in eight patients, and both sentinel and nonsentinel nodes contained metastatic disease in the remaining two patients. We concluded that identification of the sentinel lymph node is feasible in patients with vulvar cancer by the combination of a preoperatively administered ^{99m}Tc-labeled nanocolloid and intraoperatively administered blue dye (see case report and Figs. 2 and 3).

Two other feasibility studies concerning identification of the sentinel lymph node in vulvar cancer with comparable results were published [51,52]. Recently, Ansink et al. published a multicenter study to investigate the negative predictive value of the sentinel node procedure in 51 patients [53]. Only blue dye was used,

TABLE 2   Studies on Lymphatic Mapping of Squamous Cell Carcinoma of the Vulva

Study [Ref.]	Patients (*n*)	Tracer	Blue dye	Scintigraphy	SLN[a] found (groins)	False negative SLN
Levenback et al. 1995 [48]	21	no	yes	no	66%	0
DeCesare et al. 1997 [49]	10	yes	no	no	100%	0
De Cicco et al. 1997 [51]	15	yes	no	yes	100%	0
de Hullu et al. 1998 [50]	10	yes	yes	yes	100%	0
Rodier et al. 1999 [52]	8	yes	yes	yes	100%	1
Ansink et al. 1999 [53]	51	no	yes	no	56%	2

[a] SLN = sentinel lymph node.

and the identification of sentinel lymph nodes was successful in only 56% of the groins. Moreover, in two patients false-negative sentinel lymph nodes were found. (See Table 2 for a summary of the studies). In this multicenter study, five referral centers participated. However, three of the five centers included less than 10 patients, and it is generally accepted that there is a learning curve in performing the SLN procedure. Morton suggested a learning phase of at least 30 consecutive cases per center for cutaneous melanoma. In view of the fact that there are only minimal variations in the anatomy of lymph flow in vulvar cancer to the inguinofemoral lymph nodes (compared with the sometimes unpredictable lymph flow of cutaneous melanoma), the learning curve will probably be steeper, but at least the first 10 patients (with SLN procedures in 10–20 groins), should be regarded as the learning phase for the SLN procedure in vulvar cancer.

CASE REPORT

A 76-year-old woman was referred to the Groningen University Hospital for treatment of a suspicious lesion of the vulva. A tumor with a diameter of 3 cm was found on the left labium minus, encroaching on the clitoris. A punch biopsy showed squamous cell cancer with a depth of invasion of 4 mm. Because of the location of the tumor, radical local excision with bilateral completion inguinofemoral lymphadenectomy with sentinel lymphadenectomy was performed. Figure 2 shows the location of the tumor. Figure 3 shows the preoperative lymphoscintigram. One inguinofemoral sentinel lymph node is depicted on each side. At operation, both sentinel nodes were identified with the hand-held gamma probe. The sentinel node in the left groin was also stained blue. Histopathological examina-

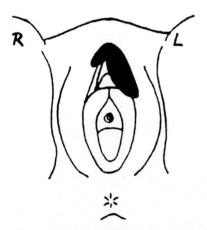

FIGURE 2   Location of the tumor of the patient described in the case report.

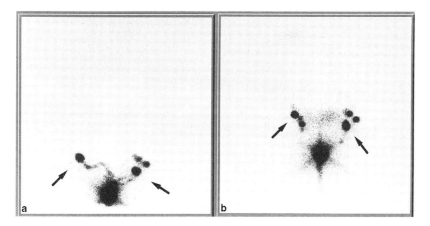

FIGURE 3   Anterior lymphoscintigraphy at 40 min postinjection (a) and after 6.5 h (b). One first-tier node is shown on either side. Several second-tier lymph nodes are also depicted. The early image depicts the lymphatic ducts.

tion of the primary lesion showed a highly differentiated squamous cell cancer. Neither the sentinel nodes nor the other 15 nonsentinel nodes contained metastatic disease. Fifteen months after the procedure there were no signs of recurrence.

DISCUSSION

Several issues are important in a discussion on lymphatic mapping in vulvar cancer. An important aspect is whether to use peritumoral blue dye as a single technique or to use blue dye in combination with a radioactive tracer. The technique with blue dye alone, as used by Levenback and co-workers, has several advantages: blue dye is cheap and its use avoids exposure of patients and medical personnel to the risk of radiation. No expensive equipment is required. The whole procedure is performed intraoperatively under general anesthesia, thereby avoiding painful preoperative perilesional injections [47,48]. However, the technique with only blue dye also has some important disadvantages: the incision has to be larger, and intraoperative mapping with only blue dye is more difficult and more time-consuming. Based on a multicenter study in 51 patients, Ansink et al. concluded that sentinel lymph node detection with only blue dye is not feasible (56% identification of the sentinel lymph node), and its negative predictive value is too low (two patients with false-negative sentinel lymph nodes) [53]. Larger experience with sentinel lymphadenectomy in melanoma and breast cancer has demonstrated that the combination of intraoperatively administered blue dye together with preoperatively performed lymphoscintigraphy and use of the intraoperative gamma probe enables one to find sentinel node in more patients than is possible with intraoperative blue dye alone [54,55]. Kapteijn and co-workers recently compared the two techniques in patients with cutaneous melanoma. They were able to find the sentinel node in 99.5% of the patients with the combined technique, whereas the node was identified in only 84% with blue dye alone [56]. The same group also showed a high reproducibility of lymphoscintigraphy in assessing the location and the number of sentinel lymph nodes in cutaneous melanoma [57].

Although the numbers from our own institution in vulvar cancer are still small, a trend can be found when our results are compared with those of Levenback. Our combined technique allowed sentinel node identification in 100% of the patients and in 88% of the groins, compared with 86% and 66%, respectively, in Levenback's series with the blue dye technique only. Another argument is that identification of the sentinel node is generally easier using the combined technique with the intraoperative gamma probe guiding the dissection. It is the experience of several authors that a learning phase of 20–40 patients is usual for the blue dye technique (Nieweg and Schraffordt Koops, personal communication). The combined technique is mastered more quickly. This is an important issue, especially in vulvar cancer because it is a rare gynecological tumor. Few gynecologists are likely to gain as much experience as the general surgeons dealing with breast cancer or melanoma. A final important argument in favor of use of the combined technique in vulvar cancer is that only one groin needs to be explored when preoperative lymphoscintigraphy shows unilateral drainage.

Another issue to be considered is the optimum time for lymphoscintigraphy. DeCesare injected the ^{99m}Tc-labeled colloid after induction of general anesthesia, thereby avoiding painful preoperative peritumoral injections. A disadvantage of the immediately preoperative radioactivity injection is the nonspecific background radiation in the groin. It takes at least 1 h before evaluation with the hand-held probe can commence. Also, dynamic imaging is impossible with this approach and identification of the first-tier node is difficult. Therefore, all radioactive nodes have to be harvested. The unavoidable overflow of radioactive tracer from a first-tier node to higher-tier (nonsentinel) nodes will result in removal of more nodes than is necessary. Our study on the identification of the sentinel node with preoperative administration of the radioactive tracer showed the feasibility of this technique. This approach avoids the above-mentioned disadvantages of intraoperative administration of the radioactive tracer. Another advantage of preoperative lymphoscintigraphy is that it allows identification of sentinel nodes that are in an unexpected extreme lateral or medial position. Such locations were occasionally observed by Levenback.

Recent studies in melanoma and breast cancer patients show very low frequencies of false-negative sentinel lymph nodes [54,55]. In the combined 115 patients in 6 studies in vulvar cancer, three false-negative sentinel lymph nodes have been reported so far [48–53]. In two patients in whom false-negative sentinel lymph nodes were found, only blue dye was used. The results with the combined technique are encouraging, but it is obvious that more data have to be collected until meaningful statistical conclusions can be reached with regard to the predictive value of a negative sentinel lymph node for the tumor status of the entire groin. This may take several years. The predictive value of a negative sentinel lymph node can be calculated to be higher than 90% (within 95% confidence interval) when in 34 patients no or only one false-negative sentinel lymph node is found. For patients with a vulvar cancer less than 2 cm in size with an estimated frequency of inguinofemoral metastases of 10%, application of the sentinel node technique with a previously proven sensitivity of more than 90% implies that in 100 patients, one inguinofemoral lymph node metastasis will be missed at the most. We are currently extending our feasibility study to 34 patients with tumor-positive groins. Identification of all these patients with metastatic disease would indicate a sensitivity of this approach of 100% with a confidence interval of 90–100%. If, indeed, sensitivity of our combined detection technique proves to be more than 90%, we will perform a subsequent study in which patients with early-stage vulvar cancer and a negative sentinel node will be spared a full inguinofemoral lymphadenectomy. At present, we certainly do not advocate application of lymphatic mapping by individual departments that do not participate in trials in which the safety of this approach is closely evaluated.

CONCLUSIONS

The clinical characteristics of vulvar cancer imply a possibly important role of lymphatic mapping in patients with this disease. Currently available studies on the identification of the sentinel lymph node in vulvar cancer are preliminary but show that so far the histopathology of the sentinel lymph node is representative of the entire inguinofemoral region if the sentinel node is free of disease. At present, we prefer identification of the sentinel node by a combined technique with a preoperatively administered ^{99m}Tc-labeled nanocolloid and intraoperative use of patent blue dye and a gamma detection probe, thereby allowing preoperative lymphoscintigraphy with the designation of sentinel lymph nodes. Further validation of the technique in patients with vulvar cancer hopefully will spare future patients with a negative sentinel node a full groin dissection with its associated short-term and long-term morbidities.

REFERENCES

1. DJS Hunter. Cancer of the vulva: a review of 361 patients. Gynecol Oncol 3:117–123, 1975.

2. O Visser, JWW Coebergh, LJ Schouten. Incidence of Cancer in the Netherlands 1993. Utrecht: Hoonte-Holland bv, 1996.
3. NF Hacker. Vulvar cancer. In: JS Berek, NF Hacker, eds. Practical Gynecologic Oncology. 2d ed. Baltimore, MD: Williams & Wilkins, 1994, pp. 403–439.
4. KC Podratz, RE Symmonds, WF Taylor, TJ Williams. Carcinoma of the vulva: analysis of treatment and survival. Obstet Gynecol 61:63–74, 1983.
5. C Rosen, H Malmström. Invasive cancer of the vulva. Gynecol Oncol 65:213–217, 1997.
6. F Rutledge, JP Smith, EW Franklin. Carcinoma of the vulva. Am J Obstet Gynecol 106:1117–1130, 1970.
7. SR Sturgeon, LA Brinton, SS Devesa, RJ Kurman. In situ and invasive vulvar cancer incidence trends (1973 to 1987). Am J Obstet Gynecol 166:1482–1485, 1992.
8. NF Hacker, JS Berek, LD Lagasse, RS Leuchter, JG Moore. Management of regional lymph nodes and their prognostic influence in vulvar cancer. Obstet Gynecol 61: 408–412, 1983.
9. JH Shepherd. Staging announcement. FIGO staging of gynecologic cancers; cervical and vulva. Int J Gynecol Cancer 5:319, 1995.
10. HD Homesley, BN Bundy, A Sedlis, E Yordan, JS Berek, A Jahshan, R Mortel. Assessment of current International Federation of Gynecology and Obstetrics staging of vulvar carcinoma relative to prognostic factors for survival (a gynecologic oncology group study). Am J Obstet 164:997–1004, 1991.
11. FJ Taussig. Cancer of the vulva: an analysis of 155 cases. Am J Obstet Gynecol 40:764–779, 1940.
12. S Way. Carcinoma of the vulva. Am J Obstet Gynecol 79:692–697, 1960.
13. D Paladini, P Cross, A Lopes, JM Monaghan. Prognostic significance of lymph node variables in squamous cell carcinoma of the vulva. Cancer 74:2491–2496, 1994.
14. J van der Velden, ACM van Lindert, FB Lammes, FJW ten Kate, DMDS Sie-Go, H Oosting, APM Heintz. Extracapsular growth of lymph node metastases in squamous cell cancer of the vulva: the impact on recurrence and survival. Cancer 75: 2885–2890, 1995.
15. GM Thomas, AJ Dembo, SCP Bryson, R Osborbe, AD DePetrillo. Changing concepts in the management of vulvar cancer. Gynecol Oncol 42:9–21, 1991.
16. NF Hacker, JS Berek, GJF Juillard, LD Lagasse. Preoperative radiation therapy for locally advanced vulvar cancer. Cancer 54:2056–2061, 1984.
17. T Iversen, JG Aalders, A Christensen, P Kolstad. Squamous cell carcinoma of the vulva: a review of 424 patients, 1956–1974. Gynecol Oncol 9:271–279, 1980.
18. PJ DiSaia, WT Creasman, WM Rich. An alternative approach to early cancer of the vulva. Am J Obstet Gynecol 133:825–830, 1979.
19. BL Andersen, NF Hacker. Psychosexual adjustment after vulvar surgery. Obstet Gynecol 62:457–462, 1983.
20. K van der Velden. Some aspects of the management of squamous cell carcinoma of the vulva. Academic thesis, Utrecht University, 1997.
21. JM Heaps, YS Fu, FJ Montz, NF Hacker, JS Berek. Surgical–pathological variables predictive of local recurrence in squamous cell carcinoma of the vulva. Gynecol Oncol 38:309–314, 1990.

22. R Farias-Eisner, FD Cirisano, D Grouse, RS Leuchter, BY Karlan, LE Lagasse, JS Berek. Conservative and individualized surgery for early squamous carcinoma of the vulva: the treatment of choice for stage I and II ($T_{1-2}N_{0-1}M_0$) disease. Gynecol Oncol 53:55–58, 1994.

23. SL Curry, JT Wharton, F Rutledge. Positive lymph nodes in vulvar squamous carcinoma. Gynecol Oncol 9:63–67, 1980.

24. NF Hacker, RK Nieberg, JS Berek, RS Leuchter, WE Lucas, HK Tamimi, JF Nolan, JG Moore, LD Lagasse. Superficially invasive vulvar cancer with nodal metastases. Gynecol Oncol 15:65–77, 1983.

25. F Stehman, B Bundy, G Thomas, M Varia, T Okagaki, J Roberts, J Bell, PB Heller. Groin dissection versus groin radiation in carcinoma of the vulva: a Gynecologic Oncology Group Study. Int J Radiat Oncol Biol Phys 24:389–396, 1992.

26. D Theodorescu, P Russo, Z Zhang, C Morash, WR Fair. Outcomes of initial surveillance of invasive squamous cell carcinoma of the penis and negative nodes. J Urol 155:1626–1631, 1996.

27. S Horenblas, H van Tinteren, JFM Delemarre, LMF Moonen, V Lustig, EW van Waardenburg. Squamous cell carcinoma of the penis. III. Treatment of regional lymph nodes. J Urol 149:492–497, 1993.

28. A Sedlis, H Homesley, BN Bundy, R Marshall, E Yordan, N Hacker, JH Lee, C Whitney. Positive groin lymph nodes in superficial squamous cell vulvar cancer. Am J Obstet Gynecol 156:1159–1164, 1987.

29. F Atamtede, D Hoogerland. Regional lymph node recurrence following local excision for microinvasive vulvar carcinoma. Gynecol Oncol 34:125–128, 1989.

30. J Van der Velden, CD Kooyman, ACM Van Lindert, APM Heintz. A stage Ia vulvar carcinoma with an inguinal lymph node recurrence after local excision. A case report and literature review. Int J Gynecol Cancer 2:157–159, 1992.

31. EW Franklin, FD Rutledge. Prognostic factors in epidermoid carcinoma of the vulva. Obstet Gynecol 37:892–901, 1971.

32. JT Wharton, S Gallager, FN Rutledge. Microinvasive carcinoma of the vulva. Am J Obstet Gynecol 118:159–162, 1974.

33. GR Dipaola, N Gomez-Rueda, L Arrighi. Relevance of microinvasion in carcinoma of the vulva. Obstet Gynecol 45:647–649, 1975.

34. JM Morris. A formula for selective lymphadenectomy. Obstet Gynecol 50:152–158, 1977.

35. HD Homesley, BN Bundy, A Sedlis, L Adcock. Radiation therapy versus pelvic node resection for carcinoma of the vulva with positive groin nodes. Obstet Gynecol 68:733–740, 1986.

36. RA Willis. The Spread of Tumours in the Human Body. 3rd ed. London: Butterworth, 1973, pp. 19–30.

37. NF Hacker, RS Leuchter, JS Berek, TW Castaldo, LD Lagasse. Radical vulvectomy and bilateral inguinal lymphadenectomy through separate groin incisions. Obstet Gynecol 58:574–579, 1981.

38. MJ Schulz, M Penalver. Recurrent vulvar carcinoma in the intervening tissue bridge in early invasive stage I disease treated by radical vulvectomy and bilateral groin dissection through separate incisions. Gynecol Oncol 35:383–386, 1989.

39. RN Grimshaw, JB Murdoch, JM Monaghan. Radical vulvectomy and bilateral ingui-

nal–femoral lymphadenectomy through separate incisions—experience with 100 cases. Int J Gynecol Cancer 3:18–23, 1993.

40. MPM Burger, H Hollema, J Bouma. The side of groin node metastases in unilateral vulvar carcinoma. Int J Gynecol Cancer 6:318–322, 1996.

41. JF Magrina, MJ Webb, TA Gaffey, RE Symmonds. Stage I squamous cell cancer of the vulva. Am J Obstet Gynecol 134:453–459, 1981.

42. PJ Mäkelä, A Leminen, M Kääriäinen, P Lehtovirta. Pretreatment sonographic evaluation of inguinal lymph nodes in patients with vulvar malignancy. J Ultrasound Med 5:255–258, 1993.

43. JA de Hullu, J Pruim, TH Qué, JGS Aalders, H Boonstra, W Vaalburg, H Hollema, AGJ van der Zee. Noninvasive detection of inguinofemoral lymph node metastases in squamous cell cancer (SCC) of the vulva by L-[1-^{11}C]-tyrosine positron emission tomography (PET). Int J Gynecol Cancer 9:141–146, 1999.

44. J Chu, HK Tamimi, DC Figge. Femoral node metastases with negative superficial inguinal nodes in early vulvar cancer. Am J Obstet Gynecol 140:337–338, 1981.

45. T Iversen, M Aas. Lymph drainage from the vulva. Gynecol Oncol 16:179–189, 1983.

46. DPJ Barton, C Berman, D Cavanagh, WS Roberts, MS Hoffman, JV Fiorica, MA Finan. Lymphoscintigraphy in vulva cancer: a pilot study. Gynecol Oncol 46:341–344, 1992.

47. C Levenback, TW Burke, DM Gershenson, M Morris, A Malpica, MI Ross. Intraoperative lymphatic mapping for vulvar cancer. Obstet Gynecol 84:163–167, 1994.

48. C Levenback, TW Burke, M Morris, A Malpica, KR Lucas, DM Gershenson. Potential applications of intraoperative lymphatic mapping in vulvar cancer. Gynecol Oncol 59:216–220, 1995.

49. SL DeCesare, JV Fiorica, WS Roberts, D Reintgen, H Arango, MS Hoffman, C Puleo, D Cavanagh. A pilot study utilizing intraoperative lymphoscintigraphy for identification of the sentinel lymph nodes in vulvar cancer. Gynecol Oncol 66:425–428, 1997.

50. JA de Hullu, MHE Doting, DA Piers, H Hollema, JG Aalders, H Schraffordt Koops, H Boonstra, AGJ van der Zee. Identification of the sentinel lymph nodes with [99m]technetium labeled nanocolloid and blue due in squamous cell cancer of the vulva. J Nucl Med 39:1381–1385, 1998.

51. C De Cicco, M Sideri, M Bartolomei, A Maggioni, N Colombo, L Bocciolone, M Chinol, L Leonardi, C Mangioni, G Paganelli. Sentinel node detection by lymphoscintigraphy and gamma detecting probe in patients with vulvar cancer (abstr). J Nucl Med 38:33P, 1997.

52. JF Rodier, JC Janser, T Routiot, E David, G Ott, O Schneegans, JP Ghnassia. Sentinel node biopsy in vulvar malignancies: a preliminary feasibility study. Oncol Rep 6:1249–1252, 1999.

53. AC Ansink, DMDS Sie-Go, J van der Velden, EA Sijmons, A de Barros Lopes, JM Monaghan, GG Kenter, JB Murdoch, FJW ten Kate, APM Heintz. Identification of sentinel lymph nodes in vulvar carcinoma patients with the aid of a patent blue V injection. Cancer 86:652–656, 1999.

54. DN Krag, SJ Meijer, DL Weaver, BW Loggie, SP Harlow, KK Tanabe, EH Laughin,

JC Alex. Minimal-access surgery for staging of malignant melanoma. Arch Surg 130:654–658, 1995.

55. JJ Albertini, GH Lyman, C Cox, R Yeatman, L Balducci, N Ku, S Shivers, C Berman, K Wells, D Rapaport, A Shons, J Horton, H Greenberg, S Nicosia, R Clark, A Cantor, DS Reintgen. Lymphatic mapping and sentinel node biopsy in the patient with breast cancer. JAMA 276:1818–1822, 1996.

56. BAE Kapteijn. Biopsy of the sentinel node in melanoma, penile carcinoma and breast carcinoma. The case for lymphatic mapping. Academic thesis, University of Amsterdam, 1997.

57. BAE Kapteijn, OE Nieweg, RA Valdés Olmos, IH Liem, RKL Baidjnath Panday, CA Hoefnagel, BBR Kroon. Reproducibility of lymphoscintigraphy for lymphatic mapping in cutaneous melanoma. J Nucl Med 37:972–975, 1997.

12

Lymphatic Mapping and Sentinel Lympadenectomy in Carcinoma of the Penis

Simon Horenblas and Willem Meinhardt
The Netherlands Cancer Institute, Amsterdam, the Netherlands

Liesbeth Jansen
Gelre Hospital, Lukas Site, Apeldoorn, the Netherlands

INTRODUCTION

The vast majority of penile cancers are squamous cell carcinomas. The incidence of this type of cancer varies across the world from 7.9/100,000 in Brazil to 0.9/100,000 in the Netherlands. Smoking, foreskin pathology, and human papilloma virus infection are generally considered causal factors. The rarity of this disease in Western countries has precluded large-scale prospective randomized clinical trials. As treatment recommendations have been based mostly on retrospective studies, some aspects of management are still controversial. Questions that remain to be answered are the safety of organ-preserving procedures and the best management of the regional nodes. Controversies include the timing and extent of regional lymph node dissection. Should a node dissection be done in every patient presenting with a penile cancer and should the node dissection be inguinal or ilio-inguinal, unilateral or bilateral?

Lymphatic mapping with sentinel lymphadenectomy can be of help in solving some of these dilemmas. In this chapter, we will present the rationale for this approach and the results that have been obtained so far.

LYMPHATIC DRAINAGE PATTERNS AND NATURAL HISTORY OF PENILE CANCER

Anatomic studies by Rouvière at the beginning of this century and subsequent studies by Daseler, as well as clinical observations, have given us insight into normal lymphatic drainage patterns of the penis [1,2]. The lymph nodes in the groin are considered to be the primary regional nodes. The pelvic (iliac) nodes are second-tier nodes.

Squamous cell carcinoma is characterized by local invasion and regional spread, with late onset of hematogenous dissemination. Lymph node metastasis is an adverse prognostic factor for survival. However, patients with minimal involvement of the nodes have an excellent prognosis after regional lymphadenectomy. By contrast, most patients with extensive inguinal metastases or spread to the pelvic nodes die of their disease, hence, the rationale to perform a lymph node dissection at the earliest possible moment to remove metastases at a time when they are still clinically occult. By definition, occult metastases cannot be detected by simple physical examination. Analysis at our institution has shown that the negative predictive value of normal findings at physical examination (probability of absence of metastasis with negative findings at physical examination) of the inguinal region is 88%. Lymphangiography, ultrasound, computerized tomography, and magnetic resonance imaging are all incapable of improving this figure [3]. This leads us to state that no test is more reliable than physical examination in assessing clinically node-negative patients with squamous cell carcinoma of the penis and that physical examination has limitations. The limited value of clinical methods in detecting occult metastasis and the excellent survival figures of patients with minimal nodal involvement have led some investigators to recommend a lymph node dissection for all patients presenting with penile cancer. However, more than 80% of these node dissections are unnecessary because of the absence of nodal involvement in the resected specimen. Some 20–40% of the patients develop short-term and/or long-term complications such as wound-healing problems and lymphedema of the limb and/or the genital area [4]. Based on studies at our and other institutions, risk profiles for nodal involvement have been established [5]. Low-risk and high-risk patients are defined according to the extent of the primary tumor and the grade of differentiation. Examining the high-risk category patients only, 40% of the elective node dissections at our institution were unnecessary because of the absence of node metastasis. The need for better detection of occult metastasis is clearly apparent.

SENTINEL NODE BIOPSY

In 1977, Cabanas published his study of lymphatic drainage of the penis using pedal and penile lymphangiography [6]. He identified a lymph node that was always visualized in the same position and named it the sentinel node. This node was considered to be the first node reached by cancerous cells. Based on the assumption of orderly progression of lymphatic tumor spread, absence of metastatic deposits in the sentinel node would obviate the need for a regional lymph node dissection. This is the first use of the phrase ''sentinel node'' in the literature.

The sentinel node was described as being situated medial to the superficial epigastric vein. Its identification was based on static anatomical landmarks. This procedure did not take into account the individual drainage pattern of each tumor and the diverse anatomy of lymphatic drainage in individual patients [7]. Cabanas's sentinel node concept for penile carcinoma has been regarded with scepticism by several other investigators and has never become universally accepted. A number of false-negative biopsies have been reported [8–12].

Morton and co-workers took the sentinel node concept one step further in patients with melanoma [13]. They identified the sentinel node with the aid of a vital dye through *individual* visualization of lymphatic channels originating in the primary tumor. We took this innovation back to penile cancer for a prospective study of this new approach. In addition to the blue dye technique, we explored the value of lymphoscintigraphy with a ^{99m}Tc nanocolloid as a tracer for preoperative evaluation and the value of a gamma detection probe for intraoperative guidance.

LYMPHATIC MAPPING AND SENTINEL LYMPHADENECTOMY STUDY

From January 1994, all clinically node-negative patients with squamous cell carcinoma of the penis were enrolled in this study with the exception of patients with T1 tumors or carcinoma *in situ*. These latter patients are assumed to be at a low risk of having occult metastases. The study group consisted of 40 consecutive patients with a median age of 65 years (range: 28–87 years). Four of these patients presented with a recurrent tumor of the penis after previous penis-conserving therapy. Two patients with palpable unilateral lymph node metastases, proven by fine-needle-aspiration cytology, were included in the study for the clinically unaffected side.

Scintigraphy of lymphatic drainage was performed the day before surgery. An amount of 60 MBq of a technetium-99m (^{99m}Tc)-labeled nanocolloid (Nanocoll®, Sorin Radiofarmaci S.r.I., Saluggia, Italy in a volume of 0.3–0.4 mL was injected around the tumor. Immediately after injection, dynamic acquisition was started for a period of 20 minutes using a gamma camera (ADAC Vertex, Milpitas, CA) to visualize the lymphatic flow. Subsequently, anterior and lateral static views were obtained for an acquisition duration of 5 min each (Fig. 1) and repeated 2 h after injection. Sentinel nodes were defined as nodes receiving direct drainage from the site of injection. The location of each sentinel node was marked on the skin with a dye. The following day, 1 mL of patent blue dye (Blue Patenté

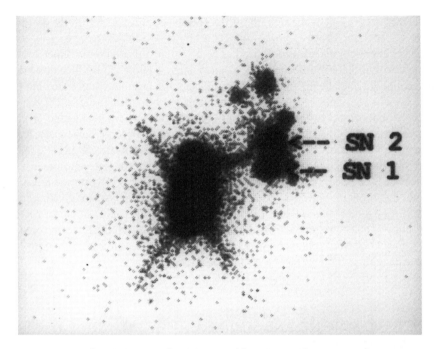

FIGURE 1 Lymphoscintigram of a 66-year-old patient with a T2 penile carcinoma. From the site of injection (tumor), there is drainage to two sentinel nodes (marked) in the left groin. Several nonsentinel nodes are also clearly seen.

V, Guerbet, Aulney-Sous-Bois, France) was injected intradermally around the tumor in the same way as injection of the radiopharmaceutical (Fig. 2). A few minutes later, a small incision was made over the skin mark. The sentinel node was identified by tracing blue lymphatic channels leading to blue lymph nodes and by using a gamma detection probe (Neoprobe 1000®, Neoprobe Corporation, Dublin, OH). Once identified, the sentinel node was removed and the wound was scanned for remaining radioactivity. Pathological examination consisted of routine paraffin sections and hematoxylin & eosin staining. Immunohistochemical staining using antibodies against pankeratin (Dako, Copenhagen, Denmark) and CAM 5.2 (Becton Dickinson, San Jose, CA) was used only recently. The grade of differentiation was determined according to Broders [14].

Regional lymph node dissection was reserved for patients with a tumor-positive sentinel node. All patients were followed at 2-month intervals during the first 2 years after surgery. The median period of follow-up for all patients was 9 months (range: 18 days to 45 months). One patient was lost to follow-up.

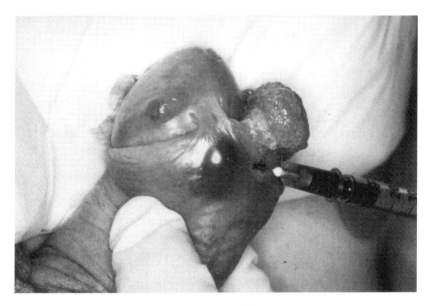

Figure 2   Injection of patent blue dye around the tumor.

RESULTS

Preoperative lymphoscintigraphy showed bilateral drainage in 30 patients and unilateral drainage in 8 patients, and no sentinel node was visualized in 2 patients. A total of 92 sentinel nodes were visualized in 78 inguinal regions. Forty-five regions contained 1 sentinel node, 22 contained 2 sentinel nodes, and 1 region contained 3 sentinel nodes.

Intraoperative localization and removal was successful for 83 of the 92 visualized sentinel nodes (90%). In seven cases, we harvested one sentinel node but were unable to identify the second sentinel node that was depicted on the lymphoscintigram. In one case, only one sentinel node was found although three had been visualized on the images. In five cases, one unexpected additional sentinel node was identified because of remaining radioactivity after removal of the initial sentinel node. These 5 additional nodes were also harvested, resulting in the removal of a total of 88 sentinel nodes. Of these 88 sentinel nodes, 62 (70%) were identified with both the probe and blue dye and 26 (30%) were located with the probe only. The mean duration of exploration was 12 minutes (range: 2–37 minutes).

Of the removed 88 sentinel nodes, 11 contained metastases in 9 patients. Dissemination was unilateral in seven patients and bilateral in two. These nine patients underwent standard regional lymph node dissection 1–2 weeks later. The inguinal lymph node specimens revealed additional lymph node metastases in two patients only. These patients underwent ipsilateral iliac node dissection according to our treatment protocol [15].

Two patients returned with an ipsilateral palpable node metastasis 4 and 14 months, respectively, after a tumor-negative sentinel node had been harvested. They both underwent an inguinal lymphadenectomy. Of these two patients, the histopathology slides of the original sentinel nodes were retrieved and reviewed. One of the sentinel nodes was found to contain tumor after all and had thus been erroneously considered to be tumor-free. In the other patient, no metastatic involvement was found on review and his procedure has to be considered false negative. There were no complications following the sentinel node procedure.

DISCUSSION

Cabanas developed the sentinel node concept in an attempt to solve the controversy surrounding inguinal lymph node dissection in clinically node-negative patients with penile carcinoma [6]. The original procedure was based on identification of a specific lymph node by lymphangiography of the dorsal lymphatics of the penis and did not take into account the individual drainage pattern of each tumor and the diversity of the anatomy of lymphatic drainage [7]. This original sentinel node concept for penile carcinoma has been regarded with scepticism and has never been accepted as a standard procedure in the management of the disease.

The work of Morton and co-workers in melanoma patients resulted in the recognition of an individualized specific pattern of lymphatic drainage in each patient. In a large study of melanoma patients, they identified the sentinel node in 82% of 237 lymph node basins with metastatic basins remaining unidentified in less than 1% of the entire group of patients [13]. The addition of preoperative lymphoscintigraphy and intraoperative use of a gamma detection probe improved the ability to identify the sentinel node to over 95% [16,17]. Encouraged by the favorable results in melanoma, the sentinel node concept is now being explored in other types of malignancies like breast cancer and carcinoma of the vulva [18,19]. The results in carcinoma of the vulva deserve to be mentioned because of the similarities in the natural history of this disease when compared with carcinoma of the penis. Levenback and co-workers studied patients with vulvar cancer and identified the sentinel node in 19 of 29 groins (66%) using only the blue dye technique. The inguinal lymph node dissection was used as the gold standard and no false-negative results were obtained. The reader seeking more information on lymphatic mapping in carcinoma of the vulva is referred to Chapter 11. In our own study of patients with penile carcinoma, we identified 90% of sentinel nodes. There was only a limited concordance between numbers of sentinel nodes found on preoperative lymphoscintigraphy and found on exploration. Several reasons can be given for these discrepancies. The limited resolution of the gamma camera may have given rise to incorrect labeling of second-tier nodes as sentinel nodes. Due to spill of the tracer from the first-tier node to other nodes, not all ''hot spots'' on lymphoscintigraphy necessarily represent sentinel nodes. When multiple nodes light up, one or more can, in fact, be second-tier nodes. The limited resolution of the gamma camera may also explain why we sometimes harvest more sentinel nodes than expected, as one large hot spot may represent two hot sentinel nodes situated closely together. Early lymphoscintigraphy reveals the individual drainage pattern of the tumor in a dynamic way, but we are not fully informed about the reproducibility of the technique. A study involving 25 melanoma patients showed reproducibility in 22 patients (88%) [20]. The pitfalls of cutaneous lymphoscintigraphy are discussed in detail in Chapter 3.

All the nodes in this study were identified with the aid of a gamma probe. Had we not used the probe but only blue dye, we would have missed almost one-third of the nodes (26 of 88). Moreover, five additional sentinel nodes were identified during the operation through use of the probe. These findings could be interpreted as inferiority of the blue dye technique compared with the approach using a radioactive tracer and the probe. However, in our experience, the blue dye can give important clues by clearly visualizing lymphatic channels and thus mapping the lymphatic drainage pattern. This is useful when lymphoscintigraphy does not distinguish first-tier nodes from second-tier nodes. The sentinel node was found to contain metastatic disease in nine patients. One patient with known unilateral palpable metastasis had a tumor-positive sentinel node on the contralateral side. So, the presence of unilateral metastatic involvement does not have to be a contraindication for lymphatic mapping and, in fact, is helpful for selecting patients in need of contralateral lymph node dissection. The sentinel node procedure is also feasible when there is local penile cancer recurrence, as demonstrated in one of our cases.

Until now, the sentinel node procedure has resulted in an unsatisfactory outcome in two patients, who presented with clinically palpable inguinal recurrences 4 and 14 months after a dynamic sentinel node procedure. On review of the slides, one of the sentinel nodes did harbor a metastatic deposit after all and had been incorrectly reported to be tumor negative at the time of its removal. This finding led us to a change the routine pathology analysis. The sentinel node is now completely step-sectioned and immunohistochemistry is added to routine staining. The probability of a false-negative result underscores the need for a strict follow-up scheme. During the first 2 years after a sentinel node procedure, patients are seen every second month. Salvage procedures can then be undertaken at the earliest opportune moment.

The occurrence of a false-negative sentinel node may partially be explained by the presence of a metastatic tumor deposit that blocks the lymph flow [21].

The tracer is then diverted to another node that is falsely labeled as a sentinel node. It is not clear from our experience whether this occurs in grossly metastatic invasion only or whether microscopic invasion may do the same. More clinical research is needed to answer this important question.

The conclusions that we can draw from our study are somewhat limited because of the lack of a gold standard in the form of a routine completion lymph node dissection. Elective lymph node dissection has never been our policy. Lymph node dissection has been restricted to patients considered to be at high risk for occult metastasis, as explained earlier [3,5,15]. Despite the lack of routine complete node dissections, our findings will become more relevant with passing time. Also, metastases may be missed in nodes removed at elective node dissections! Our patients are followed closely. Patients rarely miss a follow-up visit because of the small size of the country, easy accessibility of our institution, and the health insurance policy. Only one of them was lost to follow-up because of emigration.

PITFALLS

The following pitfalls have been encountered so far: failure to visualize sentinel nodes with lymphoscintigraphy, a discrepancy between lymphoscintigraphy and surgical findings, false-negative sentinel lymphadenectomy because of false-negative histopathological examination, and, finally, a ''true'' false-negative sentinel node procedure. It is unclear why imaging failed in two of the patients. The discrepancies between lymphoscintigraphy and surgery can largely be explained by the resolution limitations of the gamma camera. More specific tracers and/or improving imaging capability may address this problem in the near future. In order to prevent false-negative histopathological findings, staining with immuno-histochemistry is mandatory. Some microscopic deposits may be detected only in this fashion. The rate of false-negative sentinel node biopsy in our hands is around 3%. Frequent follow-up is essential in order to treat a recurrence at the earliest possible moment. Based on patterns of recurrence, twice-monthly visits during 2 years are strongly advised. Patients who cannot comply with the follow-up requirements should not undergo lymphatic mapping.

CONCLUSIONS

In an attempt to solve some of the controversial aspects of the management of penile cancer, we prospectively assessed the value of lymphatic mapping and sentinel lymphadenectomy based on the individual drainage pattern of the tumor. The technique is minimally invasive and allows selection of the majority of patients with clinically occult metastasis for early regional node dissection. Lymphoscintigraphy is an essential element to localize the sentinel node before surgery, whereas use of a handheld gamma detector is mandatory during exploration. Based on experience so far, there is reason to believe that the number of unnecessary lymph node dissections can be reduced substantially and that complete lymph node dissections can be reserved for patients with proven metastasis.

REFERENCES

1. H Rouvière (MJ Tobias, transl.). Anatomy of the Human Lymphatic System. Ann Arbor, MI: Edwards Bros., 1938.
2. E Daseler, B Anson, A Riemann. Radical excision of the inguinal and iliac lymph glands. Surg Gynecol Obstet 87:679–694, 1948.
3. S Horenblas, H Van Tinteren, JFM Delemarre, LMF Moonen, V Lustig, R Kröger. Squamous cell carcinoma of the penis: accuracy of tumor, nodes and metastasis classification system, and role of lymphangiography, computerized tomography scan and fine needle aspiration cytology. J Urol 146:1279–1283, 1991.
4. S Horenblas, H Van Tinteren, JFM Delemarre, LMF Moonen, V Lustig, EW Van Waardenburg. Squamous cell carcinoma of the penis. III. Treatment of the regional nodes. J Urol 149:492–497, 1993.
5. S Horenblas, H Van Tinteren. Squamous cell carcinoma of the penis. IV. Prognostic factors of survival: analysis of tumor, nodes and metastasis classification system. J Urol 151:1239–1243, 1994.
6. RM Cabanas. An approach for the treatment of penile carcinoma. Cancer 39:456–466, 1977.
7. RM Cabanas. Anatomy and biopsy of sentinel lymph nodes. Urol Clin North Am 19:267–276, 1992.
8. CA Pettaway, LL Pisters, DPN Dinney, F Jularbal, DA Swanson, AC Von Eschenbach, A Ayala. Sentinel lymph node dissection for penile carcinoma: The M.D. Anderson Cancer Center experience. J Urol 154:1999–2003, 1995.
9. E Perinetti, DB Crane, WJ Catalona. Unreliability of sentinel lymph node biopsy for staging penile carcinoma. J Urol 124:734–735, 1980.
10. JE Fowler. Sentinel lymph node biopsy for staging penile cancer. Urology 23:352–354, 1984.
11. E Wespes, J Simon, CC Schulman. Cabanas approach: is sentinel node biopsy reliable for staging penile carcinoma? Urology 28:278–279, 1986.
12. SD Fossa, KS Hall, NB Johannessen, Th Urnes, O Kaalhus. Cancer of the penis, experience at the Norwegian Radium Hospital 1974–1985. Eur Urol 13:372–377, 1987.
13. DL Morton, D Wen, JH Wong, JS Economou, LA Cagle, FK Storm, LJ Foshag, AJ Cochran. Technical details of intraoperative lymphatic mapping for early stage melanoma. Arch Surg 127:392–399, 1992.
14. AC Broders. Carcinoma, grading and practical application. Arch Pathol Lab Med 2:376–381, 1926.
15. S Horenblas. Squamous cell carcinoma of the penis: update on diagnosis, staging and management. Eur Urol Update Series 3:58–63, 1994.
16. JF Thompson, WH McCarthy, CMJ Bosch, CJ O'Brien, MJ Quinn, S Paramaes-

varan, K Crotty, SW McCarthy, RF Uren, R Howman-Giles. Sentinel lymph node status as an indicator of the presence of metastatic melanoma in regional lymph nodes. Melanoma Res 5:255–260, 1995.

17. BAE Kapteijn, OE Nieweg, IH Liem, WJ Mooi, AJM Balm, SH Muller, JL Peterse, RA Valdes Olmos, CA Hoefnagel, BBR Kroon. Localizing the sentinel node in cutaneous melanoma: gamma probe detection versus blue dye. Ann Surg Oncol 4: 156–160, 1997.

18. AE Giuliano, DM Kirgan, JM Guenther, DL Morton. Lymphatic mapping and sentinel lymphadenectomy for breast cancer. Ann Surg 220:391–401, 1994.

19. C Levenback, TW Burke, DM Gershenson, M Morris, A Malpica, KR Lucas, DM Gershenson. Potential applications of intraoperative lymphatic mapping in vulvar cancer. Gynecol Oncol 59:216–220, 1995.

20. BAE Kapteijn, OE Nieweg, RA Valdés Olmos, IH Liem, RKL Baidjnath Panday, CA Hoefnagel, BBR Kroon. Reproducibility of lymphoscintigraphy for lymphatic mapping in cutaneous melanoma. J Nucl Med 37:972–975, 1996.

21. S Horenblas MJC Nuyten, CA Hoefnagel, LMF Moonen, JFM Delemarre. Detection of lymph node invasion in prostatic carcinoma with iliopelvic lymphoscintigraphy. Br J Urol 69:180–182, 1992.

13

Radiation Protection in the Sentinel Node Procedure

Rik Pijpers, Sybren Meijer, Peter H. Dignum, Otto S. Hoekstra,
Paul J. Borgstein, Arthur van Lingen, and Gerrit J. J. Teule
Vrije Universiteit Medical Center, Amsterdam, the Netherlands

INTRODUCTION

The first description of probe-guided surgery was given by Selverstone et al. in 1949 [1]. Until recently, however, the use of intraoperative probes was limited to a small number of indications [2–4]. With the validation of the sentinel node concept in melanoma [5–8] and in breast cancer [9–12], an application for the gamma probe has been introduced that will undoubtedly result in a widespread introduction of gamma probe–guided surgery. In the earliest studies on sentinel lymphadenectomy [5], the surgeon used dye guidance only. Soon, the additional value of radiolabeling of the sentinel lymph nodes followed by gamma probe–guided search was described [6–9,11–14]. As a result of this procedure, personnel in surgery and pathology departments will be exposed to small quantities of radiation on a regular basis. Moreover, excised radioactive tissue specimens (i.e., tumor and sentinel node) have to be transported from the operating room to the pathology department, which may demand guidelines additional to those already existing for surgical procedures.

This chapter deals with the radiation dose for patients and personnel during the sentinel node procedure, and with methods to reduce the exposure to radiation. The basis of transportation regulations will be introduced briefly.

GENERAL COMMENTS ON RADIATION PROTECTION

Radiation protection is basically founded on three principles, which have been described by the International Commission on Radiological Protection (ICRP) [15] and are still used as the basis for legislation in many countries.

> *Justification*: The application of radiation is only justified when the benefit to the exposed individual predominates over the negative consequences. This most often applies to the phase of a new practice in which various design options are being considered.
>
> *Optimization*: If the use of radioactive material is justified, the next aim is to ensure that the radiation dose to the patient and the general public is ''As Low As Reasonably Achievable'' (ALARA), taking social and economic factors into account.
>
> *Limitation*: Limitation of dose is used to place bounds on risks to individuals and to ensure that the risks do not exceed values considered to be acceptable. This principle also underlies the individual dose limits for exposure to radiation for radiological workers and the general public [15,16].

Justification and optimization can be applied to every member of society. Dose limits are applicable to patients only to a certain extent. When part of a treatment, it can be justified to expose a patient to higher radiation doses if the expected gain in health outweighs the risks associated with the radiation.

PRINCIPLES UNDERLYING DOSE LIMITS

Radiation protection deals with the protection of individuals, their offspring, and the general population against potentially harmful effects of radiation. There are two types of cellular damage that may occur following exposure to ionizing radiation: deterministic and stochastic damage [15].

Deterministic effects occur above a certain threshold. The probability of damage resulting in cell death or loss of reproductive potential will increase with the radiation dose. The extent of damage will also increase with the dose.

If cells are ''modified'' instead of killed, the outcome is different. In the clones of cells resulting from the reproduction of the modified cells, a malignant tumor may develop. This may occur even after a prolonged delay. The probability of tumor development following radiation increases with the increment of the radiation dose. However, the severity of the tumor is not related to this dose. This effect is called stochastic. Stochastic damage can be transmitted to later generations when it occurs in germ cells. The radiation dose used for determination of the stochastic risk is calculated in the following way. The ''absorbed dose'' (D) is the basic dosimetric unity. It is expressed in energy per unit mass (joules per kilogram, J/kg) and is called the Gray (Gy), where 1 J/kg is equivalent to 1 Gy. The probability of biological damage depends not only on the amount of Gy but also on the type of radiation and the organ or tissue that is irradiated.

The influence of the type of radiation on biological damage is expressed as a "radiation weighting factor," W_R. For example, gamma rays ($W_R = 1$) cause less damage than alpha particles ($W_R = 20$) when the absorbed dose is the same. When this weighting factor is taken into account, the result is the "equivalent dose" (H), which is expressed in Sievert (Sv). The equivalent dose in an organ or tissue (H_T) is the sum (Σ) of the weighted doses of all radiation types:

$$H_T = \sum_R W_R \, D_{T.R}$$

where $D_{T.R}$ is the absorbed dose in the organ T due to radiation R. The radionuclide technetium-99m (^{99}Tc), as used in the tracers for sentinel node labeling, emits only gamma rays and has a weighting factor of 1.

The "effective dose" is the dosimetric unit that takes into account the sensitivity to radiation damage of the different organs and tissues of the body. For example, the gonads are more susceptible to stochastic radiation damage than the skin. If the body is irradiated uniformly, the contribution of each tissue T to the total detriment resulting from the exposure is represented by a "tissue weighting factor," W_T. The effective dose (E) is the sum (Σ) of all weighted equivalent doses to all tissues and organs:

$$E = \sum_T W_T \, H_T$$

where H_T is the equivalent dose in a tissue or organ. The effective dose is, like the equivalent dose, expressed in Sv. The effective dose limit for the general population is accepted to be 1 mSv/year [15,16].

DOSE LIMITS FOR THE GENERAL PUBLIC

The average annual effective radiation dose from natural sources amounts to 2.4 mSv [17]. This is supplemented by an average of 0.4 mSv/year that is caused by man-made sources like radiographs and nuclear medicine procedures. The natural annual radiation dose differs according to geographical location and altitude. The ICRP recommends that any exposure to amounts over the natural background radiation levels should be as low as reasonably achievable (ALARA), but always below individual dose limits. Separate dose limits have been established for radiological personnel (e.g., those working in radiology and nuclear medicine departments) [16]. Employees in surgery and pathology departments also are to be considered as members of the general public with according dose

TABLE 1 Annual Recommended Dose Limits for Members of the General Public, According to ICRP-60

Effective dose	1 mSv
Without prejudice to the effective dose limit, separate annual dose limits have been instituted:	
For the lens of the eye	15 mSv
For the skin	50 mSv
For the extremities	50 mSv

Source: Refs. 15 and 16.

limits. In addition to the effective dose limit of 1 mSv/year, deterministic dose limits are applied to the skin, the extremities, and the lens of the eye, independent of the effective dose (Table 1). The importance of these deterministic dose limits will be clarified later in this chapter.

RADIATION EXPOSURE OF STAFF

Various hospital staff members are exposed to radiation during the sentinel node procedure. Because the surgeon is in closest contact with both tumor and sentinel node, dose calculations will be focused primarily on this person. Radiation exposure of others (e.g., nurses and pathology personnel) can be deduced from the values that apply to the surgeon. The skin of the surgeon's hands is expected to receive the highest dose and therefore serves as the dose-limiting organ. The radiation exposure of the surgeon during the operation is determined by the amount of tracer that is retained around the tumor, the distance from the injection depot to the surgeon's hands, and the duration of exposure. The amount of tracer uptake in the sentinel node is small and will not exceed a few percent of the total injected dose [18,19].

The amount of remaining activity at the moment of surgery is determined by the injected tracer dose and the time delay since injection. The physical decay of ^{99m}Tc can be calculated as

$$A_t = A_0 e^{-\lambda t}$$

where A_t is the remaining activity at surgery, A_0 is the amount of radioactivity at the moment of injection, λ is the decay constant of ^{99m}Tc (0.11 h^{-1}), and t is the time interval between injection and surgery. Every 6.02 h the radioactivity will be halved. To a lesser extent, the remaining activity is related to the amount of transported and excreted tracer, which is relatively small. Finally, a deeper injection results in more shielding by the overlying soft tissues and, consequently, in a lower exposure rate outside the body.

We performed dose-rate measurements in phantoms and in patients to calculate the radiation dose for exposed personnel.

PHANTOM MEASUREMENTS

The dose calculations were based on the assumption that 10 megabecquerels (MBq) of tracer is retained at the injection depot at the moment of surgery. The effects of two variables were estimated: the depth of the depot, which was placed in tissue equivalent material (i.e., water), and the distance from the depot to the dose-rate monitor.

A sphere with a diameter of 2 cm was filled with 10 MBq of ^{99m}Tc pertechnetate and submersed in water at a depth of 1, 2, and 4 cm as a model for peritumoral injections in breast cancer. A 1-mL syringe filled with 10 MBq of ^{99m}Tc pertechnetate in 0.4 mL of saline served as a model for intracutaneous injections such as used in sentinel lymphadenectomy in melanoma. Triple-dose-rate measurements were performed at distances of 10, 15, 25, 50, and 100 cm with a Berthold LB123 monitor (Berthold GmbH, Bad Wildbad, Germany).

We found that the distance from the source to the dose-rate monitor is the single most important determining factor (Fig. 1). From 50 cm to 10 cm distance, the average dose rate increased by a factor of 16.7 for the spherical phantom and 16.8 for the melanoma phantom.

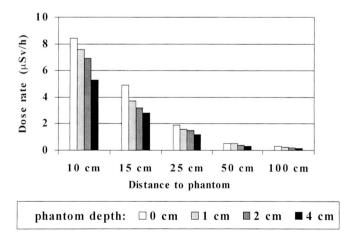

FIGURE 1   Dose rates (in μSv/h/10 MBq) at different distances from a breast and melanoma phantom.

TABLE 2   Dose Rates (in μSv/h/10 MBq) as Function of Distance from the Source in Breast Cancer (*n* = 10, average ± SD) and melanoma patients (*n* = 10, average ± SD) and phantoms

	10 cm	15 cm	25 cm	50 cm	100 cm
Breast phantom	6.9	3.2	1.5	0.4	0.2
Melanoma phantom	8.4	5.0	1.9	0.7	0.3
Breast patient	11.7[a]	5.8[a]	1.9 ± 0.4	0.7 ± 0.3	0.25 ± 0.07
(range)			(1.4–2.8)	(0.4–1.3)	(0.16–0.39)
Melanoma patient	9.8 ± 2.4	4.7 ± 1.1	2.0 ± 0.8	0.6 ± 0.3	0.28 ± 0.12
(range)	(7.9–12.5)	(3.7–6.0)	(1.0–3.5)	(0.2–0.9)	(0.16–0.50)

[a] Calculated values, based on phantom measurements.

PATIENT MEASUREMENTS IN BREAST CANCER

Ten consecutive breast cancer patients, who were eligible for a sentinel node procedure according to the standard protocol of our hospital [11,14] were asked to cooperate with the measurements. Dose rates were registered at distances of 25, 50, and 100 cm from the injection site within 3 h after a peritumoral injection of 50±5 MBq ^{99m}Tc colloidal albumin (Nanocoll®, Sorin Radiofarmaci S.r.I., Saluggia, Italy) in 4 mL of saline. Due to injecting the tracer at different depths, the depots will have a varying geometric relation to the dose-rate meter, which may influence the measured dose-rate at short distances. Therefore, the dose rates at 10 and 15 cm were calculated from measurements at 50 cm with multiplication factors of 16.7 and 8.3, respectively. These multiplication factors were obtained from the breast phantom results. The dose rates thus obtained are displayed in Table 2.

PATIENT MEASUREMENTS IN MELANOMA

The measurements in 10 melanoma patients were performed according to the same protocol as in the breast cancer patients. Because the tracer was injected intracutaneously, dose rates at short distances of 10 and 15 cm could be obtained in these patients. The injected dose in the melanoma patients amounted to 19± 6 MBq ^{99m}Tc nanocolloid in a total volume of 0.4 mL saline. Due to more rapid transportation of the tracer, measurements were obtained within 30 min after injection. Results are displayed in Table 2.

DISCUSSION OF PHANTOM AND PATIENT MEASUREMENTS

The dose rates as measured in melanoma patients were not significantly different from those in breast cancer patients (Student's *t*-test, $p > 0.5$). The higher dose rates obtained in the patient studies compared with the phantom results (Table 2) may have been caused by differences in geometric relations of the source to the dose-rate meter. The highest dose rates are used for further calculations, as is standard practice in radiation safety and protection protocols.

It can be assumed that, in clinical practice, the surgeon's hands will be at an average distance of 10 cm from the tumor. The dose rate to the surgeon's hands, with a breast tumor at a depth of 2 cm, will not exceed 11.7 µSv/h/10 MBq. In the case of a melanoma, this will be 9.8 µSv/h/10 MBq.

EXPOSURE OF THE SURGEON

The total radiation dose received by a surgeon working in a community hospital as a result of sentinel node biopsies in melanoma probably will be minor. In the first place, the incidence of melanoma is far less compared with breast cancer. Second, the time required for excision of the injection site in melanoma is less than for excision of a breast tumor. Moreover, it remains to be established which melanoma patients benefit from sentinel lymphadenectomy [20].

According to the results from the above measurements on phantoms and patients, dose rates to the surgeon's hands will be within the acceptable annual limits. If a surgeon performs sentinel node biopsies for 100 h during a year, with 10 MBq of ^{99m}Tc-labeled tracer retained at the injection site, the dose to the skin of the hands will be approximately 1 mSv. This is well below the deterministic annual dose limit for the skin of 50 mSv [15,16].

EXPOSURE OF OTHER PERSONNEL

The distance from patient to personnel has a strong effect on the absorbed radiation dose. According to the inverse square law, exposure to radiation diminishes with the square of the distance. So, doubling the distance from the source will result in a reduction of exposure by 75%. According to international regulations, no additional safety measures are required if the dose rate is below 0.5 µSv/h. At that rate, the annual dose will remain below 1 mSv (0.5 µSv/h × 40 h × 50 weeks = 1000 µSv = 1 mSv). Except for the surgeon and, possibly, his first assistant, other employees in the operating room will usually be at a distance of more than 1 m from the patient and will fall within this dose rate (Table 2). The radiation dose to the pathologist will also be low compared with that of the surgeon because of only a brief contact with the specimen, and usually after a delay of many hours following operation.

EXPOSURE OF PREGNANT PERSONNEL

The ICRP considers that the fetus of a pregnant employee should be treated as a member of the public [15,16]. In practice, this means that the dose to the abdominal surface of the maternal abdomen should be below 2 mSv during pregnancy [15,21]. During an operation, even the surgeon's abdomen will be at a distance of 25 cm or more from the patient. Although our measurements give no reason for concern (Table 2), it nevertheless seems sensible, from the ALARA principle, that a pregnant surgeon does not perform sentinel node procedures. Others can assist in the procedure because their distance from the patient usually exceeds 1 m.

PATIENT DOSIMETRY

Radiolabeled colloids are well suited for sentinel node detection. The amount of injected tracer ranges from 7 MBq [12] up to 60 MBq [8]. Compared with other nuclear medicine studies, these tracer doses are low [22]. Estimation of the patient's radiation dose after intracutaneous or subcutaneous injection of colloidal solutions is difficult. Because only a small fraction of the tracer is transported, the effective dose is largely determined by the amount of tracer that is retained in the injection depot. Strand et al. calculated that after subcutaneous injection of ^{99m}Tc–antimony trisulfide (^{99m}Tc–Sb_2S_3), the dose at the injection site is related to the extent of local diffusion [23]. Tracer washout and uptake in the lymph nodes depends on the size of the colloidal particles (Table 3). In the most widely used tracers, lymph node uptake varies between 0.04% and 5% [18,19,24]. Because the injection depot is usually excised during surgery, shortening of the interval between injection and operation will help to decrease the local radiation dose.

The radiation dose absorbed by a patient after subcutaneous injection of a tracer is given in Table 3. Following intracutaneous injection, employed in senti-

TABLE 3 Absorbed Dose in Injection Site and Lymph Nodes and Effective Dose for the Total Body After Subcutaneous Injection of Different Colloidal Tracers

	^{99m}Tc colloidal albumin[a]	^{99m}Tc–Sb_2S_3[b]	Filtered ^{99m}Tc sulfur colloid[c]
Injection site (mGy/MBq)	12	10	6.5–30.7
Lymph nodes (mGy/MBq)	0.59	1.0	0.01–0.9
Total body (mSv/MBq)	0.0046	0.005	0.0035–0.046
% Nodal uptake	0.3–1.6%[d]	0.2–5%	0.04–1.1%[d] (unfiltered)

[a] Data from Ref. 25.
[b] Data from Ref. 24.
[c] Data from Ref. 26.
[d] Percentage nodal uptake following intracutaneous injection [19].

nel node detection in melanoma, the radiation dose is probably not essentially different. After subcutaneous injection of 40 MBq ^{99m}Tc colloidal tracer, the effective total-body dose is of the order of 0.2 mSv, which is less than 10% of the dose received from, for example, bone scintigraphy [22]. Despite differences in retention of the ^{99m}Tc colloidal tracers at the injection site and lymph nodes, the total-body dose is of the same order of magnitude. Local reactions resulting from radiation damage by ^{99m}Tc-labeled tracers have not been described in the literature and are highly unlikely, considering studies performed in animals [27].

TRANSPORTATION OF RADIOACTIVE TISSUES

If surgery and pathology departments are located in the same hospital, transportation of the radioactive tissues can be supervised by the local nuclear medicine physician or radiation safety officer. If radioactive tissues are transported between hospitals, there are additional legal requirements. Depending on the amount of ^{99m}Tc at the moment of transportation, adequate packaging, package labeling, and shipping papers are required. In general, the amounts of the ^{99m}Tc colloid in the tissue specimens do not exceed several megabecquerels, and chances of contamination are low because the radioactivity is totally embedded.

In most countries, transportation legislation is based on International Atomic Energy Agency (IAEA) standards [28]. The basic principles of transportation regulation in the United States and the European Union are described below. If transportation cannot be executed according to the local regulations, it may be necessary to store the tissues until the ^{99m}Tc has decayed. In all cases, it is sensible for the nuclear medicine physician or radiation safety officer to be aware of exceptions and changes to national regulations.

TRANSPORTATION REGULATIONS IN THE UNITED STATES

Transportation of radioactive material is regulated by the Nuclear Regulatory Commission and Department of Transport. Material is defined as radioactive when the specific activity exceeds 70 Bq/g. The activity in tumor and sentinel node, directly following the surgical removal is usually less than 10 MBq and therefore can be considered to be a ''limited quantity'' [29]. Transportation in a strong and tight package will be sufficient in most cases. The package in which the material is transported needs external labeling to indicate the type and amount of radioactivity. Provided that the radiation levels at the surface of the package are below 5 μSv/h, a marking of ''radioactive'' on the exterior of the package is sufficient.

TRANSPORTATION REGULATIONS IN THE EUROPEAN UNION

National regulations in the member states of the European Union show only minimal differences from those of the United States. Tissue is considered to be radioactive when the tracer concentration exceeds 100 Bq/g. Limited quantities—less than 10 MBq of ^{99m}Tc per package with little risk of spill in case of an accident—are allowed to be transported in a strong, tight container. Radiation levels at the surface of the package should not exceed 5 μSv/h. The package and transport documents should be labeled "radioactive, limited quantity."

CONCLUDING REMARKS

The radiation dose to the surgeon is well within the annual dose limits, even when a considerable number of sentinel node procedures is performed. In clinical practice, the remaining radioactivity at the moment of surgery is usually less than 10 MBq with a consequently lower dose rate.

Pregnancy is not a reason to exclude staff from being present in the operating room during sentinel node procedures. Given the ALARA principle, it is proper to give pregnant personnel the opportunity to keep a distance of at least 1 m from the patient.

Before introducing the sentinel node procedure, all involved personnel should be informed about radiation levels and safety procedures to avoid unnecessary concern. Transportation of radioactive tissues between hospitals can be executed with relatively simple precautions. The person responsible for radiation safety should ensure that the transportation procedures conform to local regulations before actual implementation.

ACKNOWLEDGMENTS

The authors thank Ms. Anouk Bosma for performing the phantom measurements and Ms. Cora Brouwer for her assistance in translation of the manuscript.

REFERENCES

1. B Selverstone, WH Sweet, CV Robinson. The clinical use of radioactive phosphorus in the surgery of brain tumors. Ann Surg 136:643–651, 1949.
2. AC Morris, TR Barclay, R Tanida, JV Nemeck. A miniaturized probe for detecting radioactivity at thyroid surgery. Phys Med Biol 16:397–404, 1971.
3. JA Kim, PL Triozzi, EW Martin. Radioimmunoguided surgery for colorectal cancer. Oncology 7:55–64, 1993.

4. AC Perkins, JG Hardy. Intraoperative nuclear medicine in surgical practice. Nucl Med Commun 17:1006–1015, 1996.
5. DL Morton, DR Wen, JH Wong, JS Economou, LA Cagle, FK Storm, LJ Foshag, AJ Cochran. Technical details of intraoperative lymphatic mapping for early stage melanoma. Arch Surg 127:392–399, 1992.
6. DN Krag, S Meijer, DL Weaver, BW Loggie, SP Harlow, KK Tanabe, EH Laughlin, JC Alex. Minimal-access surgery for staging of malignant melanoma. Arch Surg 130:654–658, 1995.
7. R Pijpers, GJ Collet, S Meijer, OS Hoekstra. The impact of dynamic lymphoscintigraphy and gamma probe guidance on sentinel node biopsy in melanoma. Eur J Nucl Med 22:1238–1241, 1995.
8. BAE Kapteijn, OE Nieweg, SH Muller, IH Liem, CA Hoefnagel, EJTh Rutgers, BBR Kroon. Validation of gamma probe detection of the sentinel node in melanoma. J Nucl Med 38:362–366, 1997.
9. DN Krag, DL Weaver, JC Alex, JT Fairbank. Surgical resection and radiolocalization of the sentinel lymph node in breast cancer using a gamma probe. Surg Oncol 2:335–340, 1993.
10. AE Giuliano, RC Jones, M Brennan, R Statman. Sentinel lymphadenectomy in breast cancer. J Clin Oncol 15:2345–2350, 1997.
11. R Pijpers, S Meijer, OS Hoekstra, GJ Collet, EFI Comans, RPA Boom, PJ van Diest, GJJ Teule. Impact of lymphoscintigraphy on sentinel node identification with Tc-99m colloidal albumin in breast cancer. J Nucl Med 38:366–368, 1997.
12. U Veronesi, G Paganelli, V Galimberti, G Viale, S Zurrida, M Bedoni, A Costa, C de Cicco, JG Geraghty, A Luini, V Sacchini, P Veronesi. Sentinel node biopsy to avoid axillary dissection in breast cancer with clinically negative lymph nodes. Lancet 349:1864–1867, 1997.
13. JJ Albertini, GH Lyman, O Cox, T Yeatman, L Balducci, N Ku, S Shivers, C Berman, K Wells, D Rapaport, A Shons, J Horton, H Greenberg, S Nicosia, R Clark, A Cantor, DS Reintgen. Lymphatic mapping and sentinel node biopsy in the patient with breast cancer. JAMA 276:1818–1822, 1996.
14. PJ Borgstein, R Pijpers, EFI Comans, PJ van Diest, RPA Boom, S Meijer. Sentinel lymph node biopsy in breast cancer: guidelines and pitfalls of lymphoscintigraphy and gamma probe detection. J Am Coll Surg 186:275–283, 1998.
15. International Commission on Radiological Protection. 1990 Recommendations of the ICRP. Oxford: Pergamon Press; ICRP Publication 60; Ann. ICRP 21(1–3); 1991.
16. RH Clarke, JW Stather. Implementation of the 1990 recommendations of ICRP in the countries of the European Community. Radiat Environ Biophys 32:151–161, 1993.
17. J Cormack, JEC Towson, M Flower. Radiation protection and dosimetry in clinical practice. In: IPC Murray and PJ Ell, eds. Nuclear Medicine in Clinical Diagnosis and Treatment. Edinburgh: Churchill Livingstone, 1998:1373–1374.
18. R Pijpers, D Krag, P Borgstein, H Greuter, G Teule, S Meijer. Influence of the applied tracer on nodal uptake in sentinel node biopsy in melanoma (abstr). Eur J Nucl Med 24:992, 1997.
19. R Pijpers, P Borgstein, H Greuter, G Teule, S Meijer. Influence of nodal metastasis

on absolute tracer uptake in sentinel node biopsy in breast cancer (abstr). Eur J Nucl Med 24:994, 1997.

20. OE Nieweg, BAE Kapteijn, JF Thompson, BBR Kroon. Lymphatic mapping and selective lymphadenectomy for melanoma: not yet standard therapy. Eur J Surg Oncol 23:397–398, 1997.

21. LK Harding, WH Thomson. Where do we stand with ICRP 60? Eur J Nucl Med 20:787–791, 1993.

22. JT Bushberg, MG Stabin. Radiopharmaceutical dosimetry. In: MP Sandler, JA Patton, RE Coleman, A Gottschalk, FJTh Wackers, PB Hoffer, eds. Diagnostic Nuclear Medicine. 3rd ed. Baltimore, MD: Williams & Wilkins, 1996, pp. 304–305.

23. SE Strand, L Bergqvist. Radiolabeled colloids and macromolecules in the lymphatic system. Crit Rev Ther Drug Carrier Syst 6:211–238, 1989.

24. L Bergqvist, SE Strand, B Persson, L Hafström, PE Jönsson. Dosimetry in lymphoscintigraphy of Tc-99m antimony sulfide colloid. J Nucl Med 23:698–705, 1982.

25. Instruction leaflet of manufacturer. Sorin Radiofarmaci S.r.I., 13040 Saluggia (VC), Italy, April 1998.

26. JC Hung, GA Wiseman, HW Wahner, BP Mullan, TR Taggart, WL Dunn. Filtered technetium-99m-sulfur colloid evaluated for lymphoscintigraphy. J Nucl Med 36: 1895–1901, 1995.

27. FP Castronovo, KA McKusick, HW Strauss. The infiltrated radiopharmaceutical injection: Dosimetric considerations. Eur J Nucl Med 14:93–97, 1988.

28. Safety Series No 6. IAEA Safety Standards. Vienna: IAEA, 1979, p. 35.

29. Title 49 of the Code of Federal Regulations. Washington, DC: U.S. Government Printing Office, 1996, Part 173, Section 425. pp. 554–555.

14

Implementation of Lymphatic Mapping in a Community Hospital

D. Michael Rose and Richard Essner
John Wayne Cancer Institute at Saint John's Health Center,
Santa Monica, California

Armando E. Giuliano
Joyce Eisenberg-Keefer Breast Center and John Wayne Cancer Institute at Saint
John's Health Center, Santa Monica, California

INTRODUCTION

As lymphatic mapping with sentinel lymph node dissection has become an increasingly popular alternative to complete nodal dissection, more centers have begun to incorporate this technique into routine patient management. Multiple reports have documented the feasibility and accuracy of lymphatic mapping for identifying regional lymph node metastases in patients with melanoma or breast cancer. However, the majority of these reports have been generated at large centers with high patient volumes, allowing a greater training opportunity to those learning this approach. As these reports become more widely disseminated and the validity of the sentinel node hypothesis is accepted, health-care providers in community hospitals will also begin to perform these procedures. Patients themselves are already beginning to request sentinel node biopsy as an alternative to complete nodal dissection. In fact, pressure from better informed and more sophisticated health-care consumers has led many community surgeons to explore the addition of lymphatic mapping to their practices. The transfer of sentinel node technology from the larger tertiary referral centers to the community hospital has many similarities to the dissemination of laparoscopic technology. During the early 1990s, a patient-driven demand for minimally invasive techniques and "painless and bloodless" surgery forced surgeons to change long-established approaches to biliary disease. Many surgeons began performing laparoscopic procedures after brief training courses and with little clinical experience. The complication rate was notably higher after laparoscopic cholecystectomy than after traditional open procedures. However, this significantly decreased after completion of a well-defined learning phase [1,2].

Lymphatic mapping with sentinel node biopsy is an alternative procedure for staging the regional lymph nodes. Like laparoscopic cholecystectomy, it can be technologically challenging and requires the mastery of new skills during the learning phase. Laparoscopic techniques have been extensively implemented into surgical residency training, and the majority of recent graduates from surgical training programs in this country have performed more laparoscopic than open cholecystectomies. This has not yet become the case for lymphatic mapping, which has just recently begun to be introduced into training programs. Other differences include the multidisciplinary nature of sentinel node technology and the clinical differences between sentinel node dissection and standard nodal clearance. Although the technical feasibility and validity of the new approach have been addressed in patients with melanoma or breast cancer, the clinical implications of selective rather than complete nodal dissection have not yet been fully explored. In addition, because lymphatic mapping is applied to malignant disease, its failure may have a substantially greater impact than failure of a laparoscopic technique used in benign conditions. Achieving the goal of laparoscopic cholecystectomy is immediately known, as is the failure of the procedure. Achieving the goal of lymphatic mapping is only absolutely known if a completion lymph node dissection is performed, and failure can present as recurrent disease years after the procedure.

Because of the lack of long-term clinical data and the current lack of technique standardization, some investigators have suggested that lymphatic mapping should not be routinely used in a community hospital outside the setting of a clinical trial [3]. Although the new technique should not replace traditional management of patients with melanoma or breast cancer, it can be integrated into the community surgeon's practice under the auspices of a controlled clinical trial. The informed consent process for lymphatic mapping should clearly convey the current deficiencies in available data on this technique. A review of the currently available data as well as considerations on the community application of lymphatic mapping in melanoma and breast cancer follows.

MELANOMA

Lymphatic mapping with sentinel node biopsy for cutaneous melanoma was originally described by Morton and colleagues in 1990 as a potential solution to the controversy surrounding elective lymph node dissection [4]. The manuscript took 2 years to publish because of the reviewers' skepticism to the validity of the technique. However, since Morton's original article, approximately 300 reports on this approach have appeared in the literature. All major centers use presurgical cutaneous lymphoscintigraphy and a combination of radioisotope and blue dye for intrasurgical localization; however, the details at each institution vary significantly. The *Journal of Surgical Oncology* reported a comparison of techniques in the "How I Do It" section in 1997. Contributing authors included D. L. Morton from the John Wayne Cancer Institute [5], J. F. Thompson from the Sydney Melanoma Unit [6], M. I. Ross from the M.D. Anderson Cancer Center [7], D. S. Reintgen from the Moffitt Cancer Center [8], and C. P. Karakousis from the State University of New York, Buffalo [9]. Each surgeon reported excellent results but none used the same technique for sentinel node identification. This variation among the experts underscores the importance of a learning phase during which the procedure is always followed by completion lymphadenectomy.

Currently there is no national standard on credentialing for new surgical procedures or technology; however, guidelines for appropriate training are available in other formats. A symposium on lymphatic mapping and sentinel node biopsy in patients with breast cancer and melanoma was published in *Contemporary Surgery* in 1998 [3]. A panel of experts, including Morton, Reintgen, D. F. Roses, Ross, and Thompson, agreed that a surgeon should perform 30 sentinel node procedures in patients with melanoma in order to achieve proficiency. These learning cases must be followed by completion lymphadenectomy to assess the accuracy and, most importantly, the false-negative rate of the individual surgeon. Thompson noted that the number of required cases was arbitrary and 30 cases was probably adequate in a center where the procedure is already performed and expert guidance is available. He remarked that even after several hundred procedures, he was still learning. Morton concluded the panel discussion by emphasizing not only the importance of experience with the technical details of sentinel lymph node dissection, but also the multidisciplinary nature of this technique. Accuracy in sentinel node identification is generally reached after performing 30 cases [5]. Most surgeons should perform at least 30 cases with complete lymph node dissections and should be able to achieve 98% accuracy after experience with 100 cases [5].

Another guideline for appropriate surgical training in lymphatic mapping can be found in the definition of the learning phase of the Multicenter Selective Lymphadenectomy Trial. This multicenter international trial compares wide excision alone versus wide excision with sentinel node biopsy in patients with intermediate thickness melanoma. Proof of technical competence is required to enroll patients in the randomized phase of the study. Each clinic must accumulate at least 30 cases and have at least one surgeon who has performed 15 cases with an 85% identification rate. All participating surgeons must have completed 15 cases.

From the available data it is apparent that a surgeon should perform at least 30 cases followed by completion lymphadenectomy in order to safely begin performing sentinel node biopsy in patients with melanoma. Ideally, this should be done in an environment with experienced assistance available. At the least, a formal didactic and technical training course should be taken in order to introduce the surgeon to the multiple pitfalls and difficulties associated with these techniques.

A recent report has examined the accuracy of lymphatic mapping in patients enrolled in the Multicenter Selective Lymphadenectomy Trial [10]. By December 1998, the 16 participating centers had enrolled 1135 patients, of whom 570 had complete data for review. The total success rate for sentinel node identification among all centers was 96.7%. After each center completed the required 30-case learning phase, the success rate of sentinel node identification was independent of case volume or experience, with no difference noted between the initial and more recent procedures. The investigators concluded that in this extensive multicenter experience, a multidisciplinary approach and a learning phase of 30 consecutive cases per center are sufficient for mastery of lymphatic mapping for cutaneous melanoma.

In addition to surgical expertise, nuclear medicine and pathology support are critically important in the establishment of a successful program. Presurgical lymphoscintigraphy is an essential component of successful sentinel lymphadenectomy. It is used to identify all nodal basins at risk, determine the number and location of the sentinel nodes, and identify any possible in-transit sentinel nodes or nodes in basins not predicted by the anatomy. Unfortunately, the nuclear medicine literature contains no standardized guidelines for lymphoscintigraphy. Success rates are operator-dependent and subject to a learning curve. Pathological examination of the sentinel node is also important in establishing the validity of sentinel lymphadenectomy. With only one or two nodes to examine, the pathologist can study multiple sections rather than bivalving multiple nodes. In addition to hematoxylin and eosin staining, most centers currently recommend both serial sectioning and immunohistochemical staining using monoclonal antibodies targeting S-100 and HMB-45 proteins. The majority of pathological laboratories have this capability; however, this needs to be in place before any lymphatic mapping procedures. The previously outlined requirements for participation in the Multicenter Selective Lymphadenectomy Trial are important to consider because they are a test of the entire clinical system, including the success of lymphoscintigraphy and pathological examination.

In a commentary published in *The Cancer Journal from Scientific American,* Morton addressed the current status of sentinel node technology with respect to community standard care [11]. He emphasized the learning curve with these techniques and stated that an acceptable level of success in melanoma patients (90% accuracy in identifying the sentinel node) can only be achieved by performing 30 to 50 cases of mapping, which exceeds the expected case load of most community-based surgeons. Clearly, the successful implementation of a sentinel node program for melanoma requires a high-volume center with a dedicated goal of incorporating lymphatic mapping into the care of their patients.

BREAST CARCINOMA

Adapting the methodology of sentinel lymphadenectomy for melanoma, Giuliano and colleagues began investigating the possibility of dye-based lymphatic mapping for patients with breast cancer in 1991 and published their first report of 174 cases in 1994 [12]. Since that time, multiple studies have reported the feasibility, accuracy, and technique of sentinel lymph node dissection in patients with breast cancer. Although complete level I and II axillary node dissection remains the standard of care for patients with breast cancer, sentinel node biopsy is a less-extensive operation with decreased morbidity, decreased time to full activity, and no need for drain placement. Both patients and clinicians are increasingly interested in this modality as a replacement for traditional complete Level I and II nodal dissection. McMasters et al., however, warn that although sentinel node technique may be considered ''state of the art'' in experienced hands, it should not be performed without completion axillary node dissection until more data exist [13]. False-negative rates from multicenter trials need to be determined, as does the characterization of patients with false-negative nodes, and a consensus needs to be reached on acceptable false-negative rates. At present, most data on accuracy and false negativity rates are from single institutions, and little agreement exists within the literature.

The technical challenge of lymphatic mapping for breast carcinoma is reflected by the accuracy and false-negative rates reported in the literature. The original data from Giuliano et al. in 1994 revealed a 66% sentinel node identification rate and an 11.9% false-negative rate [12]. However, this included all patients, even those in the developmental stage of this previously untested procedure. With increased experience these investigators reported a 93% identification rate and no false negatives [14]. The improved accuracy rates and shortened learning phase were confirmed by Cody et al. at the Memorial Sloan-Kettering Cancer Center, who recently reviewed their experience of 500 breast sentinel node cases performed by eight surgeons [15]. The success rate was 94% for the three most experienced surgeons and only 86% for the five less experienced individuals. Of note, there were four failed procedures in the last 100 cases; increasing experience did not eliminate the chance of failure. In those 104 patients who also underwent completion axillary node dissection (completion node dissection was not routine in this study), a false-negative rate of 10.6% was found, with a reported range of 7–20% between surgeons. Most false-negative cases occurred early in the surgeons' experience. Excluding the first 15 cases of each surgeon decreased the false-negative rate to 2%. These findings prompted the suggestion that lymphatic mapping for breast cancer may have a true false-negative rate as low as 2%; however, others have reported lower false-negative rates.

Variability among individual surgeons was also seen in the multicenter validation study of lymphatic mapping in breast cancer reported by Krag et al. [16]. Eleven surgeons prospectively enrolled 443 patients with breast cancer and clinically node-negative axillae. The success rate for identification of the sentinel node was 93.2% overall but this ranged from 79–98% for individual surgeons. The overall false-negative rate was 11.4% with a range of 0–28.6%. Clearly, there is a significant amount of individual variability in outcomes after lymphatic mapping. Achieving the highest success rate and lowest false-negative rate is the goal of any individual planning to perform these techniques.

Similar to melanoma, the numbers "required" for adequate training in breast cancer are controversial. In a symposium on lymphatic mapping for breast cancer, M. I. Ross suggested that between 50 to 100 cases were required to become comfortable with the technique [17]. Other investigators felt this was too "elitist" and an exaggeration of the likely required numbers; Giuliano recommended 25 consecutive cases with subsequent completion axillary node dissection to assess accuracy and determine the false-negative rate. A later report used a decision analysis model to evaluate the clinical implications of sentinel node dissection versus traditional level I and II nodal dissection during a learning phase estimated at 60 to 80 cases [18]. This estimate was based on the initial report of sentinel lymphadenectomy in breast cancer and a subsequent report in a community-managed–care setting [12,19]. The investigators simulated a randomized trial of 20,000 patients and concluded that only after documentation of accuracy of sentinel node biopsy (sensitivity >90%) should full axillary node dissection be omitted.

Additional guidelines for appropriate training for lymphatic mapping in breast cancer patients can be found in the surgeon skill-verification requirements for a trial recently opened by the American College of Surgeons Oncology Group. The study evaluates the prognostic significance of sentinel node and bone marrow micrometastases in women with clinical T1 or T2N0M0 breast cancer. A specified degree of accuracy and satisfactory performance by a contributing site's investigators are required to enroll patients in the study. This includes documentation of 30 cases of sentinel node dissection followed by a completion axillary dissection with a ≥85% successful identification rate and a false-negative rate of <5%, or a single false-negative sentinel node in the series with at least 10 tumor-involved sentinel nodes.

A recent publication specifically examined learning curves and success rates of surgeons performing sentinel node biopsies for breat cancer [20]. Seven hundred cases were studied and the learning curves of five surgeons revealed similar findings of a high initial-failure rate and a subsequent rapid decrease after

20 cases. The mean of the five surgeons' learning curves indicated that an average of 23 and 53 cases led to success rates of 90% and 95%, respectively. The number of cases required to achieve a 90% success rate ranged from 13 to 40, a range that included the estimate of 25 cases offered by Giuliano [21]. Currently at the John Wayne Cancer Institute, the performance of sentinel node dissection requires documentation of special training and experience, including 25 cases with subsequent axillary node dissection to evaluate success rate and false-negative rate.

Another recent report introduced several guidelines for lymphatic mapping in patients with breast cancer [22]. Recommendations included completion dissection when a sentinel node was not identified or contained tumor, the implementation of institutional review board protocol for lymphatic mapping as an investigational procedure, radiation safety protocols, appropriate training, ongoing data collection, and evaluation of sensitivity, specificity, and follow-up in all cases. In a commentary on the current status and future of sentinel node technique, Giuliano warned that the ''beginner is often unaware of . . . subtle technical variations and may be tempted to mix different techniques'' [23]. He cautioned that ''any surgeon interested in providing sentinel lymph node dissection as an alternative to axillary lymph node dissection in node-negative women must establish an institutional protocol to accurately perform sentinel lymph node dissection, organize a committed team of pathologists, nuclear medicine physicians, and surgeons; and apply rigorous controls at every stage of the technique.''

As in any application of sentinel node technology, the interaction with nuclear medicine and pathology is essential. Breast lymphoscintigraphy for sentinel node localization is a demanding technique that requires time and effort to master [24]. Of note, sentinel node techniques for breast cancer have been reported to be more challenging than for melanoma, although users have consistently reported higher success rates with experience. The use of presurgical and intrasurgical lymphatic mapping using radioisotope versus using blue dye alone has been extensively debated with most experienced centers reporting excellent results with each technique. Currently, at the John Wayne Cancer Institute, breast lymphoscintigraphy is used in patients with medial hemisphere lesions to evaluate the possible presence of internal mammary drainage and to ascertain the first draining node in cases with mammary and axillary nodal drainage. Similar to the surgical techniques, no credentialing is required for lymphoscintigraphy; however, experience with many of the nuances of this procedure is required for successful localization.

The pathological examination of the sentinel node in breast cancer requires both serial sectioning and immunohistochemical examination of sections for cytokeratin. Focused histopathological examination of the sentinel node has identified more metastases than standard examination of routine level I and II nodal dissections. Turner et al. described optimal evaluation of the sentinel node by obtaining permanent sections from at least two levels of the tissue block, at 40-μm intervals, for hematoxylin and eosin staining and cytokeratin immunohisto-chemistry [25]. Each pathological department will need to standardize its protocol for sentinel node evaluation.

The implementation of breast lymphatic mapping and sentinel node dissection is a significant consideration for any medical center because the status of axillary lymph nodes affects treatment decisions. Reaching an appropriate level of technical expertise is critical to minimize the false-negative rate and maximize the success rate. Each individual institution must be responsible for local credentialing of surgeons. Patient incentives to pursue this technology are multiple; however, the decision to abandon traditional axillary nodal dissection in favor of the sentinel node biopsy must be done in a structured and formalized fashion. Achieving surgical expertise, obtaining an experienced nuclear medicine and pathology staff, and a dedication to the critical analysis of individual outcomes are all necessary components.

LYMPHATIC MAPPING IN OTHER NEOPLASMS

With the increased experience with sentinel node technology in melanoma and breast cancer, investigators have begun to apply this technique to the staging of other solid neoplasms. Bilchik et al. reported their experience with the universal application of lymphatic mapping at the John Wayne Cancer Institute [26]. The investigators evaluated their experience with lymphatic mapping in Merkel cell tumors, squamous cell carcinoma of the head and neck, thyroid cancer, gastrointestinal malignancies (including small bowel, pancreas, and colon primaries), and vulvar neoplasms. They found the technique to be feasible for solid tumors other than breast and melanoma. Lymphatic mapping may ultimately replace conventional dissection with more accurate staging. Other investigators have confirmed the feasibility of the technique in colon and oral squamous cell carcinoma [27,28]. However, there have been no larger prospective studies in malignancies other than melanoma and breast cancer. At this point, the use of lymphatic mapping in other solid neoplasms should be considered investigational and should only be performed in the context of a clinical trial. These applications are not yet appropriate for transfer to the community setting.

CONCLUSIONS

In a 1997 editorial on the credentialing of surgery in the United States, Reintgen noted that lymphatic mapping was only beginning to be incorporated into the everyday practice of the surgeon [29]. He stated that the process for credentialing surgeons with new technology is probably inadequate and recommended that surgeons be required to take a formal training course and show their local credentialing committees that they have proper nuclear medicine and pathology support.

From the available data, surgeons should probably perform 25 to 30 cases for melanoma and breast cancer before abandoning traditional complete lymph node dissection. These numbers are only rough guidelines and each individual surgeon should prove an appropriate accuracy and low false-negative rate before adopting these techniques. Morton has stated that the success of lymphatic mapping requires the facilities, personnel, and training for a multidisciplinary approach [11]. Lymphatic mapping with sentinel node biopsy has the potential to provide critical pathological staging data for patients with melanoma, breast cancer, and other solid tumors with a decreased morbidity. However, this technology can be implemented only after a proven success rate by both the surgeon and the institution.

REFERENCES

1. The Southern Surgeons Club. A prospective analysis of 1518 laparoscopic cholecystectomies. N Engl J Med 324:1073–1078, 1991.
2. The Southern Surgeons Club. The learning curve for laparoscopic cholecystectomy. Am J Surg 170:55–59, 1995.
3. DL Morton, AE Giuliano, DS Reintgen, DF Roses, MI Ross, JF Thompson. Symposium: lymphatic mapping and sentinel node biopsy in patients with breast cancer and melanoma—part 2. Contemp Surg 53:353–361, 1998.
4. DL Morton, LA Cagle, JH Wong, JS Economou, LJ Foshag, D-R Wen, AJ Cochran. Intraoperative lymphatic mapping and selective lymphadenectomy: technical details of a new procedure for clinical stage I melanoma. Presented at the Society of Surgical Oncology, Washington, D.C., March 1990.
5. DL Morton. How I Do It: introduction: sentinel lymphadenectomy for patients with clinical stage I melanoma. J Surg Oncol 66:267–269, 1997.
6. JF Thompson. How I Do It: sentinel node biopsy. J Surg Oncol 66:270–272, 1997.
7. MI Ross. How I Do It: lymphatic mapping and sentinel node biopsy for early stage melanoma: how we do it at the M.D. Anderson Cancer Center. J Surg Oncol 66: 273–276, 1997.
8. D Reintgen. How I Do It: lymphatic mapping and sentinel node harvest for malignant melanoma. J Surg Oncol 66:277–281, 1997.
9. CP Karakousis, S Najibi, J Trunk. How I Do It: sentinel node biopsy in malignant melanoma. J Surg Oncol 66:282–284, 1997.
10. DL Morton, JF Thompson, R Essner, R Elashoff, SL Stern, OE Nieweg, DF Roses, CP Karakousis, N Mozillo, D Reintgen, H Wang, EC Glass, AJ Cochran, and the Multicenter Selective Lymphadenectomy Trial Group. Multicenter Selective Lymphadenectomy Trial Group. Validation of the accuracy of intraoperative lymphatic mapping and sentinel lymphadenectomy for early-stage melanoma: a multicenter trial. Ann Surg 230:453–465, 1999.
11. DL Morton. Intraoperative lymphatic mapping and sentinel lymphadenectomy: community standard care or clinical investigation? Cancer J Sci Am 3:328–330, 1997.
12. AE Giuliano, DM Kirgan, JM Guenther, DL Morton. Lymphatic mapping and sentinel lymphadenectomy for breast cancer. Ann Surg 220:391–401, 1994.

13. KM McMasters, AE Giuliano, MI Ross, DS Reintgen, KK Hunt, DR Byrd, VS Klimberg, PW Whitworth, LC Tafra, MJ Edwards. Sentinel lymph node biopsy for breast cancer—not yet the standard of care. N Engl J Med 339:990–995, 1998.

14. AE Giuliano, RC Jones, M Brennan, R Statman. Sentinel lymphadenectomy in breast cancer. J Clin Oncol 15:2345–2350, 1997.

15. HS Cody, ADK Hill, KN Tran, MF Brennan, PI Borgen. Credentialing for breast lymphatic mapping: how many cases are enough? Ann Surg 229:723–728, 1999.

16. D Krag, D Weaver, T Ashikaga, F Moffat, VS Klimberg, C Shriver, S Feldman, R Kusminsky, M Gadd, J Kuhn, S Harlow, P Beitsch. The sentinel node in breast cancer: a multicenter validation study. N Engl J Med 339:941–946, 1998.

17. DL Morton, AE Giuliano, DS Reintgen, DF Roses, MI Ross, JF Thompson. Symposium: lymphatic mapping and sentinel node biopsy in patients with breast cancer and melanoma—part 1. Contemp Surg 53:281–298, 1998.

18. RK Orr, JL Hoehn, NF Col. The learning curve for sentinel node biopsy in breast cancer: practical considerations. Arch Surg 134:764–767, 1999.

19. JM Guenther, M Krishnamoorthy, LR Tan. Sentinel lymphadenectomy for breast cancer in a community managed care setting. Cancer J Sci Am 3:336–340, 1997.

20. CE Cox, SS Bass, D Boulware, NN Ku, C Berman, DS Reintgen. Implementation of a new surgical technology: outcome measures for lymphatic mapping of breast carcinoma. Ann Surg Oncol 39:843–856, 1999.

21. AE Giuliano. See one, do twenty-five, teach one: the implementation of sentinel node dissection in breast cancer [editorial]. Ann Surg Oncol 6:520–521, 1999.

22. CE Cox, S Pendas, JM Cox, E Joseph, AR Shons, T Yeatman, NN Ku, GH Lyman, C Berman, F Haddad, DS Reingten. Guidelines for sentinel node biopsy and lymphatic mapping of patients with breast cancer. Ann Surg 227:645–653, 1998.

23. AE Giuliano. Mapping a pathway for axillary staging: a personal perspective on the current status of sentinel lymph node dissection for breast cancer. Arch Surg 134: 195–199, 1999.

24. EC Glass, R Essner, AE Giuliano. Sentinel node localizaton in breast cancer. Semin Nucl Med 29:57–68, 1999.

25. RR Turner, DW Ollila, S Stern, AE Giuliano. Optimal histopathologic examination of the sentinel lymph node for breast carcinoma staging. Am J Surg Pathol 23:263–267, 1999.

26. AJ Bilchik, A Giuliano, R Essner, et al. Universal application of intraoperative lymphatic mapping and sentinel lymphadenectomy in solid neoplasms. Cancer J Sci Am 4:351–358, 1998.

27. S Saha, M Espinosa, J Badin, D Wiese, T Beutler, D Nora, BK Ganatra, D Desai, J Bhagat, E Gomez, M Latchana. Micrometastases in colorectal cancer (CRCa)—accuracy of diagnosis by sentinel lymph node (SLN) mapping: an update. Presented at the Society of Surgical Oncology, Orlando, March 1998.

28. WM Koch, MA Choti, AC Civelek, DW Eisele, JR Saunders. Gamma probe-directed biopsy of the sentinel node in oral squamous cell carcinoma. Arch Otolaryngol Head Neck Surg 124:455–459, 1998.

29. D Reintgen. The credentialing of American surgery. Ann Surg Oncol 4:99–101, 1997.

15

Minimally Invasive Radioguided Parathyroidectomy

Colleen Jaffray and James Norman
University of South Florida, Tampa, Florida

INTRODUCTION

Historically, the inability of presurgical testing to accurately distinguish patients with sporadic primary hyperparathyroidism involving a single gland from those with the much less common (8–13%) occurrence of multiple adenomas or four-gland hyperplasia has challenged surgeons. The advent of technetium-99m (^{99m}Tc) labeled sestamibi scintigraphy in the early 1990's has changed the management of primary hyperparathyroidism for the majority of surgeons, because most nuclear medicine departments have become more proficient in performing and interpreting this test. A recent meta-analysis of more than 6,000 patients showed that presurgical sestamibi scanning has a sensitivity of approximately 90% and a specificity approaching 100% in identifying patients with a single adenoma when appropriately applied to patients with sporadic primary hyperparathyroidism [1]. The key is utilizing the information provided by the sestamibi scan to benefit the highest number of patients without increasing the risk of incomplete surgeries on the remainder.

We developed radioguided parathyroidectomy several years ago in an attempt to improve parathyroid surgery through application of the data afforded by a clearly positive sestamibi scan in patients with sporadic primary hyperparathyroidism. The goal was to allow a quick outpatient procedure to be performed under local anesthesia on most patients with primary hyperparathyroidism. Our experience, after performing over 500 of these cases over the past three years and teaching this technique to several hundred surgeons, has brought to light a few important points about radioguided parathyroidectomy that are described in this chapter. First, this procedure is only applicable to patients with *sporadic*, *primary* hyperparathyroidism. Secondly, the operating surgeon must be able to work closely with his/her nuclear medicine physician. Furthermore, a new generation hand-held gamma-ray detection probe must be used. Finally, to be able to interpret the information correctly, the surgeon must know how to use and set up the probe, which is different for each probe manufacturer and very different from sentinel lymph node mapping.

The probe is a simple tool yet it can provide invaluable information. It will not make an expert out of every surgeon; however, if appropriately applied to the correct patient population, the surgery can be simplified tremendously. This technique allows for a smaller incision, which is appealing to patients and referring physicians alike. The use of local anesthesia also has a positive influence on the patient's view of the surgery beforehand and, perhaps more importantly, readily allows for the patient to be discharged almost immediately after the procedure. Our experience supports that approximately 85% of all patients with sporadic primary hyperparathyroidism can have a minimally invasive radioguided parathyroidectomy with examination of one gland only. A few more can be adequately treated with a unilateral exploration, examining two glands, with only 10% or so requiring a bilateral exploration.

SELECTION OF SURGICAL PROCEDURE

With the diagnosis of primary hyperparathyroidism, patients are counseled regarding the standard versus radioguided approach. Sestamibi scintigraphy or any other localizing studies are not performed until the day of the surgery. Patients are scheduled for an operation and the surgical technique used (standard vs. radioguided parathyroidectomy) is dictated by the results of the sestamibi scintigraphy performed an hour or two before the procedure. Because of the importance of timing, it is our recommendation that surgeons learning this technique begin by selecting patients for radioguided parathyroidectomy who have had a sestamibi scan, deemed clearly positive, a week or two before the surgery. Subsequently, once the technique has been learned, the goal is to scan patients only once, 1 or 2 h before surgery. If a single adenoma is found on the presurgical scan, then radioguided parathyroidectomy is performed. If no localization occurs, a standard bilateral exploration will be performed (Fig. 1).

Because of the tremendous variability in the quality of sestamibi scans from institution to institution, the percentage of patients who are able to undergo radioguided parathyroidectomy will vary at each hospital. The dosage of ^{99m}Tc-sestamibi that we use is 740-925 MBq (20-25 mCi) [2]. In working closely with our nuclear medicine department, we are able to get a positive sestamibi scan on 86.9% of all patients referred. Interestingly, only about 6% of patients referred

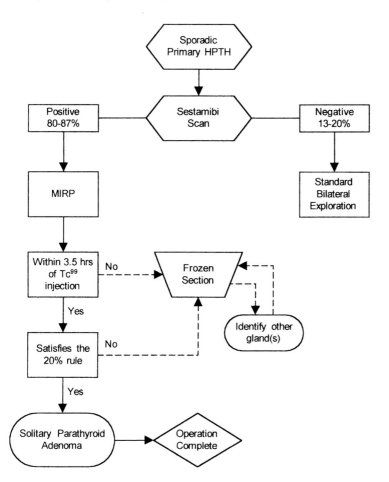

FIGURE 1 Perisurgical management scheme based on ^{99m}Tc-sestamibi scanning and minimally invasive radioguided parathyroidectomy (MIRP).

to us have had scans previously, with the majority having negative scans. The weight rests on the surgeon, not just the nuclear medicine physician, to review the films closely and be confident that the scan is positive. Our definition of a positive sestamibi scan is one that has been performed on a patient with sporadic primary hyperparathyroidism that shows a single focus of increased radioactivity which is distinct and separate from the thyroid. In order to achieve the latter part of this definition, more than just anterior-posterior views must be obtained. We strongly believe that simple oblique views are the only other views that are needed, and in fact are essential to clearly delineate the focus of radioactivity separate from the thyroid. Interestingly, lateral views are almost universally use-less.

THE IMPORTANCE OF TIMING BETWEEN SESTAMIBI AND OPERATIVE EXPLORATION

In order to perform a successful radioguided parathyroidectomy, two elements are critical [2-5]. The first is the quality of the presurgical sestamibi, which allows for a clearly positive scan to be obtained, as defined previously. The second critical determinant for success became obvious only after we had accumulated

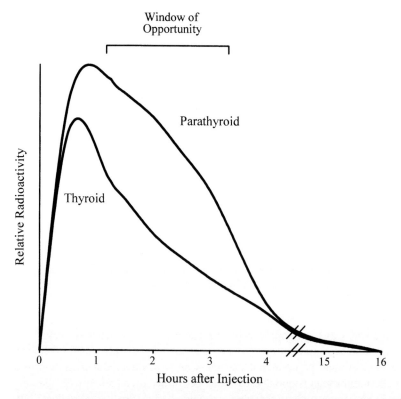

FIGURE 2   Window of opportunity. Based on the relative speeds at which the thyroid and parathyroid "wash out" ^{99m}Tc-sestamibi and keeping in mind the 6.2 h half-life of ^{99m}Tc, the optimal situation to identify parathyroid adenomas with the probe occurs when the thyroid has washed out and the parathyroid remains radioactive. This window of opportunity occurs between 1.5 and 3.0 h.

sufficient experience with this technique to realize that there was a "window" of optimal timing between injection of the radiopharmaceutical and using the probe in the surgery room.

This surgical window is a function of the relative speeds at which the thyroid and parathyroid "wash out" their nuclear tag. Because the thyroid will lose its initial uptake of ^{99m}Tc-sestamibi at a faster rate than a hyperactive parathyroid gland, the optimal situation occurs when the thyroid has washed out and the parathyroid remains radioactive (shown in Figure 2 as "optimal window"). Only when there is differential activity between the thyroid and the parathyroid adenoma can the gamma probe be helpful. We have found that this situation occurs between 1.5 and 3.0 h. Typically, 1.5–2.5 h after radiopharmaceutical injection is ideal for the vast majority of patients, and an elapsed time over 3.5 h usually will not work. The 6.2-h physical half-life of ^{99m}Tc allows the use of the indicated window.

SURGICAL TECHNIQUE

When positioned on the surgery room table, a small new-generation (9-14 mm) gamma-ray detection probe is used to measure radioactivity in four quadrants of the neck defined by the upper and lower poles of the thyroid on each side. Note that the first-generation probes are not useful for this operation. These were large in diameter and lacked the directionality because they were unshielded and non-collimated. The initial incision is placed according to the expected location of the adenoma as determined by both the sestamibi images and the measurement of gamma-ray emission on the skin. This may necessitate that the incision is placed slightly higher or lower than usual, but should always be oriented transversely to allow extension as needed, or even conversion to a bilateral exploration if necessary. Superficial adenomas (at the level of the thyroid lobe) can be removed through a 2.0–2.5 cm incision. Adenomas lying in the tracheo-esophageal groove, however, may require a 3.0 cm incision.

The skin and subcutaneous tissues are infiltrated with a local anesthetic and the patient is given intravenous sedation. We do not perform a cervical block to avoid the risk of wasting time during a period when timing is most critical. There is no other reason that this technique would not work just fine. Subplatysmal flaps are created, the gamma probe is placed into the wound, and background radioactivity counts are quantified in all four quadrants of the neck. The strap muscles are now separated along the midline and another self-retaining retractor is placed to hold these muscles apart. The dissection is carried deeper as directed by the increasing count rate to locate the radioactive gland. Beyond this point, blunt dissection should be used exclusively to prevent damage to small vascular or nervous structures. Cautery below the strap muscles can usually be avoided completely, but when needed, any deep cautery should be of the bipolar type.

The recurrent laryngeal nerve, if within the surgical field, is examined, and although we never make a specific point to locate the nerve, we are constantly aware of anatomical relationships in this regard.

The adenoma is located by continued and frequent use of the probe to direct the dissection. It is very important to use the probe in the "counts per second" mode and not the timed mode, as is often used for lymphatic mapping. When placing the probe deep in the neck, it must be remembered not to aim it towards the chest because this may give a false-positive reading. The reason is that ^{99m}Tc-sestamibi is accumulated in the heart and is, in fact, also used as a cardiac imaging agent. Once identified, the adenoma is teased from its surrounding tissues bluntly and elevated to show its single pedicle that is ligated with a hemoclip and transected. At no time should safety be compromised by a hesitancy to extend the incision or even convert to general anesthesia if necessary. When using the probe to its full potential there will be very little unnecessary dissection. Our experience has shown that as many as 30% of all parathyroid adenomas can be removed without even exposing the thyroid gland. The average operative time for radioguided parathyroidectomy is now about 25 min with a chief resident performing the majority of these cases. Although the speed at which an operation is performed is not important in itself, we believe these times are a reflection of the simplicity of this technique.

Detailed monitoring of the potential radiation hazards has shown this procedure to pose no significant risk to patients, operating room personnel, surgeons, or pathologists [3]. The soiled linens and sponges do not require special handling and can be discarded as per routine. Because sestamibi is concentrated in the heart and right upper quadrant of the abdomen, we routinely place a lead apron over the patient once they have been placed on the operating room table. This decreases radioactivity emission and thereby allows the surgeon and operating room personnel to avoid wearing radiation monitoring devices. We have estimated that the surgeon would have to perform more than 700 of these cases per year to exceed radiation exposure limits. We routinely send radioguided parathyroidectomy patients home within an hour of the procedure. Those patients with significant underlying medical problems are kept overnight, but this is rarely necessary. All patients are sent home on supplemental calcium, approximately 1.5 g/day for 2 weeks.

THE 20% RULE

There are several important points after removal of the radioactive tissue that combine to confirm that the tissue that has been removed is the anticipated parathyroid adenoma [2-4]. From our experience, we have learned that an ex vivo adenoma will almost always have a count rate that is at least 20%, and usually

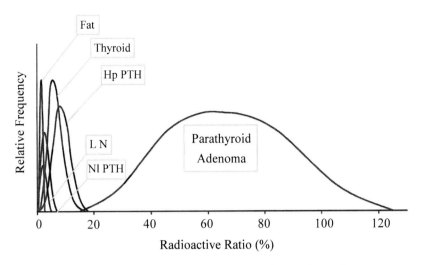

FIGURE 3 The 20% rule. An ex-vivo adenoma will almost always have a count rate of at least 20% of the postexcision background reading (horizontal axis). Conversely, all other neck tissues including fat, lymph nodes (LN), thyroid, normal parathyroids (Nl PTH), and hyperplastic parathyroids (Hp PTH) always contain less than 20% of the background reading. Therefore, any excised tissue containing more than 20% of background radioactivity is guaranteed a parathyroid adenoma.

more than 50%, of the count rate of the postexcision background (Fig 3). After analyzing thousands of tissues removed from the neck during all types of parathyroid explorations, we are confident that fat, lymph nodes, and even thyroid nodules will not be confused with a parathyroid adenoma as typical ex vivo count rates from these tissues are consistently less than 3% of background [5,6] Ex vivo radioactivity reading has proven to be 100% accurate in distinguishing parathyroid adenomas from all other neck tissues when the excised tissue has a count rate of at least 20% of the post excision background. This observation has reduced the number of diagnostic frozen sections dramatically with less that 6% of all adenomas falling below this threshold radioactivity level and thereby necessitating frozen section analysis. Because of the systemic administration of the radiopharmaceutical, ex vivo counts must be performed several feet from the patient with the probe aimed away.

DISCUSSION AND CONCLUDING REMARKS

Timing is an integral part of this procedure and therefore surgeries performed more than 3 h after sestamibi injection result in a less radioactive adenoma. This information must be kept in mind when measuring ex vivo radioactivity and if there is any doubt, a frozen section examination should be performed. Figure 1 details our intrasurgical decision-making process with respect to the radioactivity of the excised adenoma.

Several points should be kept in mind. It must be remembered that the 20% rule refers to 20% of postexcision background, not 120%. In addition, radioactivity should be monitored at 1 sec intervals. Removal of the radioactive gland will be associated with dramatically decreased gamma-ray emission within that area of the neck. The loss of this main focus of radioactivity within the neck will give rise to the third observation: the radioactivity in all four quadrants should equalize after removal of the offending parathyroid tissue [2-4].

With appropriate patient selection and high-quality sestamibi scans, the majority of patients with primary hyperparathyroidism can be successfully treated by radioguided parathyroidectomy. The use of local anesthesia and the limited scope of the dissection afforded by probe guided mapping may decrease the incidence of failed explorations and other potential complications associated with this procedure. Although intrasurgical nuclear mapping can be a very simple, useful tool to minimize the efforts necessary to localize a diseased parathyroid, prior experience in parathyroid surgery remains mandatory as clinical judgement will continue to play the dominant role in determining when the procedure is complete or when a bilateral exploration is required.

To conclude, we believe that there are four key points to a successful surgery:

1. The operation must be performed within 3.5 h of the radiopharmaceutical injection.
2. Radioactivity emitted by the heart should not be interpreted as coming from a substernal parathyroid gland, especially when the scan shows the adenoma to be in the neck.
3. Blunt dissection with meticulous hemostasis should be performed below the strap muscles.
4. If a resected adenoma has more than 20% of background reading (counts/sec) and the patient has primary sporadic hyperparathyroidism with a positive sestamibi scan, then the surgery is complete.

REFERENCES

1. D Denham, J Norman. Cost-effectiveness of preoperative sestamibi scan for primary hyperparathyroidism is dependent solely upon surgeon's choice of operative procedure. J Am Coll Surg 186:293–304, 1998.
2. J Norman, D Denham. Minimally invasive radioguided parathyroidectomy in the reoperative neck. Surgery 124:1088–1093, 1998.

3. J Norman, H Chheda. Minimally invasive parathyroidectomy facilitated by intraoperative nuclear mapping. Surgery 22:998–1004, 1997.
4. J Norman. The technique of intraoperative nuclear mapping to facilitate minimally invasive parathyroidectomy. Cancer Control 4:500–504, 1997.
5. J Norman, C Jaffray, N Chheda. The false v-positive parathyroid sestamibi: a real or perceived problem and a case for radioguided parathyroidectomy. Ann Surg 231:31–37, 2000.
6. C Murphy-Jaffray, C Farrell, C Norman. The 20 percent rule: a simple instantaneous radioactivity measurement defines cure and allows elimination of frozen sections and hormone assays during parathyroidectomy. Surgery 1999 (in press).

16

Radioimmunoguided Surgery

Schlomo Schneebaum, Anton Troitsa, Shmuel Avital, Riad Haddad, Eli Brazovsky, Gilad Gitstein, Joseph Papo, and Yehuda Skornick
Tel Aviv Sourasky Medical Center, Tel Aviv, Israel

INTRODUCTION

Cancer of the colon and rectum is the most common gastrointestinal cancer in the Western world. It is estimated that approximately 500,000 new cases of colorectal cancer are diagnosed annually. Surgery is the most effective treatment. The surgical technique evolved over the first half of the 20th century and has not undergone any significant changes since. The extent of the surgery is based on the empirical knowledge of the pattern of tumor spread, gross findings at laparotomy, and histological confirmation of tumor-free margins. The intent of surgery is curative. However, in this day and age, it is incomprehensible that the surgeon's assessment should still be based on inspection and palpation during surgery and that tissue is excised merely on the basis of its color or consistency, with no way of knowing whether any residual tumor has been left in the abdomen. Any tool that can help the surgeon and assist in staging the disease would be a welcome addition to the armamentarium. This chapter reviews the status of radioimmunoguided surgery (RIGS) in colorectal cancer.

RIGS is a surgical technique whereby the patient is injected with a radiolabeled monoclonal antibody (MoAb) before surgery. With the aid of a gamma-ray detection probe during the operation, the surgeon may better assess the abdomen and stage the disease more accurately. The purpose of developing this technology was fourfold: (1) to confirm the presence or absence of disease; (2) to delineate the surgical margins of resection; (3) to detect clinically occult tumor (tissue not seen by preoperative imaging nor found by the surgeon without the probe); and (4) to confirm the surgical margins of resection [1].

245

The currently used MoAb is CC49, an antitumor-associated glycoprotein (anti-TAG-72) [2]. It is labeled with iodine-125 (^{125}I). RIGS using CC49 for primary and recurrent colorectal cancer has resulted in tumor localization of 92% to 97% of recurrent tumors [3–5]. A number of studies have been conducted with the anti-TAG MoAb, most of them at Ohio State University and James Cancer and Research Institute in Columbus, OH, where several benefits of this technology were demonstrated [4,6–9]. The surgeon was able to locate cancer and find micrometastasis in lymph nodes that were negative for tumor after routine hematoxylin and eosin (H&E) pathological examination. RIGS technology showed patterns of tumor dissemination [10,11]. RIGS provided additional information that resulted in a change in traditional surgical decision-making and in a better selection of patients with resectable disease and enhanced survival [3,7,8].

RIGS adds another tool to the traditional methods used by the surgeon. This addition requires learning and adaptation of the surgeon's perception in realizing that a gamma-ray detection probe may locate suspicious tissue neither observed nor palpated traditionally. Not only does the surgeon have to change his traditional behavior, but the pathologist does as well. The conventional method of bivalving the node and then staining it with H&E is not accurate enough. The tissue may need a more sophisticated pathology method such as immunohistochemistry or reverse-transcriptase polymerase chain reaction (RT-PCR) to detect cancer markers.

RIGS was invented by a surgeon, E.W. Martin, and a nuclear engineer, M. Thurston, and we know today that one of the important factors of its development and implementation is team work between the nuclear medicine physician, the surgeon, and the pathologist.

PRINCIPLES OF RIGS

To create a system that would function as efficiently as possible and to have the maximum sensitivity, four aspects had to be considered in the development of the RIGS system: probe design, choice of targeting agent, choice of radionuclide, and data processing.

Gamma-Ray Detection Probe

The idea of using a hand-held probe for the localization of diseased tissue was first reported by William G. Myers in 1960 [12]. The first reported use of the probe for RIGS was in 1984 [13].

The design of the probe is based on the use of a semiconductor detector in a hand-held instrument. The probe uses a built-in 12-mm cadmium telluride detector, together with a preamplifier, and has the ability to detect gamma rays from a radioactive tracer. The gamma photons detected by the crystal are con-

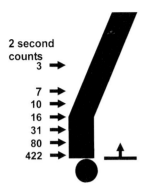

2 second
counts
   3 ➡
   7 ➡
  10 ➡
  16 ➡
  31 ➡
  80 ➡
 422 ➡

FIGURE 1   Probe over 50 nCi node (2-second count). The count rate decreases proportionately to the square of the distance between the two. (From Ref. 14. Copyright 1999 Springer-Verlag. Reprinted by permission of Springer-Verlag GmbH & Co.)

verted into electric pulses and presented as both a digital numerical display and an auditory signal.

The efficacy of detection is the ratio between the area of the detector and the area of the sphere of radiation. The ratio between these two areas increases proportionately to the square of the distance between the two (Fig. 1) according to the inverse square law [14]. The probe serves as a homing device by directing the surgeon to the tissue with the high-count rate.

The Neoprobe 1000 and later models (Neoprobe 1500 and 2000; Neoprobe Corporation, Dublin, OH) have a special "squelch" mode character. This is a mathematical character of the computer that calculates the mean count of a given point (5-second count), calculates the standard deviation (square root), and starts to emit a sound only when the count is three standard deviations greater than the mean count (denoting significantly higher radiation). This feature enables the surgeon to survey an area and guide himself to the possibly diseased radioactive tissue [15].

The surgical technique is based on careful survey of the area in question. Slow scanning is mandatory. An important point in this technology is the three-point counting principle. First, an in vivo count is performed, then the tissue is excised, and an ex vivo count is performed to verify that the correct tissue was excised. Subsequently, the bed of resection is probed again to verify that no radioactive tissue is left behind. Table 1 describes several scenarios using this three-point principle.

Isotope

In RIGS, the radiolabeled MoAb is injected 3 to 4 weeks before surgery. The antibody becomes attached to the tumor while the body secretes the surplus anti-

TABLE 1   The Three-Point Counting Principle

Scenario	In vivo	Ex vivo	Bed of resection	
1	+	+	−	Right tissue, completely excised
2	+	−	+	Wrong tissue excised
3	+	+	+	Right tissue, not completely excised
4	+	−	−	Technical error with resulting high in vivo count

Source: Ref. 14. Copyright 1999 Springer-Verlag. Reprinted by permission of Springer-Verlag GmbH & Co.

body. The concentration in the blood decreases, and a ratio builds up between the tumor and the blood, enabling the surgeon to detect the tumor when using the gamma-detecting probe (Fig. 2) [16].

Several isotopes were tested in the development of the technique: [125]I, ^{131}I, indium-111 (^{111}In), and technetium-99m (^{99m}Tc). [125]I was chosen because it combines the advantages of low Compton scattering, which obviates the need for collimation; high tissue attenuation, which improves the tumor-to-background

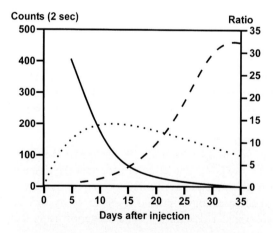

FIGURE 2   Tumor and background concentration in an animal model injected with monoclonal antibody labeled with [125]I. Background, continuous line; tumors; dotted line; background to tumor ratio, broken line. (From Ref. 14. Copyright 1999 Springer-Verlag. Reprinted by permission of Springer-Verlag GmbH & Co.)

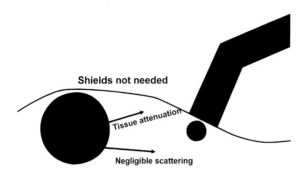

FIGURE 3   Advantage of low-energy radiation with ^{125}I: no collimation needed, tissue attenuation, and negligible Compton scattering. (From Ref. 14. Copyright 1999 Springer-Verlag. Reprinted by permission of Springer-Verlag GmbH & Co.)

ratio; a good detector efficiency; and a half-life long enough to accommodate the slow clearing of the complete antibody (Figs. 3 and 4) [17,18].

Carrier Substance

Different antibodies have been tested before the currently used antibody CC49 was chosen, a second-generation anti-TAG-72 tumor-associated glycoprotein. TAG-72 is a pancarcinoma antigen found in colorectal tumors, breast cancer, prostate cancer, and ovarian cancer, as well as in secretory endometrium [19]. The antigen for CC49 has a molecular weight of 200 to 400 kDa^2 and is purified

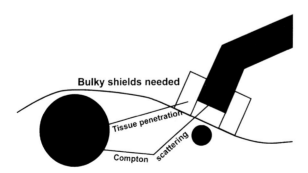

FIGURE 4   Disadvantage of high-energy radiation: collimation needed, tissue penetration, and Compton scattering. (From Ref. 14. Copyright 1999 Springer-Verlag. Reprinted by permission of Springer-Verlag GmbH & Co.)

from a human colon cancer xenograft used as an immunogen to generate a series of second-generation MoAbs [2].

Surgical Procedure

Patients enrolled in the RIGS study were all diagnosed with recurrent or metastatic colorectal cancer by clinical findings, abdominal computed tomography (CT), or elevated carcinoembryonic antigen (CEA) blood levels in patients who previously underwent surgery for colorectal cancer.

Before enrollment, all patients underwent a CT of the chest to exclude extra-abdominal disease, a CT of the abdomen and pelvis, and colonoscopy. All patients signed an informed consent form approved by the local institutional review board. All patients took a thyroid-blocking agent starting 2 hours before injection and then daily until surgery. This was either a saturated solution of potassium iodide or Thyro-block tablets (Wallace Laboratories, Cranbury, NJ). Patients were injected with 1 mg CC49 (anti-TAG-72 tumor-associated glycoprotein MoAb) radiolabeled with [125]I. The patients were taken to surgery with a precordial count rate of no more than 20 counts per 2 seconds. Such a count rate is usually obtained 3 to 4 weeks after injection and enables good intra-abdominal discrimination between the blood pool background and small tumors, based on 95% correlation between precordial counts and intra-abdominal aortic counts.

Surgery started with traditional exploration of inspection and palpation. To standardize exploration and abdominal assessment, the abdomen was divided into four zones: zone I is the liver; zone II concerns the upper abdomen and includes stomach, spleen, and periportal and celiac lymph nodes (Fig. 5); zone III concerns the midabdomen, including colon, small bowel, kidneys, and lymph nodes along the aorta and vena cava as far as the bifurcation; and zone IV contains the pelvis, including rectum, lymph nodes along both iliac artery and vein, female reproductive organs, and urinary bladder (Fig. 6). CT evaluation before surgery was also performed following the same zonal configuration. In all patients, the liver was examined with intraoperative ultrasound as part of the traditional evaluation. After exploration, the surgeon reported his findings, resectability status, and surgical plan. This was followed by survey with the gamma-detecting probe, Neoprobe 1000.

At the start of the operation, the surgeon "squelches" on the aortic bifurcation or any intra-abdominal major blood vessel with a count rate that correlates with the precordial count rate [20]. The blood vessel serves as a reference point "blood pool background" for the lymph nodes. For parenchymatous organs such as the liver, the surgeon may also squelch on an adjacent normal-appearing area as a reference point. The surgeon then surveys the abdomen with the probe, and whenever the device emits a continuous sound, he stops and takes three 2-second count readings. Readings that are twice as high as the reference point and greater

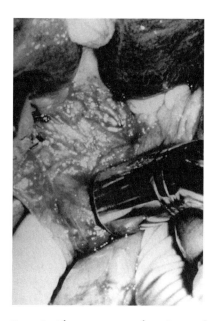

FIGURE 5   The gamma-ray detection probe is brought into contact with the lymph node in the periportal area. The surgeon's finger is inserted in the Winslow's foramen. (From Ref. 30. Copyright 1995 American Cancer Society. Reprinted by permission of Wiley-Liss, Inc., a subsidiary of John Wiley & Sons, Inc.)

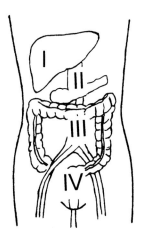

FIGURE 6   Abdominal zones. (From Ref. 21. Copyright 1999 Springer-Verlag. Reprinted by permission of Springer-Verlag GmbH & Co.)

than 20 are considered to be positive. At the end of the survey, the surgeon again reports the surgical findings, resectability status of the patient, and surgical plan. Every suspicious tissue undergoes biopsy or is resected because lymph node involvement in certain cases may cause the surgeon to abandon the intended resection. As shown in previous studies [4], certain RIGS-positive lymph nodes are not always confirmed by H&E staining. Resection was not abandoned based on RIGS-positive lymph nodes without frozen H&E confirmation. Data were analyzed according to abdominal zones and H&E confirmation.

TEL AVIV SOURASKY MEDICAL CENTER EXPERIENCE

Because the RIGS methodology was introduced at the Tel Aviv Sourasky Medical Center after the initiation of the phase III study, all surgery was performed according to this protocol. Sixty-six patients with recurrent colorectal cancer were enrolled in phase III multicenter studies (Neo2-14, Neo2-12, and single-center study Neo2-04 and compassionate use protocol Neo2-81) [21].

Eight of the 66 patients enrolled were not assessable because they did not undergo surgery. Three of the patients were injected but underwent emergency surgery for various reasons without using the probe. Thus, 58 patients were assessable and are the subjects of this study. Localization of CC49 in the tumor was observed in 54 of the 66 intent-to-treat patients (81.8%) or in 54 of the 58 assessable patients (96.4%).

In Table 2, the tumor findings are categorized according to the four zones, preoperative CT findings, surgeon's findings with traditional exploration and then

TABLE 2   CT, Surgical (Traditional), and RIGS-Positive and H&E-Positive Findings of Excised Tumor Sites.

Zone	CT	Surgeon	RIGS	Pathology
I	19	34	35	35
II	2	5	23	5
III	13	42	68	48
IV	22	36	51	45
Total	56	117	177	133

CT, tumor sites identified before surgery; Surgeon, tumor sites identified by the surgeon using traditional methods; RIGS, tumor sites identified in surgery using the gamma-detecting probe; Pathology, excised tissue confirmed by pathology to be H&E-positive.
Source: Ref. 21. Copyright 1999 Springer-Verlag. Reprinted by permission of Springer-Verlag GmbH & Co.

the use of the RIGS methodology, and H&E pathology confirmation. The performance differed between the four zones. Using intraoperative ultrasound, the detection capability of the surgeon is high in zone I. CT performance is poor in zones II and III, but there were also some false-positive findings by RIGS. In zone IV, RIGS identified many tumors, most of them H&E-positive. Altogether, CT identified 56 tumor sites, the surgeon identified 117 using traditional exploration and 177 with the RIGS methodology, and pathology confirmed 133 tumor sites.

A summary of the RIGS findings by anatomical sites is presented in Table 3. In 17 of 58 patients (28.2%), RIGS exploration resulted in new findings that led to a change in the surgical plan in 16 patients. In five of these patients, a planned resection was abandoned: four liver resections were abandoned because of periportal lymph node metastasis, and one planned pelvic exenteration had to be abandoned because of extrapelvic disease. Additional tissue was removed in 11 patients. In the one remaining patient whose disease was already found to be unresectable by traditional exploration, such an additional finding did not cause a change in surgical plan.

The results were also analyzed according to criteria of true positive, false positive, true negative, and false negative. Calculations of sensitivity, specificity, positive predictive value, and negative predictive values of all tumor sites are presented in Table 4 for the 54 patients in whom the disease was localized by the MoAb and for the whole group of 58 patients. These calculations were also made for the lymph nodes and for nonlymphatic tissue that was removed during surgery (Table 5). In nonlymphatic tissue, the sensitivity was 95.6% and the

TABLE 3 Summary of Biopsied RIGS-Positive Findings in 58 Patients with Metastatic Colorectal Cancer

Tumor site	No. of RIGS-positive tumors
Liver	34
Anastomotic recurrence	9
Pelvic tumor	19
Peritoneal metastasis	11
Uterus	6
Periaortic nodes	90
Ovary	6
Small bowel	2

Source: Ref. 21. Copyright 1999 Springer-Verlag. Reprinted by permission of Springer-Verlag GmbH & Co.

Table 4   RIGS Performance in the Whole Group of
58 Patients and in the 54 Patients in Whom
Disease Was Localized With This Technique

	Total (%)	Localizing patients (%)
Sensitivity	95	96.8
Specificity	42.7	44
Positive predictive value	67.2	67.9
Negative predictive value	88	91

Source: Ref. 21. Copyright 1999 Springer-Verlag. Reprinted by
permission of Springer-Verlag GmbH & Co.

specificity 90%. In the lymph nodes, the sensitivity was 100% with a very low
specificity of 7%. The latter finding was caused by a high false-positive rate and
the fact that no negative lymph nodes underwent biopsy. On the other hand, the
negative predictive value of lymphatic tissue was 100% because of the fact that
no false-negative nodes were identified. This means that a RIGS-negative lymph
node implies no tumor in a patient with localizing disease. The only false-positive
nonlymphatic tissue was in patients with nonlocalizing disease (four tumor sites)
and in those with peritoneal spread (two tumor sites). There was no false-positive
tissue in a liver, pelvis, or parenchymatous organs. All true-negative tissue was
tissue that was suspected by the surgeon, was RIGS-negative, and that underwent
biopsy. The average number of tumor sites was 2.7 per patient.

Subgroups According to Anatomic Location

RIGS was developed to guide the surgeon during CEA-directed second-look surgery and to detect clinically occult tumor that was causing an elevated CEA but

Table 5   RIGS Performance in 58 Patients (Lymph
Nodes and Nonlymphatic Tissues)

	Nonlymphatic tissue (%)	Lymph nodes (%)
Sensitivity	95.6	100
Specificity	90	7
Positive predictive value	95.6	40
Negative predictive value	90	100

Source: Ref. 21. Copyright 1999 Springer-Verlag. Reprinted by
permission of Springer-Verlag GmbH & Co.

that was not found by the surgeon. Its use was then extended to patients with recurrent or metastatic colorectal cancer as surgeons noticed the ability of RIGS to detect more cancer as well as its value in assessing margins of resection. A natural question under investigation is what constitutes the clinical scenario in which RIGS would be most beneficial or have the capacity to improve survival. Although a two-arm study was never conducted and in every study each patient was his own control (traditional exploration was followed by a RIGS survey), there are some clinical scenarios in which RIGS information can dramatically influence the decision-making process of the surgeon: liver surgery and pelvic surgery.

Phase III Study Results: Liver Metastasis

One hundred fifty-five patients were enrolled in the Neoprobe Multicenter Phase III Study (Neo2-14) for recurrent and metastatic colorectal cancer in the United States, Europe, and Israel. Sixty patients were diagnosed with liver metastasis based on preoperative CT [22].

Tumor was pathologically proven in 56 of the 60 patients (93.3%), while localization of antibody in tumor was observed in 52 of these patients (92.9%). After the traditional intraoperative assessment, the disease in 35 of the 60 patients was found to be resectable. Ten of these 35 patients had RIGScan (surgeon uses the RIGS methodology with CC49 MoAb) occult tumor (28.5%) versus 25 patients with no RIGScan occult tumor. Seven of the 10 patients with occult tumor (70%) died with a median survival time of 412 days, whereas seven of the 25 patients with no occult tumor died (28.0%). The median for this group could not be computed because of the small proportion of observed deaths. The log-rank test was significant at a *P* value of .046 (Fig. 7).

Because the prognosis of these patients is dependent on the occurrence of extrahepatic tumor, and in particular tumor deposits in lymph nodes, an analysis of survival was performed only in patients with biopsied lymph nodes. Twenty-two patients were eligible for this analysis: 10 in the occult group and 12 in the nonoccult group. Seven of the 10 patients with occult tumor died (70%), whereas only two of the 12 with no occult tumor died (16.7%). The resultant *P* value from the log-rank statistic was .025 (Fig. 8). The efficacy of the RIGS methodology was also tested in patients whose liver resection margins underwent biopsy or were excised during surgery, correctly identifying five positive and 33 negative resection margins.

Pelvic Recurrence

At the Tel Aviv Sourasky Medical Center, 21 patients diagnosed with recurrent pelvic cancer underwent surgery using the RIGS methodology [23]. In their primary surgery, 14 of these patients had undergone anterior resection, and seven had undergone abdominoperineal resection.

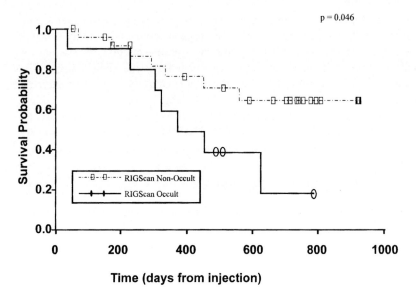

FIGURE 7 Survival differences for patients with surgically resectable disease with hepatic lesions identified preoperatively by CT scan (clinical study Neo2-14). Patients with RIGScan-identified nonoccult metastasis versus those with RIGScan-identified occult metastasis. Long-rank *P* value = .046. (From Ref. 22.)

Traditional exploration identified eight intracolorectal recurrences, nine extracolonic pelvic recurrences, and five extrapelvic lymph node metastases. RIGS exploration confirmed all intracolorectal recurrences except in one patient with no MoAb localization. RIGS identified 13 extracolonic pelvic recurrences and 10 lymph node metastases. In all, seven patients (33%) had lesions identified by RIGS that were previously unknown. These findings resulted in a more extensive surgical procedure than was originally planned in six patients. In the remaining patient, newly identified extrapelvic disease led to a decision to abandon the intended pelvic resection. RIGS positivity at the end of surgery was also monitored. Of the 20 patients who localized, 12 were RIGS-positive and eight were RIGS-negative. At 36-month follow-up, actual survival of RIGS-negative patients was significantly better than that of RIGS-positive patients ($P = .034$).

Elevated CEA

Surgeons are usually reluctant to operate solely on the basis of an elevated CEA blood level with no supporting evidence of tumor location in any of the imaging modalities. This attitude is based on the knowledge that exploration may be diffi-

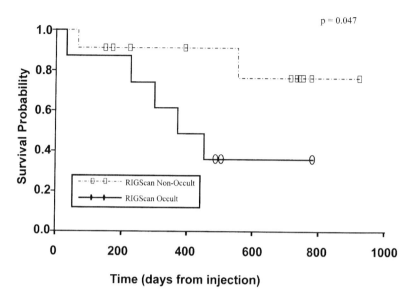

FIGURE 8   Survival differences for patients with surgically resectable disease with hepatic lesions identified preoperatively by CT scan, and lymph nodes that underwent biopsy (clinical study Neo2-14). Patients with RIGScan-identified nonoccult versus RIGScan-identified occult metastasis. Log-rank *P* value = .047. (From Ref. 22.)

cult and may prove futile. RIGS is an appealing concept in such patients. Preoperative scintigraphy with anti-CEA MoAb is an attractive solution, especially because it may indicate the existence of extra-abdominal disease and may prevent unnecessary abdominal exploration. Patients with colorectal disease are monitored by a medical oncologist after adjuvant therapy, and many undergo such a scan before being referred for RIGS.

At the Tel-Aviv Sourasky Medical Center 19 patients underwent RIGS for a suspected tumor recurrence based solely on an elevated CEA level [24]. All patients underwent scintigraphy with an anti-CEA MoAb labeled with ^{99m}Tc or ^{111}In. Traditional exploration identified 26 recurrent tumors: seven in the liver, eight in the pelvis, six in the retroperitoneum, three in the colon, one in the spleen, and one in the anastomosis. RIGS exploration confirmed the presence of all of these tumors and identified additional tumor sites in seven patients (36.8%). These findings led to a change in the surgical plan in seven patients: two resections were abandoned, and in five patients additional tissue was removed. CEA scintigraphy correlated with intra-abdominal findings in six patients. Additional findings not detected by the scan were intraoperatively discovered in eight patients. There was a discrepancy between the scintigraphy findings and the intraoperative findings in three patients, and the CEA scintigraphy results were inconclusive in another two.

These results support the assumption that patients with elevated CEA level and no other findings should undergo surgery using RIGS because this can provide the surgeon with more accurate knowledge of the extent of the disease.

Primary Colorectal Cancer

Although RIGS was developed for recurrent colorectal cancer, it was a natural follow-through to use it in patients with primary colorectal cancer. With the first MoAbs used, the localization rate was low, and this was attributed to the desquamation of cells during the interval between injection and surgery. Use of CC49 for patients with primary lesions resulted in a 90% localization rate. In the first report by Arnold et al. [6], additional RIGS-positive tissue was found in 50% of the patients, but the tissue was not analyzed pathologically. In later studies, however, it became evident that type III tissue (RIGS-positive, H&E-negative) was common in extraregional lymph nodes. In yet another report studying the pattern of RIGS-positive tissue dissemination, it was shown that this tissue was more common in patients with primary colorectal cancer than in those with recurrent disease [10,25]. A further observation when analyzing the survival of some groups of patients was that patients left with RIGS-positive tissue at the end of surgery had a worse prognosis than those who were RIGS-negative [26].

There are several problems in using RIGS for primary cancer that deserve to be mentioned. (1) Surgery performed for early colorectal cancer is anatomically oriented. The colon is resected with its draining lymphatic field along the arterial blood supply, which usually results in fairly rigid wide margins, e.g., right hemicolectomy, left hemicolectomy, etc. (2) The decision concerning postoperative treatment is based on knowledge of the lymph node status. This has led to the belief that the only value of using RIGS in early colon cancer resection is that it obtains information during the operation, whereas pathology results are obtained afterward. However, RIGS can also identify the lymph nodes to be examined by the pathologist and provide information about tissues that are not resected. The prognostic value of this information can only be studied prospectively. The Neo2-13 phase III study was an attempt to include only early cases as those with more advanced disease and suspected extracolonic involvement were enrolled in the Neo2-14 study. The situation is different in patients with rectal cancer, where the margins are narrow and known to determine the incidence of local recurrence. The use of techniques such as total mesorectal excision reduces the risk of a local recurrence [27], and this risk is reduced even further by administering adjuvant radiotherapy, but the question remains whether every patient is a candidate for these treatment modalities. At present, the answer is in the affirmative because there is no superior way to select patients. RIGS may have a role in selecting patients for adjuvant treatment. Ensuring completeness of removal because of its almost 100% negative predictive value, RIGS may even direct the surgeon to use a more aggressive procedure in some patients. Preliminary results of the phase III study seem to confirm this assumption.

The Neoprobe phase III study, Neo2-13, had an unplanned interim analysis including the first 62 patients and was never reported. Thirty-five of these patients had rectal cancer.

The localization ratio with RIGS was 86%. As part of the study, lymph nodes that were RIGS-positive but H&E-negative (type III) were submitted to a central laboratory for multiple cuts and immunohistochemistry with anticytokeratin antibody. Regional lymph nodes resected with the primary specimen were included in this approach. These nodes were also tested with the probe in the pathology laboratory. Twenty-three patients with stage II disease underwent a full pathology evaluation (H&E and immunohistochemistry). Eleven patients had at least one positive lymph node by immunohistochemistry, upstaging 48% of the patients. Twenty-nine patients with rectal cancer had a complete evaluation. Twelve of these patients had stage II disease, and eight of them were upstaged (67%). A total of 146 regional lymph nodes were submitted for serial sectioning and immunohistochemistry. Ninety-one of these lymph nodes were RIGS-positive, and 55 were RIGS-negative. Twenty of the RIGS-positive lymph nodes (22%) and three of the 55 RIGS-negative lymph nodes (5.5%) were found to harbor tumor cells ($P < .01$; unpublished data, personal communication).

Performance evaluation of the extraregional lymph nodes in these patients with rectal cancer showed a high sensitivity, a negative predictive value of 100%, and a low specificity because of the high rate of false-positive nodes.

The study evaluating the regional tissue was discontinued because of financial reasons and the belief that the regulatory authorities would evaluate these data as unimportant because the tissue had to be removed anyway.

COMMENTS

An important prognostic variable in colorectal cancer is the presence or absence of tumor in lymph nodes [28]. However, the clinical assessment of lymph node involvement is not easy because size and consistency, the two parameters used by the surgeon in traditional exploration, are not reliable indicators for the presence of metastasis [29].

RIGS has proven to be a technology capable of detecting lymph node metastasis in areas such as along the vena cava and hepatoduodenal ligament [3,4,30]. Biopsy of lymph nodes during surgery is part of colorectal cancer surgery, but random biopsies have a low yield. Even when concentrating on distinct areas, such as the periportal region, biopsy of only firm or enlarged (> 1 cm) lymph nodes results in only 11% positive findings [31]. In a recent study by

Gibbs et al. [32], periportal and celiac lymph node sampling resulted in 11% positive findings.

RIGS identifies lymph nodes with cancer, but using an anti-TAG MoAb may result in a high ratio of RIGScan-positive lymph nodes that cannot be confirmed by H&E. The problem of RIGS-positive lymph nodes that are H&E-negative was first reported by Arnold et al. [10] when using the MoAb CC49. They found that these pathologically uninvolved lymph nodes have similar tumor–to–normal tissue ratios as pathologically proven metastatic nodes. It is accepted today that routine analysis with one-cut H&E can miss micrometastases, and that when dealing with sentinel nodes, for example, more sophisticated pathology such as immunohistochemistry and RT-PCR is advisable [33]. Arnold et al. [4] have named such lymph nodes type III (RIGS-positive/H&E-negative). Type I is RIGS-negative/H&E-negative, type II is RIGS-negative/H&E-positive, and type IV is obvious tumor RIGS-positive/H&E-positive. In a study conducted by Cote et al. [34], 57 lymph nodes were evaluated by routine analysis with H&E staining. Seventeen nodes were H&E-positive, and 40 were H&E-negative. Thirty-nine of the 57 were RIGS-positive, but only 14 of these were H&E-positive. Of the 39 RIGS-positive nodes, 25 were type III (RIGS-positive/H&E-negative). These 25 type III lymph nodes were subjected to multiple H&E sections and immunohistochemistry staining with cytokeratin. Occult metastasis was found in 10 of these 25 nodes (40%). Therefore, routine analysis identified tumor in 17 of 27 nodes (63%), whereas the probe identified the presence of tumor in 24 of these 27 nodes (89%). The clinical significance of these lymph nodes with metastasis identified by immunohistochemistry with anticytokeratin was demonstrated in a study reported by Greenson et al. [35] in which 448 lymph nodes of 41 patients with Dukes' B disease were analyzed by immunohistochemistry with anticytokeratin antibodies. After a 5-year follow-up period, seven of 14 patients with cytokeratin-positive lymph nodes died of disease, whereas only one of the 27 patients with cytokeratin-uninvolved lymph nodes died. In a study that concentrated on periportal lymph nodes, type III lymph nodes from 34 patients were subjected to multiple sections and immunohistochemistry analysis [30]. Multiple sectioning identified tumor in 24% of the patients, immunohistochemistry with cytokeratin in 48%, and immunohistochemistry with both cytokeratin and CC49 found tumor and tumor antigen in 70%.

Further proof of the clinical significance of these findings can be observed in some of the data generated in the phase III study, in which prognostic variable data were analyzed only in patients with resectable disease after traditional survey [36]. The prognostic outcome of RIGS findings in lymph nodes was examined by looking at survival data for three distinct groups: (1) patients with RIGS-positive/pathology-positive lymph nodes; (2) patients with RIGS-positive/pathology-negative lymph nodes; and (3) patients with RIGS-negative/pathology-negative lymph nodes. Because patients may have presented with all three RIGS/

pathology combinations, assignment to the groups was made in the following manner: patients with ≥ 1 RIGS-positive/pathology-positive node were classified as (+)/(+) patients; patients with no pathology-positive nodes but ≥ 1 RIGS-positive nodes were classified as (+)/(−); and patients in whom all nodes were RIGS-negative/pathology-negative were classified as (−)/(−) group (Table 6 and Fig. 9). The difference between RIGS-positive/pathology-positive and RIGS-negative/pathology-negative groups makes sense. RIGS is associated with high negative predictive value, especially in lymph nodes (94%). This outcome of the RIGS performance, coupled with the aforementioned analysis, tends to suggest that RIGS-negative findings reliably predict the absence of tumor and may be of prognostic value. This high negative predictive value is of major importance in surgery, where decisions are made whether or not to resect hepatic metastasis or perform extensive pelvic surgery. Although not usually appreciated by the regulatory authorities, this advantage is unique to the RIGS technology, and its importance should not be underestimated because a surgeon is often faced with this question, and frozen section may be problematic because sampling errors cannot be ruled out. This unique attribute of RIGS enables the surgeon to carry out the surgical plan with more confidence. Our experience has taught us that extensive lymph node dissection in patients with widespread abdominal lymph node involvement does not translate into cure. The reason is probably the existence of extra-abdominal spread not previously evaluated or detected by RIGS because these patients invariably develop thoracic metastasis within a short time.

The data shown and reviewed suggest that RIGS-negative lymph nodes in a patient with localizing disease signify no tumor. Major decisions based on RIGS-positive lymph nodes need H&E confirmation. RIGS-positive lymph nodes signify a dismal prognosis but do not necessarily mean regional cancer. Using RIGS, the surgeon is better able to detect lymph node metastasis. RIGS provides the surgeon with additional information that results in better staging, better prognostication, and better intraoperative and postoperative decision-making.

TABLE 6 RIGS Findings in Biopsied/Resected Lymph Nodes in Patients with Traditionally Resectable Disease (Clinical Study Neo2-14) [36]

	RIGS (+) Pathology (+)	RIGS (+) Pathology (−)	RIGS (−) Pathology (−)
No. of patients	12	29	7
No. of deaths	8	12	0
% deaths	66.7	42.4	0.0
Median survival time (days)	460	699	—[a]

Log-rank *P* value = .002; Wilcoxon *P* value = .006.

[a] Median not computed because of small number of deaths.

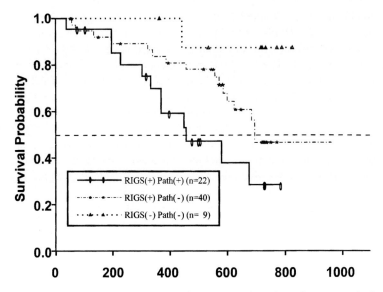

FIGURE 9   Overall survival RIGS performance in lymph nodes (n = 71), clinical study Neo2-14. RIGS-positive/pathology-positive versus RIGS-positive/pathology-negative versus RIGS-negative/pathology-negative. Log-rank *P* value = .002. (From Ref. 36.)

The advantage of RIGS in these cases is overwhelming, and although the surgical indications have to be weighed before any decisions are made, the data generated in the phase III study strongly support the use of RIGS once the decision to operate has been made.

Shortcomings in traditional pathology evaluation of lymph nodes identified by RIGS were found in several studies. RIGS directed the pathologist to lymph nodes that proved to be tumor-positive when examined with immunohistochemistry [27,28]. However, more studies using molecular biology techniques are needed to determine the biological significance of such nodes, some of which may carry tumor antigen but no viable tumor cells.

THE FUTURE OF RIGS

RIGS started as a diagnostic method to locate occult cancer in patients with an elevated CEA level and has evolved into a method that not only helps the surgeon to delineate margins of resection, but also to find occult tumor and assess the completeness of a resection. It also provides the knowledge of patterns of tumor spread in the early stages of disease that previously could only be obtained by autopsy. The ability to locate occult tumor involvement and the high negative predictive value of 100% enable the surgeon to select patients for resection with more confidence and to make more accurate intraoperative and postoperative treatment decisions.

The currently used antibody has been tried for other gastrointestinal tumors, such as carcinoma of the pancreas, with promising results of 100% localization and a 17% detection rate of occult disease [37]. Other anti-TAG MoAbs as well as several anti-CEA MoAbs have been tested in patients with ovarian cancer [38], prostatic cancer [39], or breast cancer [40,41]. Trying to find the MoAb of the future involves experiments with single chains [42,43] and new humanized MoAb to overcome the development of human antimouse antibody production. MoAbs that shorten the interval between injection and surgery are also being investigated. An example of a new MoAb is a C_H2 domain–deleted molecule. Peptides such as ^{125}I-TYR(3)-octreotide are under investigation for neuroendocrine tumors [44,45], neuroblastomas, and breast tumors [46].

Gamma-guided surgery has encouraged pathologists to investigate the tissue with the highest chance of metastasis by immunohistochemistry or PCR and has raised the question of the relevance of micrometastasis. RIGS technology has now been incorporated in clinical studies, and its significance will be better understood in the future. Smaller probes and special probes for minimally invasive surgery, such as laparoscopy, are currently being developed.

Teaching through telesurgery is underway and could become part of our daily practice in the future. RIGS will result in better surgery, better pathology, and, it is hoped, improved patient survival.

REFERENCES

1. Thurston MO, Mojzisik CM. History and development of radioimmunoguided surgery. Semin Colon Rectal Surg 1995; 6:185–191.
2. Muraro R, Kuroki M, Wunderlich D, Poole DJ, Colcher D, Thor A, Greiner JW, Simpson JF, Molinolo A, Noguchi P, Schlom J. Generation and characterization of second generation (B72.3) monoclonal antibodies reactive with the TAG-72 antigen. Cancer Res 1988; 48:4588–4596.
3. Schneebaum S, Papo M, Graif M, Baratz M, Baron J, Skornik Y. Radioguided surgery benefits for recurrent colorectal cancer. Ann Surg Oncol 1997; 4:371–376.
4. Arnold MW, Schneebaum S, Berens A, Petty L, Mojzisik C, Hinkle G, Martin EW Jr. Intraoperative detection of colorectal cancer with radioimmunoguided surgery and CC49, a second-generation monoclonal antibody. Ann Surg 1992; 216:627–632.
5. Daly JM, Burak W Jr, Chevinsky A, Lavery IC, Martin EW, Schneebaum S. Radioimmunoguided surgery for large bowel cancer: results of prospective multi-institutional trials. American College of Surgeons 82nd Annual Clinical Congress, 1996 (abstract), October 6–11, San Francisco, CA.

6. Arnold MW, Schneebaum S, Berens A, Mojzisik C, Hinkle G, Martin EW Jr. Radio-immunoguided surgery challenges traditional decision making in patients with primary colorectal cancer. Surgery 1992; 112:624–630.
7. Martin EW Jr, Carey LC. Second-look surgery for colorectal cancer. Ann Surg 1991; 214:321–325.
8. Bertsch DJ, Burak WE, Young DC, Arnold MW, Martin EW Jr. Radioimmuno-guided surgery system improves survival for patients with recurrent colorectal cancer. Surgery 1995; 118:634–639.
9. Cohen AM, Martin EW, Lavery I, Daly J, Sardi A, Aitken D, Bland K, Mojzisik C, Hinkle G. Radioimmunoguided surgery using iodine 125 B72.3 in patients with colorectal cancer. Arch Surg 1991; 126:349–352.
10. Arnold MW, Hitchcock CL, Young DC, Burak WE, Bertsch DJ, Martin EW. Intra-abdominal patterns of disease dissemination in colorectal cancer identified using radioimmunoguided surgery. Dis Colon Rectum 1996; 39:509–513.
11. Bertsch DJ, Burak WE, Young DC, Arnold MW, Martin EW Jr. Radioimmuno-guided surgery for colorectal cancer. Ann Surg Oncol 1996; 3:310–316.
12. Myers WG, Vanderleeden JC. Radioiodine-125. J Nucl Med 1960; 1:149–164.
13. Aitken DR, Hinkle GH, Thurston MO, Tuttle SE, Martin DT, Olsen JO, Haagensen DE Jr, Houchens D, Martin EW Jr. Gamma-detecting probe for radioimmune detection of CEA-producing tumors. Dis Colon Rectum 1984; 27:279–282.
14. Schneebaum S, Even-Sapir E, Cohen M, Shacham-Lehrman H, Gat A, Brazovsky E, Livshitz G, Stadler J, Skornick Y. Clinical applications of gamma-detecting probes—radioguided surgery. Eur J Nucl Med 1999; 26:S26–S35.
15. Thurston MO. Development of the gamma-detecting probe for radioimmunoguided surgery. In: Martin EW Jr, ed. Radioimmunoguided Surgery (RIGS) in the Detection and Treatment of Colorectal Cancer. Austin: Landes RG Co, 1994; pp 42–65.
16. Martin EW Jr, Barnes JA, Thurston MO. Introduction: The RIGS concept. In: Martin EW Jr, ed. Radioimmunoguided Surgery (RIGS) in the Detection and Treatment of Colorectal Cancer. Austin: Landes RG Co, 1994; pp 1–6.
17. Hinkle GH, Mojzisik CM, Loesch JA, Hill TL, Thurston MO, Sampsel J, Olsen J, Martin EW Jr. The evolution of the radioimmunoguided surgery™ system: an innovative technique for the intraoperative detection of tumor. Antibody Immunoconj Radiopharm 1991; 4:339–358.
18. Thurston MO, Kaehr JW, Martin EW III, Martin EW Jr. Radionuclide of choice for use with an intraoperative probe. Antibody Immunocon Radiopharm 1991; 4:595–601.
19. Thor A, Ohuchi N, Szpak CA, Johnston WW, Schlom J. Distribution of oncofetal antigen tumor-associated glycoprotein-72 defined by monoclonal antibody B72.3. Cancer Res 1986; 46:3118–3124.
20. Mojzisik CM, Cook CH, Schneebaum S. Safety and performance factors in the development and clinical use of the RIGS system. In: Martin EW Jr, ed. Radioimmuno-guided Surgery (RIGS) in the Detection and Treatment of Colorectal Cancer. Austin: Landes RG Co, 1994; pp 81–105.
21. Schneebaum S, Troitsa A, Haddad R, Avital S, Kashtan H, Baratz M, Brazovsky E, Papo J, Skornick Y. Immunoguided lymph node dissection in colorectal cancer: a new challenge? World J Surg, in press.

22. Schneebaum S, Daly JM, Burak W, Lavery I, Chevinsky A, Martin EW, The RIGS Study Group. RIGS efficacy in patients with colorectal cancer liver metastasis. 9th Congress of European Society of Surgical Oncology, June 3–6, Lausanne, 1998 (abstract).

23. Haddad R, Avital S, Baratz M, Brazovsky E, Skornick Y, Schneebaum S. Benefits of radioimmunoguided surgery for pelvic recurrence. 3rd Meeting of the Israel Society of Colon and Rectal Surgery, Dead Sea, November 11–14, 1998 (abstract).

24. Avital S, Haddad R, Troitsa A, Kashtan H, Brazovsky E, Gitstein G, Skornick Y, Schneebaum S. Radioimmunoguided surgery for recurrent colorectal cancer manifested by isolated CEA elevation. Eur J Cancer 1999; 35(suppl 4):76 (abstract).

25. Schneebaum S, Arnold MW, Martin EW Jr. The utility of radioimmunoguided surgery in colorectal cancer. In: Mazier, Levien, Luehtenfeld, Senagore, eds. Surgery of the Colon, Rectum and Anus. Philadelphia: W.B. Saunders Company, 1995, pp 460–469.

26. Arnold MW, Young DC, Hitchcock CL, Schneebaum S, Martin EW. Radioimmunoguided surgery in primary colorectal colorectal carcinoma: an intraoperative prognostic tool and adjuvant to traditional staging. Am J Surg 1995; 170:315–318.

27. Heald RJ, Karanja ND. Mesenteric considerations for adequate resection. In: Wanebo RJ, ed. Colorectal Cancer. St. Louis: Mosby, 1993, pp 389–404.

28. Cohen AM, Minsky BD, Schilsky RL. Cancer of the Colon. In: De Vita VT Jr, Hellman S, Rosenberg S, eds. Cancer Principles and Practice of Oncology. 5th Ed. Philadelphia, New York: Lippincott-Raven, 1997, pp 1144–1197.

29. Herrera-Ornelas L, Justiniano J, Castillo N, Petrelli NJ, Stule JP, Mittelman A. Metastases in small lymph nodes from colon cancer. Arch Surg 1987; 122:1253–1256.

30. Schneebaum S, Arnold MW, Houchens DP, Greenson JK, Cote RJ, Hitchcock CL, Young DC, Mojzisik CM, Martin EW Jr. The significance of intraoperative periportal lymph node metastasis identification in patients with colorectal carcinoma. Cancer 1995; 75:2809–2817.

31. Fuhrman GM, Curley SA, Hohn DC, Roh MS. Improved survival after resection of colorectal liver metastases. Ann Surg Oncol 1995; 6:537–541.

32. Gibbs JF, Weber TK, Rodriguez-Bigas MA, Driscoll DL, Petrelli NJ. Intraoperative determinants of unresectability for patients with colorectal hepatic metastases. Cancer 1998; 82:1244–1249.

33. Reintgen D, Albertini J, Berman C, Cruse CW, Fenske N, Glass F, Puleo C, Wang X, Wells K, Rapaport D, DeConti R, Messina J, Heller R. Accurate nodal staging of malignant melanoma. Cancer Control 1995; 2:405–414.

34. Cote RJ, Houchens DP, Saad AD, Nines RG, Greenson JK, Schneebaum S, Arnold MW, Martin EW. Intraoperative detection of occult colon cancer micrometastases using ^{125}I-radiolabeled monoclonal antibody CC49. Cancer 1996; 77:613–620.

35. Greenson JK, Isenhart CE, Rice R, Mojzisik C, Houchens D, Martin EW Jr. Identification of occult micrometastasis in pericolic lymph nodes of Dukes' B colorectal cancer patients using monoclonal antibodies against cytokeratin and CC49. Cancer 1994; 73:563–569.

36. Schneebaum S, Troitsa A, Avital S, Haddad R, Kashtan H, Gitstein G, Baratz M, Brazovsky E, Papo J, Skornick Y. Identification of lymph node metastases in recur-

rent colorectal cancer. In: Schlag PM, ed. Recent Results in Cancer Research, Proceedings of the International Conference Lymphatic Metastasis and Sentinel Lymphadenectomy. Berlin: Springer-Verlag, in press.

37. LaValle GJ, Martinez DA, Sobel D, DeYoung B, Martin EW Jr. Assessment of disseminated pancreatic cancer: a comparison of traditional exploratory laparotomy and radioimmunoguided surgery. Surgery 1997; 122:867–873.

38. Badalament RA, Burgers JK, Petty LR, Mojzisik CM, Berens A, Marsh W, Hinkle GH, Martin EW. Radioimmunoguided radical prostatectomy and lymphadenectomy. Cancer 1993; 71:2268–2275.

39. Bell J, Mojzisik C, Hinkle G, Derman H, Schlom J, Martin E. Intraoperative radioimmunodetection of ovarian cancer using monoclonal antibody B72.3 and a portable gamma-detecting probe. Obstet Gynecol 1990; 76:607–611.

40. Nieroda CA, Mojzisik C, Sardi A, Farrar WB, Hinkle G, Siddiqi MA, Ferrara PJ, James A, Schlom J, Thurston MO, Martin EW Jr. Staging of carcinoma of the breast using a hand-held gamma detecting probe and monoclonal antibody B72.3. Surg Gynecol Obstet 1989; 169:35–40.

41. Percivale P, Bertoglio S, Meszaros P, Canavese G, Cafiero F, Gipponi M, Campora E, Gasco M, Badellino F. Radioimmunoguided surgery after primary treatment of locally advanced breast cancer. J Clin Oncol 1996; 14:1599–1603.

42. Nieroda CA, Milenic DE, Colcher D, Schlom J. Monoclonal antibodies for use in radioimmunoguided surgery (RIGS). In: Martin EW Jr, ed. Radioimmunoguided Surgery (RIGS) in the Detection and Treatment of Colorectal Cancer. Austin: Landes RG Co, 1994, pp 7–27.

43. Begent RHJ, Verhaar MJ, Chester KA, Casey JL, Green AJ, Napier MP, Hope-Stone LD, Cushen N, Keep PA, Johnson CJ, Hawkins RE, Hilson AJW, Robson L. Clinical evidence of efficient tumor targeting based on single-chain Fv antibody selected from a combinatorial library. Nature Med 1996; 2:979–984.

44. Schirmer WJ, O'Dorisio TM, Schirmer TP, Mojzisik CM, Hinkle GH, Martin EW. Intraoperative localization of neuroendocrine tumors with ^{125}I-TYR(3)-octreotide and a hand-held gamma-detecting probe. Surgery 1993; 114:745–752.

45. Ahlman H. Radioisotope-guided surgery in patients with neuroendocrine tumours. Digestion 1996; 57:88–89.

46. Martinez DA, O'Dorisio S, O'Dorisio TM, Qualman SJ, Caniano DA, Teich S, Besner GE, King DR. Intraoperative detection and resection of occult neuroblastoma: a technique exploiting somatostatin receptor expression. J Pediatr Surg 1995; 30: 1580–1589.

17

Radioguided Open Bone Biopsy

Lary A. Robinson
H. Lee Moffitt Cancer Center and Research Institute, University of South Florida College of Medicine, Tampa, Florida

INTRODUCTION

An important aspect of the evaluation of any malignancy is the determination of the stage of the disease. Almost any solid tumor may metastasize to bone, which classifies that malignancy as having bloodborne spread, thereby designated as Stage IV disease [1]. The stage of the malignancy plays a pivotal role in determining therapy. Surgery is eliminated as a curative option when bony metastases are documented. Generally, a Stage IV malignancy mandates a systemic therapy-only approach, occasionally with radiotherapy added for symptomatic lesions. The patient's prognosis is also directly linked to staging. Accurate staging is therefore critical in the evaluation of any malignancy.

Although one 1976 study showed that as many as 15% of patients with primary extraosseous malignancies have a solitary abnormality on their bone scan [2], 36–71% of these bone lesions will prove to be benign on biopsy [2,3]. With modern, more sensitive gamma cameras, it is likely that a higher percentage of routine bone scintigraphy studies will have at least one abnormal focus, leading to an even higher false positive rate of suspected bone metastasis. This high false positive rate in solitary bone scintigraphy abnormalities could potentially lead to overstaging of a malignancy. Histological confirmation of suspected osseous metastases is imperative, especially when potential lesions are discovered only on bone scintigrams and are not corroborated by other imaging modalities.

Metastases to bone may be strongly suggested by symptoms and confirmed by imaging studies, thereby allowing the clinician comfort in making a Stage IV diagnosis. However, on other occasions symptoms and signs are minimal or absent and the imaging studies, such as radioisotope bone studies, are suggestive but not definitive. In these cases of absence of plain radiographic abnormalities, confirmatory biopsy of a suspected osseous metastasis becomes a challenging problem for the surgeon in terms of localization of the exact area of abnormal tracer activity at the time of open biopsy. This chapter describes various techniques used to evaluate bone lesions with emphasis on the radioguided approach with a gamma ray detection probe. My experience after performing 28 of these cases is presented.

BONE METASTASES

Tumors arising primarily in bone are relatively rare while bony metastases are rather common, especially in patients over the age of 45. Metastases tend to arise in areas of persistent red marrow, especially in the axial skeleton, presumably because of increased blood flow [4]. From a series of 2001 patients [5], the most frequent sites of bony metastases are shown in Table 1 [5].

Malignancies with the highest frequency of osseous metastases include breast cancer and prostate cancer, with cancers of the kidney, thyroid, and lung following with less frequency. Malignancies from the gastrointestinal tract and the remainder of the genitourinary tract as well as sarcomas rarely metastasize to bone [4]. Eventually, up to 67% of patients with breast cancer, 50% of those with prostate cancer, and 25% of lung and kidney cancer patients will develop bony metastases in their lifetime [4].

New-onset bone pain may be the presenting complaint in patients with bony metastases, and may sometimes be accompanied by swelling. Occasionally a "pathological" fracture may occur in the weakened bone. Most osseous metastases cause osteolytic destruction, although rarely osteoblastic metastases do occur. Elevation of the serum alkaline phosphatase may occur with bony metastases, but

TABLE 1   Most Common Sites of Osseous Metastases in Order of Decreasing Frequency

Vertebrae
Pelvis
Femur and sacrum
Ribs
Skull
Humerus
Scapula
Sternum

Source: Ref. 5.

abnormal elevated values of this enzyme are seen with multiple other problems including hyperparathyroidism, osteomalacia, osteitis deformans, osteogenic sarcoma, rickets, healing fractures, pregnancy, normal growth, and various hepatobiliary conditions [6]. Bone metastases may initially not produce any symptoms and be clinically silent. In some malignancies, routine bone scintigraphy is performed in the staging work-up, occasionally leading to the discovery of silent bone abnormalities. For malignancies such as non–small cell lung cancer, bone scintigraphy is recommended only if there are some clinical indicators such as bone pain, elevated serum alkaline phosphatase, or elevated serum calcium. Rarely are bone metastases found in the early-stage lung cancer patient in the absence of these clinical findings [7,8]. Bone metastases usually show destructive, osteolytic changes that are manifested by discrete areas of decreased bone density on plain bone radiographs. Focal areas of increased density are uncommon, and these osteoblastic or osteosclerotic changes are usually associated with prostate cancer or metastatic breast cancer after hormone treatment [5]. Nevertheless, plain bone radiographs are rather insensitive indicators of metastases because at least 50% of the trabecular bone must be destroyed before it is radiographically visible [4].

BONE SCINTIGRAPHY

The most sensitive indicator of metastatic disease is bone scintigraphy, which appears positive when as little as 5–15% of the trabecular bone is destroyed by tumor [4]. This technique is much more sensitive than plain bone radiographs and shows metastases to bone much earlier. Indeed, only 3% of bone metastases will be seen on plain bone radiographs in the face of a normal bone scan. The mechanism involved in the uptake of the radiopharmaceutical used in bone scintigraphy is not well understood. Usually technetium-99m (^{99m}Tc)–labeled diphosphonate is used. This radiopharmaceutical will localize on the images to show an area of increased bone formation or blood flow, resulting in a ''hot spot'' on the images [9]. When metastatic tumor invades bone it causes local bone destruction, but new bone formation will simultaneously occur as a response. The radiopharmaceutical appears to bind to the hydroxyapatite crystal of this new bone and not to the tumor cells themselves.

Rarely, there may be areas of decreased blood flow or decreased or absent new bone formation in the face of metastatic tumor in the bone that will result in a localized area of decreased tracer uptake, known as a photopenic lesion [9]. Rapid bone resorption without new bone formation may rarely occur with an aggressive, highly destructive metastatic tumor. In this case, the ^{99m}Tc-diphosphonate may not be taken up in the area of bone destruction. However, most lesions are visualized through increased tracer uptake.

TABLE 2 Conditions Causing Increased Uptake of ^{99m}Tc-Diphosphonate on Bone Scintigraphy

Increased blood flow and bone formation
  Arthritis
  Aseptic necrosis, cysts
  Bone infarct
  Eosinophilic granuloma
  Fibrous dysplasia
  Fracture (recent or healing)
  Heterotopic bone growth
  Hyperostosis frontalis interna
  Osteitis pubis
  Osteoid osteoma
  Osteomyelitis, osteitis
  Paget's disease
  Postsurgical bony changes
  Renal osteodystrophy
  Rheostosis
  Sudeck's atrophy
Soft-tissue abnormalities
  Calcific tendinitis or myositis
  Dental abscess
  Hydronephrosis or hydroureter
  Injection site
  Postsurgical scar
  Soft-tissue osseous metaplasia
Primary malignant bone tumors
  Chondrosarcoma
  Ewing's sarcoma
  Osteosarcoma
Benign bone tumors
  Fibroma
  Chondroma and enchondroma
Normal structures
  Alae of sacrum
  Base of skull
  Epiphyses of youth
  Facial bones
  Inferior tip of scapula
  Kidneys and bladder
  Sternomanubrial and corpus-manubrial joints
  Thyroid cartilage
  Variant anatomy
Artifacts from spillage of isotope during injection
  Antecubital fossa
  Lateral chest wall
Metastatic tumors

Source: From Ref. 9.

Bone scintigraphy is undoubtedly quite sensitive but not very specific for definitively confirming metastatic tumor. A wide variety of benign and malignant conditions other than metastatic disease may result in increased uptake of the tracer, as listed in Table 2. Because there are so many causes of tracer accumulation, there is a real possibility that a ''positive'' bone scan is in fact a false positive result when the images are used in the staging of a malignancy, especially if considered without other modality studies. Therefore, the presence of a positive (although nonspecific) bone scan mandates biopsy of the suspected lesion for histological confirmation of a possible metastasis, especially in the absence of definite, abnormal plain bone radiographs. Only after a diagnostic biopsy can the stage of the disease be reliably established.

MAGNETIC RESONANCE IMAGING

In patients who are symptomatic with localized bone pain, the diagnosis of osseous metastases is readily apparent. Plain bone radiographs of the areas of pain or swelling are usually obtained and are commonly positive. When results of these radiographs are negative or equivocal, bone scintigraphy is usually performed. Bone scintigrams may also be obtained to look for areas of asymptomatic metastases in patients with known bone metastases. Locating metastases in weight-bearing bones such as the femur is important in order to treat them early and avoid a pathological fracture.

Magnetic resonance imaging (MRI) with gadolinium contrast is the preferred method with which to look for suspected metastases in the spine or pelvis because it is a very sensitive and reliable technique to document bony involvement [4]. MRI is especially useful for patients with neurological abnormalities or vertebral body collapse in looking for spinal cord impingement. In the patient with advanced cancer and suspicious new-onset back pain, it may be much more time and cost efficient to go straight to a ''screening'' MRI of the spine first to avoid the usual progression of initial plain radiographs followed by bone scintigraphy and then a subsequent MRI [10].

PERCUTANEOUS NEEDLE BIOPSY

Sometimes it is possible to perform a percutaneous needle biopsy of a suspected bony metastasis for histological confirmation of tumor when there is a soft-tissue mass or large lytic lesion in the bone. A computed tomographic (CT)–guided biopsy of a spine lesion is also possible on occasion. Nevertheless, there is always the possibility of a sampling error when the needle biopsy is nondiagnostic.

An open surgical biopsy may be needed when the staging and ultimate treatment recommendation hinge on the histological confirmation of osseous lesions. Localizing the precise area to biopsy intraoperatively is usually easy if

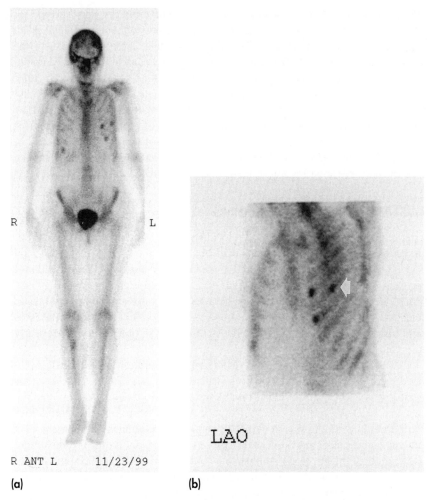

R   L

R ANT L   11/23/99

LAO

(a)   (b)

FIGURE 1   (a) Anterior view of scintigraphy of the entire skeleton of patient number 26 with adenocarcinoma of the lung. Asymptomatic areas of increased tracer activity (the dark areas on the ribs bilaterally in the image) are seen in the anterolateral area of the left 4th, 5th, and 6th ribs and the right 7th rib. (b) Coned down left anterior oblique view of just the thorax show the three ribs with increased tracer uptake. Plain rib detail radiographs of these suspected rib metastases were normal. The left 5th rib (arrow) was biopsied using gamma probe guidance. Benign hypercellularity and bone remodeling were found, probably from a healing fracture.

there are localizing symptoms and corresponding plain bone radiograph abnormalities, particularly when the target bone is a rib and the patient is thin. It is more challenging to find the correct area for biopsy in an obese or muscular patient, and it generally requires using a much larger incision and numerous intraoperative localizing radiographs. The real difficulty occurs when the asymptomatic patient with cancer has a bone scan with one or more abnormalities while the plain radiographs of the corresponding areas are normal. Most bone radiologists will report that the lesions depicted on the scintigraphy images in this setting probably represent metastatic disease [2]. A typical example of this situation is found in Figure 1 which shows the images of an asymptomatic patient with known adenocarcinoma of the lung who had a screening bone scan and was found to have multiple lesions in the ribs but normal plain bone radiographs.

The scintigrams in Figure 1 were initially read as showing probable bone metastases, but this reading was proven incorrect with a subsequent open rib biopsy that showed benign bone remodeling. The commonly held belief that the presence of metastases is proven with a positive bone scan in this setting is frequently incorrect because of the high incidence of other lesions being visualized, ranging from 47–71% in various studies [3,8,11,12]. With such a high incidence of benign bone lesions accounting for the bone scan abnormalities, a comfirmatory biopsy is a necessity. However, a needle biopsy is not feasible when only a bone scan serves as the guide.

STANDARD OPEN SURGICAL BIOPSY

The surgeon faces a real clinical problem when asked to perform an open bone biopsy in an asymptomatic cancer patient who has only an abnormal bone scan with normal plain bone radiographs of the corresponding areas. Ribs are the most surgically accessible bones to biopsy. But when using only bone scintigraphy as a guide, intraoperative localization of the exact site to biopsy is quite challenging. Depending on the clarity of the image, it may be difficult to define which numbered rib is hot.

Pinpointing the precise anterior-posterior location of the lesion on a rib may be even more of a problem. Faced with this situation, the surgeon may be forced to make a substantial incision to excise a large portion of the rib and possibly the adjacent rib as well to be sure the abnormality is included in the surgical specimen. It is difficult to precisely count the exact rib to biopsy when the patient is obese or very muscular. For this reason, it is necessary to obtain one or more intraoperative radiographs (usually including a cross-table lateral view) with a radio-opaque marker such as a needle imbedded in the bone to mark the correct rib to biopsy. The radiograph must be centered correctly such that the first or twelfth rib is seen on the same radiograph to allow counting to the marked target rib. It is commonly necessary to repeat the imaging several times in order to catch the appropriate anatomy on the radiograph taken of the anesthetized patient, who is in the lateral decubitus position. The area of the hot spot on the bone scintigram usually appears grossly normal intraoperatively and the bone is uniformly too dense to allow frozen section analysis. Therefore, it is virtually impossible during a standard bone biopsy to tell if the exact targeted lesion was excised. The final pathological diagnosis awaits 7 to 10 days of decalcification and processing. If the final diagnosis rendered is ''normal'' bone, then there is even more uncertainty whether the correct site was biopsied, because some abnormality must be present in the bone to cause the increased radionuclide uptake.

METHYLENE-BLUE RIB TARGETING TECHNIQUE

In 1983, Little and colleagues developed a targeting technique to mark the proper rib and facilitate biopsy by the surgeon [11]. ^{99m}Tc-diphosphonate is injected intravenously into the patient 6–12 h before the operation. Then, in the nuclear medicine department, the patient is positioned below the gamma camera to image the appropriate area. While the patient is imaged on the real-time scintiview screen, a radioactive point source is moved over the patient and simultaneously visualized. When the external point source overlaps the hot spot on the screen, the skin in that location is marked with indelible ink. After local anesthesia with lidocaine, a needle is inserted down to the rib in that area and a small amount of the tracer is injected to mark the hot spot deeper. The needle is left in place while the patient is repositioned and viewed from different angles under the gamma camera to be sure that the percutaneously injected tracer is superimposed over the bone scan abnormality. Several injections may be needed until the correct area is marked. Subsequently, methylene blue is injected into the same needle to stain the underlying periosteum and soft tissue up to the skin. The patient is then taken promptly to the surgery room for an open biopsy of the methylene blue–stained rib before the dye diffuses away.

Using the rib marking technique, Little and associates reported success in 15 patients with known cancer to enable them to biopsy 13 ribs, one skull, and one scapula [11]. A pathological diagnosis was found in all patients, but only eight of 15 (53%) had metastatic cancer. The other patients had a variety of benign diagnoses, including hypercellular marrow (2), old rib fractures (2), Paget's disease, granuloma, and osteoporosis. This methylene-blue targeting technique appears to work in experienced hands but requires careful coordination of the nuclear medicine department and surgical schedule. That is, a surgery room should be immediately available to accept the rib biopsy patient for surgery so that the blue dye does not have time to diffuse to other ribs. The surgeon performing only an occasional bone biopsy guided by this technique might find it difficult to duplicate the excellent results of Little and colleagues.

Moores and colleagues published a later series of 33 bone biopsies using the methylene-blue technique in 1990 [12]. A histological abnormality was found in 97% of their biopsies, but only 52% of the total had metastatic cancer in the bone. Their false positive rate of 48% was very similar to that of Little and colleagues [11]. In the 17 patients with an abnormal bone scan but normal plain bone radiographs, the false positive rate was even higher at 71%.

TECHNIQUE OF INTRAOPERATIVE GAMMA-RAY DETECTION PROBE LOCALIZATION

The development of the hand-held, high-resolution gamma-ray detection probe, which provides real-time, rapid counting in the surgery room, has allowed the development of a much simpler technique for localizing bone lesions for biopsy. The gamma probe has been quite successfully used intraoperatively for radioguided identification of sentinel lymph nodes in melanoma and breast cancer [13,14]. The gamma probe has been subsequently adapted for use at the H. Lee Moffitt Cancer Center for intraoperative localization of areas of increased uptake of a ^{99m}Tc-labeled tracer in ribs and the sternum to guide the surgeon in the open biopsy of suspicious bones [3].

The surgical technique using the gamma probe for intraoperative guidance is quite straightforward and has previously been described [3]. Three to 4 h before surgery the patient receives an intravenous injection of ^{99m}Tc-oxidronate in the standard dosage for a radioisotope bone scan (1036 MBq, 28 mCi). A 3–4 h interval from injection until surgery gives the best intraoperative discrimination. After induction of general anesthesia, preparing, and draping of the patient, the hand-held small pediatric size gamma probe (Neoprobe 1000, Neoprobe Corporation, Dublin, Ohio or Navigator, Model GGS, RMD Co., for U.S. Surgical Corporation, Watertown, Massachusetts) is packed in a sterile plastic sleeve. The device is used to localize the area of greatest tracer activity (measured in counts per sec) on the skin of the chest wall in the suspicious-looking area. A moderate amount of background activity from the tracer is found in all the nearby bones. The hot-spot target has a noticeably increased amount of tracer activity compared with the surrounding area.

A 3–4 cm incision is made over this area of increased radioactivity and the targeted rib or sternum is exposed. The probe in the sterile sleeve is then used to precisely localize in the surgical wound the area of increased tracer activity in comparison with background counts elsewhere on the same rib or on nearby ribs (Fig. 2). The point of greatest activity is then marked directly on the surface of the rib with the electrocautery device just prior to removal of that section. Although this is a small wound, the tissues can easily be moved around enough to obtain a count reading on the adjacent ribs immediately above and below the target rib, as well as further away from the hot spot on the same rib.

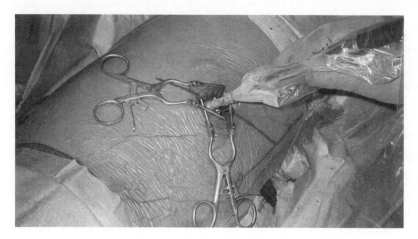

FIGURE 2   Intraoperative view of the hand-held gamma probe (the smallest, pediatric size) in a sterile sleeve being used by the surgeon to measure counts directly on the left 8th rib laterally in patient number 23. The patient is in the right lateral decubitus position with the head superiorly to the right.

In the initial few patients, an intraoperative cross-table lateral radiograph was obtained with a radio-opaque marker on the rib (a spinal needle imbedded in the periosteum is my preference) in the wound to verify that the correct numbered rib was being biopsied. Several radiographs were usually necessary to get the correct view so that the first or twelfth rib was included in the image to enable counting of the ribs from above or below. As the experience with the gamma probe grew, these time-consuming, costly radiographs were eliminated.

A 3 cm portion of the targeted rib or the outer table of the sternum is removed subperiosteally. The bone appears grossly normal in most patients with an abnormal bone scan and normal rib detail radiographs. The specimen of bone is placed in a decalcification solution and isolated 3 to 4 days to allow the ^{99m}Tc to decay. The decalcified bone subsequently undergoes histological study with particular attention paid to the area scored by the electrocautery.

The small wound is filled with saline to check for inadvertent entry into the pleura (bubbling in the wound with ventilation), which occurs about 10% of the time in our experience. If the parietal pleura has been entered, a 24 French chest tube is inserted through a separate stab wound into the pleural cavity. The tube is removed in the recovery room after a portable chest radiograph shows the absence of a pneumothorax or pleural effusion. The wound is closed in layers with absorbable sutures and a final subcuticular skin closure. Almost all patients are discharged the same day from the recovery room, with only the quite debilitated patients requiring observation overnight. The postsurgical chest radiograph also serves to document that the proper numbered rib was biopsied.

RESULTS WITH THE GAMMA-PROBE TECHNIQUE

The initial series of patients published in 1998 [3] has been updated for this chapter and now consists of 28 patients who have undergone radioguided biopsy of 31 ribs and one sternum. These 28 patients (13 men, 15 women) presented with a variety of known or suspected underlying primary cancers, as listed in Table 3. All had abnormal bone scintigrams but with normal plain radiographs. They all were either asymptomatic or had minimal, nonlocalizing symptoms.

Intraoperatively, the bone to be resected always appeared grossly normal to the surgeon. However, the surgical accuracy was 100%; all bones biopsied contained a pathological process that would account for the hot spot on the images. Table 4 lists the pathological diagnoses found with the 32 biopsies. Only seven of the 32 bones (21.9%) contained metastatic cancer (squamous cell carcinoma of the lung (2), lymphoma (2), adenocarcinoma of the lung, carcinoma of the prostate, and melanoma). The measurement of serum alkaline phosphatase was not very helpful because only two of the seven patients with osseous metastases had slightly elevated levels of this enzyme (28.6%) (see Table 4). One patient with a benign diagnosis also had a slightly elevated alkaline phosphatase level. The other 25 bones showed a variety of benign pathological processes, as shown in Table 4. Staging based solely on increased uptake on scintigraphy images would have led to a 78.1% false positive rate for diagnosing metastatic cancer.

Detection of area with increased tracer uptake was easily accomplished with the aid of the gamma-ray detection probe. The mean ratio of measured hot-spot activity on the target rib compared with adjacent ribs or the same rib away from the hot spot was a mean 2.19 ± 1.05, with a median of 1.70, and a range of 1.22–5.67. This means that the localized area of increased uptake of tracer was over twice as hot as the surrounding bones. This difference was easily discernible intraoperatively. The newer generation of gamma counters with their highly collimated probes are even more precise with increased directionality. This gives even better and easier intraoperative discrimination of the hot spot with less background interference and higher count ratios. In the most recent 11 rib biopsies in which I used the collimated probes, the mean ratio of hot spot activity to background counts was clearly higher at 3.24 ± 1.18 (median 2.89), thereby allowing an even sharper differentiation between the targeted bone lesion and the adjacent normal bone.

There was no morbidity or mortality specifically associated with the intraoperative gamma-probe technique or the actual rib biopsies. And after experience was gained with this technique on a few patients, the total surgical time for these

TABLE 3 Results of Patients Undergoing Gamma Probe–Directed Bone Biopsy

No.	Age (yr)	Sex (M/F)	Clinical diagnosis	Symptoms	Bone scan uptake	Plain bone radiographs	Alk. phos. (normal values)	PSA (normal values)	Bone biopsied	Injection to surgery (hr)	Count ratio	Rib pathology
1	65	M	Carcinoma of prostate	None	L 7th rib & skull	Normal	46 (37–107)	14.8 (0–4.0)	L 7th rib	12	1.43	Hypercellular marrow
2	44	F	Lymphoma	Vague chest pain (1 yr.)	L ribs 6, 7, & 8	Normal	294 (80–258)	—	L 6th rib	12	1.42	Lymphoma
									L 8th rib	12	1.59	Lymphoma
3	62	M	Sq. cell ca.a of lung	None	R 9th rib, L 6th rib	Normal	208 (80–258)	—	R 9th rib	6	1.69	Metastatic sq. cell carcinoma
4	74	M	Sq. cell ca. of lung	Pain in low back	Spine, mult.c ribs bilat.d	Fracture T11 spine	81 (37–147)	—	L 7th rib	6	2.00	Paget's disease
5	73	M	Sq. cell ca. of lung	None	R 10th & 11th ribs	Normal	94 (38–126)	—	L 8th rib	6	1.53	Paget's disease
									R 10th rib	6	1.57	Enchondroma
									R 11th rib	6	1.67	Enchondroma
6	70	M	Sq. cell ca. of lung	Vague chest wall pain	L 6th rib	Normal	68 (38–126)	—	L 6th rib	6	2.05	Enchondroma
7	37	F	Carcinoma of breast	None	Body of the sternum	Normal	58 (38–126)	—	Body of the sternum	6	1.22	Chondroma
8	66	M	Carcinoma of prostate	None	L 6th rib	Normal	57 (25–150)	14.3 (0.1–4.0)	L 6th rib	6	1.54	Metastatic prostate ca.
9	54	F	Sq. cell ca. of lung	Vague chest wall pain	L 6th & 9th ribs	Normal	52 (20–125)	—	L 6th rib	6	1.74	Chondroma
									L 9th rib	6	1.63	Chondroma
10	39	M	Melanoma	None	L 10th rib	Normal	52 (38–126)	—	L 10th rib	6	1.35	Localized fibrosis granulation tissue
11	64	M	Large cell ca. of lung	None	L 8th rib	Normal	62 (38–126)	—	L 8th rib	6	1.47	Hypercellular marrow
12	74	F	Carcinoma of breast	None	L 6th rib, L 9th rib	Normal	54 (38–126)	—	L 9th rib	6	1.71	Hypercell.e marrow; osteosclerosis
13	54	F	Sm. cell ca.b of lung	Vague left ant chest pain	L 8th rib	Normal	87 (38–126)	—	L 8th rib	6	1.31	Hypercell. marrow, osteosclerosis
14	76	M	Renal cell carcinoma	None	R 4th rib, L 7th rib	Normal	75 (42–121)	2.5 (0.1–4.0)	L 7th rib	6	1.83	Fibrous dysplasia

#	Age	Sex	Known malignancy	Symptoms	Rib location	Bone scan	Alk. phos. (range)	PSA (range)	Biopsy site	Count	Ratio	Histology
15	45	F	No known malignancy	Vague L chest wall pain	R 9th rib / L 5th rib	Normal	76 (38–126)	—	L 5th rib	6	2.69	Chondroma with healing fracture
16	82	M	Carcinoma of the lung	None	L 4th rib / R 7th rib	Normal	—	—	L 4th rib	6	1.62	Local fibrosis; Remote fracture
17	53	M	Melanoma	Vague chest wall pain	R 6th rib	Irregular R 6th rib	53 (38–126)	—	R 6th rib	6	1.40	Metastatic melanoma
18	55	F	Melanoma	Generalized bone pain	L 3rd rib	Normal	283 (80–253)	—	L 3rd rib	6	2.67	Benign bone remodeling
19	67	F	Adenoca.[f] of the lung	Vague chest wall pain	L 10th rib	Normal	93 (38–126)	—	L 10th rib	6	2.89	Metastatic adenocarcinoma
20	50	F	Diffuse bone pain MM?	Pain L 3rd rib	L 3rd rib / R 6th rib	Normal	87 (38–126)	—	L 3rd rib	6	4.0	Bone remodeling with fibrosis
21	69	F	Small cell ca. of lung	Diffuse chest tenderness	L 6th rib / R 11th rib	Normal	81 (38–126)	—	L 6th rib	6	3.33	Bone remodeling; Prior fracture
22	78	F	Mal. fibrous histiocytoma	Vague chest wall pain	R 5th rib	Normal	73 (48–183)	—	R 5th rib	6	5.67	Bone remodeling; Cortical fracture
23	62	M	Ca. of the prostate	None	L 8th rib / R 6th rib	Normal	57 (38–126)	36.5 (0.1–4.0)	L 8th rib	6	1.98	Bone remodeling; Old fracture
24	66	M	Ca. of the prostate	None	R 8th rib	Normal	74 (38–126)	6.1 (0.1–4.0)	R 8th rib	6	2.67	Bone remodeling; Old fracture
25	39	F	Ca. of the breast	None	L 10th rib	Normal	95 (38–126)	—	L 10th rib	4	3.43	Enchondroma
26	71	F	Adenoca. of the lung	None	Multiple bilateral ribs	Normal	87 (38–126)	—	L 5th rib	3	2.69	Hypercellularity; Bone remodeling
27	52	F	Ca. of the breast	Chest tenderness	Multiple bilateral ribs	Fracture 4th rib only	80 (38–126)	—	L 10th rib	4	4.68	Enchondroma
28	68	F	Adenoca. of the lung	Vague chest wall pain	Multiple right ribs	Old surg. changes	53 (38–126)	—	R 10th rib	4	1.58	Bone remodeling; Localized fibrosis

Abbreviations: Alk. phos., alkaline phosphatase (units/L); PSA, prostate-specific antigen (ng/mL); MM, multiple myeloma; L, left; R, right.

[a] Sq. cell ca., squamous cell carcinoma.
[b] Sm. cell ca., small cell carcinoma.
[c] Multiple.
[d] Bilateral.
[e] Hypercellular.
[f] Adenoca., adenocarcinoma.

TABLE 4 Specific Radioguided Bone Biopsy Diagnoses

Malignant	Number
Lung carcinoma (NSCLC)	3 (all had normal alk. phos.)
Lymphoma	2 (both had elevated alk. phos.)
Prostate carcinoma	1 (normal alk. phos., elevated PSA)
Melanoma	1 (normal alk. phos.)
Benign	
Enchondroma/chondroma	9
Hypercellular marrow/osteosclerosis	5
Paget's disease	2
Fibrous dysplasia	1
Localized fibrosis/remote fracture	8
Total:	32

Abbreviations: Alk. phos., alkaline phosphatase; PSA, prostate-specific antigen.
Note: Alkaline phosphatase was normal in all but one patient with a benign diagnosis.

cases decreased to only 20–40 minutes. Intraoperative radiographs were eliminated and the counting technique is precise, rapid, and reproducible.

The most common benign abnormality found in this clinical series was a chondroma or enchondroma, accounting for 9 of 32 (36%) of biopsy results. This benign cartilaginous tumor is relatively common, representing 13.4% of all benign bone tumors. The actual incidence is unknown because they occur sporadically and are asymptomatic [15]. They tend to occur most commonly in the small bones of the hands and feet, but are also found in long, thin bones such as the ribs. Unless they become very large, these lesions remain asymptomatic and are not generally visible on plain bone radiographs. They are usually found incidentally as an area of increased uptake of radioisotope on a bone scan performed during the evaluation of a patient with a malignancy. A subsequent biopsy usually follows and the diagnosis of a benign chondroma is then made.

CONCLUSIONS

In a patient with a known or suspected malignancy, the finding of an asymptomatic area of increased uptake on bone scintigraphy images but with normal plain bone radiographs does not necessarily indicate that a bone metastasis is present. In fact, such a hot spot represents a benign lesion in as many as 78% of patients. Open biopsy for histological confirmation is mandatory in this setting. Until recently, accurately locating a bone lesion for open biopsy with only the bone scan image as a guide greatly challenged the surgeon. The technique of methylene-blue ''tattooing'' of the target bone appears to be effective it is somewhat cumbersome and time consuming [11,12]. The recently described intraoperative gamma-probe technique of locating bone scan lesions offers real advantages in terms of decreased surgery time, minimal interdepartmental coordination, and 100% sensitivity [3]. With the widespread use of the gamma probe in melanoma and breast cancer surgery as well as other applications described in earlier chapters of this book, this instrument is becoming a common fixture in most active surgery rooms. As a result, the gamma probe will be readily available to guide surgeons in performing open bone biopsies.

In our study, the hand-held gamma probe was successfully used intraoperatively to guide the surgeon in locating asymptomatic rib and sternal lesions to biopsy. This same technique could no doubt be easily adapted by orthopedic surgeons to biopsy subtle lesions in other bones in the appendicular skeleton. In addition, the gamma probe could obviously be used to aid in the biopsy of symptomatic or radiographically visible bone lesions in patients whose body habitus or location of the bone lesion might make precise conventional intraoperative localization difficult. This technique is easy to learn and apply, has no apparent side effects, and should be considered for use by the surgeon in guiding the open biopsy of suspected asymptomatic bone metastases.

REFERENCES

1. OH Beahrs, DE Henson, RVP Hutter, BJ Kennedy. Handbook for Staging of Cancer. 1st ed. Philadelphia: J.B. Lippincott Co., 1993, pp 3–14.
2. RJ Corcoran, JH Thrall, RW Kyle, RJ Kaminski, MC Johnson. Solitary abnormalities in bone scans of patients with extraosseous malignancies. Radiology 1976; 121: 663–667.
3. LA Robinson, D Preksto, C Muro-Cacho, DS Hubbell. Intraoperative gamma probe-directed biopsy of asymptomatic suspected bone metastases. Ann Thorac Surg 1998; 65:1426–1432.
4. LF Rogers. Secondary malignancies of bone. In: JH Juhl, AB Crummy, eds. Paul and Juhl's Essentials of Radiological Imaging. 6th ed. Philadelphia: J.B. Lippincott Co., 1993, pp. 164–165.
5. A Clain. Secondary malignant disease of bone. Br J Cancer 1965; 19:15–29.
6. JB Henry, ed. Clinical Diagnosis and Management by Laboratory Methods. 19th ed. Philadelphia: WB Saunders Co., 1996, p 277.
7. F Michel, M Solèr, E Imhof, AP Perruchoud. Initial staging of non–small cell lung cancer: value of routine radioisotope bone scanning. Thorax 1991; 46:469–473.
8. Y Ichinose, N Hara, M Ohta, A Motohiro, T Maeda, T Nobe, K Yagawa. Preoperative examination to detect distant metastasis is not advocated for asymptomatic patients with Stages 1 and 2 non–small cell lung cancer. Chest 1989; 96:1104–1109.
9. HW Wahner, ML Brown. Role of bone scanning. In: FH Sim, ed. Diagnosis and Management of Metastatic Bone Disease. 1st ed. New York: Raven Press, 1988, pp 51–67.

10. JC Ruchdeschel. Rapid cost-effective diagnosis of spinal cord compression due to cancer. Cancer Control 1995; 2:320–323.

11. AG Little, TR DeMeester, PT Kirchner, C Iascone, N Badani, HM Golomb. Guided biopsies of abnormalities on nuclear bone scans. J Thorac Cardiovasc Surg 1983; 85:396–403.

12. DWO Moores, B Line, SW Dziuban Jr, MF McKneally Jr. Nuclear scan-guided rib biopsy. J Thorac Cardiovasc Surg 1990; 90:620–621.

13. JJ Albertini, CW Cruse, D Rapaport, K Wells, M Ross, R DeConti, CG Berman, K Jared, J Messina, G Lyman, F Glass, N Fenske, DS Reintgen. Intraoperative radio-lympho-scintigraphy improves sentinel lymph node identification for patients with melanoma. Ann Surg 1996; 223:217–224.

14. JJ Albertini, GH Lyman, C Cox, T Yeatman, L Balducci, N Ku, S Shivers, C Berman, K Wells, D Rapaport, A Shons, J Horton, H Greenberg, S Nicosia, R Clark, A Cantor, DS Reintgen. Lymphatic mapping and sentinel node biopsy in the patient with breast cancer. JAMA 1996; 276:1818–1822.

15. KK Unni. Chondroma. In: KK Unni. Dahlin's Bone Tumors. 5th ed. Philadelphia: Lippincott-Raven, 1996, pp 25–45.

18

Instructive Cases

Omgo E. Nieweg
The Netherlands Cancer Institute, Amsterdam, the Netherlands

Liesbeth Jansen
Gelre Hospital, Lukas Site, Apeldoorn, the Netherlands

Roger F. Uren
University of Sydney, Sydney, New South Wales, Australia

John F. Thompson
Royal Prince Alfred Hospital and University of Sydney, Sydney, New South Wales, Australia

MELANOMA

CASE 11. LIMITED RESOLUTION OF THE GAMMA CAMERA
CASE 12. FALSE NEGATIVE SENTINEL NODE BIOPSY
CASE 13. SENTINEL NODE CLOSE TO PRIMARY
          MELANOMA SITE (I)
CASE 14. SENTINEL NODE CLOSE TO PRIMARY
          MELANOMA SITE (II)
CASE 15. TUMOR-INVOLVED SENTINEL NODE IN THE
          GROIN: SUPERFICIAL *AND* DEEP INGUINAL
          NODE DISSECTION?
CASE 16. POSTOPERATIVE COMPLICATIONS

BREAST CANCER

CASE 1.   NORMAL DRAINAGE PATTERN
CASE 2.   LYMPHOSCINTIGRAPHY LATERAL VIEW
CASE 3.   BLUE DUCT ACCIDENTALLY DIVIDED
CASE 4.   NOT EVERY SENTINEL NODE IS RADIOACTIVE
CASE 5.   NOT EVERY SENTINEL NODE IS BLUE
CASE 6.   FALSE-NEGATIVE FROZEN-SECTION MICROSCOPY
CASE 7.   FALSE-NEGATIVE SENTINEL NODE BIOPSY,
          LEARNING PHASE
CASE 8.   LYMPHOSCINTIGRAPHY PROVIDES A ROAD
          MAP FOR THE SURGEON
CASE 9.   SENTINEL NODE IN THE INTERNAL MAMMARY
          CHAIN
CASE 10. SENTINEL NODE IN THE CONTRALATERAL
          INTERNAL MAMMARY NODE CHAIN
CASE 11. SENTINEL NODE IN INTERPECTORAL FOSSA
          (ROTTER'S SENTINEL NODE)
CASE 12. SENTINEL NODE IN THE BREAST PARENCHYMA
CASE 13. SENTINEL NODES IN MULTIPLE NODE FIELDS

OTHER NEOPLASMS

CASE 1. CARCINOMA OF THE VULVA
CASE 2. MERKEL'S CELL CARCINOMA
CASE 3. CLEAR CELL SARCOMA
CASE 4. SQUAMOUS CELL CARCINOMA OF THE PENIS

INTRODUCTION

Lymphatic mapping is an exciting undertaking. Anatomy, physiology, imaging, and technical surgical expertise go hand in hand. The routine case in which a single sentinel node is easily identified in the usual location is encountered in perhaps only 25% of patients. Sentinel nodes can be located in strange places, not described in the standard text books. Lymph drainage is much more variable than was previously assumed. Lymph vessels take unexpected turns. These variations in anatomy and physiology are captured in one image by lymphoscintigraphy. Reviewing the scintigraphy images together with the nuclear medicine physician ensures that the surgeon goes to the operating room well prepared.

Sentinel nodes are sometimes found within 1 minute after making the skin incision, practically falling into the surgeon's hand. Other times, the operation may take more than an hour and require the surgeon to use every trick in this book to find it. Blue dye outlines the drainage patterns that may be different from what the nuclear medicine images suggested. It is therefore important that the surgeon reports his operative findings back to the nuclear medicine physician. We must learn from each other. Lymphatic mapping is still being developed and refined, and a number of questions remain to be solved.

The aim of this chapter is to teach practical lessons. The techniques described have been thought over carefully, but alternative techniques may work as well or perhaps even better. The cases in this chapter have been carefully selected. The most instructive cases are possibly the ones in which the authors confess that mistakes were made. Each case carries a point, often more than one. Anatomical aberrations, variable physiology, pitfalls in the nuclear medicine suite, and technical challenges in the operating room are described.

ACKNOWLEDGMENT

Contributions were made by Cornelis A. Hoefnagel and Bin B.R. Kroon.

MELANOMA

Case 1: Normal Drainage Pattern

A 53-year-old woman was referred with a suspicious-looking mole on the sole of the right foot. The lesion had been present for many years but had recently changed in appearance: it had increased in size and become darker in color. Excision with a narrow margin was performed. Histological examination revealed a nodular melanoma with ulceration (Clark level IV, Breslow thickness 5.0 mm). Wide local excision and sentinel node biopsy were planned.

Lymphoscintigraphy

A dose of 50.2 MBq (1.4 mCi) technetium-99m (^{99m}Tc)-labeled nanocolloid (Nanocoll; Amersham Cygne, Eindhoven, the Netherlands) in a volume of 0.20 mL was injected intradermally around the biopsy scar. A radioactive flood source was placed behind the patient to outline the body contour [1]. The early images showed two lymphatic vessels running to two adjacent lymph nodes in the groin (Fig. 1). These nodes were marked on the skin with indelible ink. Several other "hot" spots higher up were visualized in a later phase. The study was reported

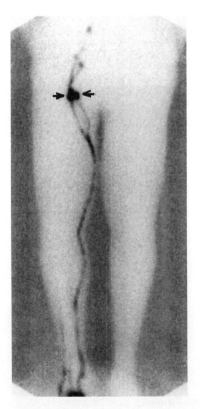

FIGURE 1   The early anterior view shows two lymphatic vessels and two sentinel nodes (arrows). Two second-tier nodes and a third-tier node are depicted higher up.

as showing two sentinel (first-tier) nodes with direct drainage from the injection site and several second-tier nodes higher up.

Surgery

The patient was taken to the operating room the next day. One milliliter of patent blue dye (Bleu Patenté V; Guerbet, Aulney-Sous-Bois, France) was administered around the biopsy site on the right foot when the patient was anesthetized, prepared, and draped. The injection site was gently massaged. The skin of the inside of the leg was massaged with strokes directed toward the groin.

Ten minutes later, a 3-cm incision was made between the skin marks placed by the nuclear medicine physician. Underneath Scarpa's subcutaneous fascia, two blue lymphatic vessels were identified. The vessels were dissected and followed to two adjacent blue nodes. Other blue ducts emerged from the nodes and ran in a cranial direction. The nodes were freed from the surrounding fat. Blood vessels and lymphatic vessels to and from the nodes were ligated and divided.

The nodes were examined with a gamma-ray detection probe (Neoprobe 1500; Neoprobe Corporation, Dublin, OH) both in the wound and after excision, and were confirmed to contain ^{99m}Tc. The nodes were submitted to the pathologist. The wound was then scanned with the probe for other hot nodes, but none was found, with the exception of the second-tier nodes that were known to be present further up the groin. The subcutaneous fat was approximated to obliterate the biopsy cavity, and the skin was closed. The operation was continued with wide local excision of the biopsy site. No completion inguinofemoral node dissection was performed.

Pathology

Hematoxylin and eosin (H&E) staining and immunohistochemistry (S-100, HMB-45) revealed no melanoma deposits in the two sentinel nodes.

Discussion

This patient demonstrates a typical drainage pattern. A melanoma on the leg usually drains to two sentinel nodes caudally from Poupart's ligament, whereas a melanoma on the arm drains more often to a single sentinel node in the axilla. Drainage on the trunk and in the head-and-neck area is more difficult to predict.

Lymphoscintigraphy nicely demonstrates the lymphatic vessels and the nodes. It is important that the surgeon reviews the images together with the nuclear medicine physician because they are not always as easy to interpret, as in this case. A thorough review of the images ensures that the surgeon knows how many nodes to expect and where to look for them.

The blue dye technique was used to identify the nodes in this patient, and the probe was used for confirmation. A surgeon obtains the best results with both techniques in the repertoire [2].

REFERENCES

1. Valdés Olmos RA, Hoefnagel CA, Nieweg OE, Jansen L, Rutgers EJTh, Borger J, Horenblas S, Kroon BBR. Lymphoscintigraphy in oncology: a rediscovered challenge. J Eur J Nucl Med 1999; 26(Suppl):S2–S10.
2. Nieweg OE, Jansen L, Kroon BBR. Technique for lymphatic mapping and sentinel node biopsy for melanoma. Eur J Surg Oncol 1998; 24:520–524.

Case 2: Definition of a Sentinel Node: Lymphatic Vessels and Time of Visualization

A 56-year-old man presented with a melanoma in the right flank. A diagnostic excision with a narrow margin was performed. Histological examination showed a superficial spreading melanoma (Breslow thickness 1.7 mm, Clark level III).

Lymphoscintigraphy

A dose of 56 MBq (1.5 mCi) ^{99m}Tc-nanocolloid in a volume of 0.25 mL was injected intradermally at four sites close to the biopsy scar on the right-flank. Early lymphoscintigraphy images were obtained 20 minutes later and showed drainage to a single sentinel node in the right axilla (Fig. 2). Two second-tier nodes were visualized more cranially.

The anterior view that was obtained 2 hours after the injection showed the same pattern. However, the late lateral view showed a second lymphatic vessel going to a second node that is situated somewhat more posteriorly. The conclusion was that there were two first-tier (sentinel) nodes and two second-tier nodes.

Surgery

The operation was performed 1 day after the lymphoscintigraphy. A quantity of 1 mL of patent blue dye was administered in two doses on either side of the biopsy scar in the right flank. Ten minutes later, a 5-cm transverse incision was made along the lower hair line in the right axilla. A blue duct was identified underneath Scarpa's fascia and traced to a blue node. The gamma-ray detection probe confirmed that the node was radioactive. A second blue duct was identified somewhat more posteriorly. This duct was dissected to a second blue radioactive node. Both sentinel nodes were removed. No other blue ducts were observed. Scanning the wound with the probe revealed increased uptake in the two second-tier nodes, but these were not pursued.

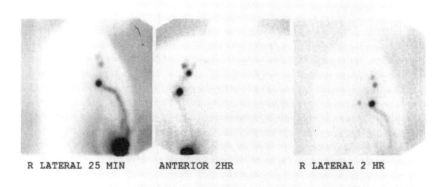

R LATERAL 25 MIN   ANTERIOR 2HR   R LATERAL 2 HR

FIGURE 2   The early lymphoscintigraphy images depict one sentinel node in the right axilla. Two second-tier nodes are visible higher up. The late anterior image gives us the impression that there is one lymphatic vessel going to one sentinel node. The lateral view makes it clear that there are two nodes on a direct drainage pathway.

Pathology and Follow-Up

Frozen sectioning, H&E staining, and immunohistochemistry (S-100, HMB-45) of the two nodes revealed no metastatic disease. No axillary node dissection was performed. The patient remained free of disease 4 years later.

Discussion

The dynamic scintigraphy images depict the lymphatic vessels and show the surgeon where to expect them. This case touches on an important point concerning the definition of a sentinel node. Some investigators in the field of nuclear medicine define the sentinel node as the first lymph node that becomes visible on the lymphoscintigraphy images [1]. Although the first node that is depicted *is* a sentinel node, this definition does not acknowledge the fact that sometimes there are more sentinel nodes than just one. Sometimes there are two lymphatic vessels originating in the region of the primary tumor running to two different lymph nodes. One of the two may be depicted on the scintigraphy images before the other. But that does not imply that the other node is not a sentinel node. Both nodes are on a direct drainage pathway, and tumor cells can travel through either duct and go to either node. Both should be collected and examined by the pathologist. Receiving drainage directly from the primary tumor site is what makes a lymph node a sentinel node [2,3]. There are several explanations for the fact that one node receives less lymph flow than another. One of the reasons is that the flow to that particular node is hampered by metastatic disease.

Another point illustrated by this cases is that lymphoscintigraphy with only one view is not good enough. A sentinel node may be located behind another sentinel node, and as a result only one hot spot is depicted.

REFERENCES

1. De Cicco C, Sideri M, Bartolomei M, Maggioni A, Colombo N, Bocciolone L, Chinol M, Leonardi L, Mangioni C, Paganelli G. Sentinel node detection by lymphoscintigraphy and gamma detecting probe in patients with vulvar cancer (abstr). J Nucl Med 1997; 38:33P.
2. Uren RF, Howman-Giles R, Thompson JF, Shaw HM, Quinn MJ, O'Brien CJ, McCarthy WH. Lymphoscintigraphy to identify sentinel lymph nodes in patients with melanoma. Melanoma Res 1994; 4:395–399.
3. Morton DL, Bostick PJ. Will the true sentinel node please stand? Ann Surg Oncol 1999; 6:12–14.

Case 3: Definition of a Sentinel Node, the Inverse Square Law of Physics

A 41-year-old woman underwent a narrow excision of a melanoma on the left calf. It was a superficial spreading lesion (Clark level IV, Breslow thickness 2.0 mm).

Lymphoscintigraphy

A dose of 58.8 MBq (1.6 mCi) ^{99m}Tc-nanocolloid in a volume of 0.25 mL was injected intradermally around the biopsy scar. Two faint lymphatic vessels were observed running toward the most proximal node. Lymphoscintigraphy was read as showing drainage to one sentinel node in the left lower inguinal region (Fig. 3). Three hot spots higher up were thought to be second-tier nodes.

Surgery

The operation was performed with the aid of vital dye and a gamma-ray detection probe. A blue lymphatic vessel was identified and traced to a blue node (Fig. 4). A little more laterally, a second blue duct was observed, which led to the most cranial node depicted on the images. This node was explored through a separate incision and found underneath Poupart's ligament (Cloquet's node). The count rate in the first node was 11.4 times as high as the count rate in the other node.

Pathology and Follow-Up

No tumor metastasis was found in either sentinel node. The patient remained free of disease 2 years later.

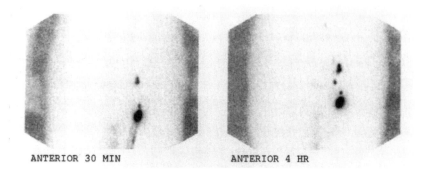

ANTERIOR 30 MIN   ANTERIOR 4 HR

FIGURE 3   The early lymphoscintigram shows a hot proximal node and several less prominent nodes higher up. The image suggests one sentinel node and three second-tier nodes. The late view shows a fourth second-tier node.

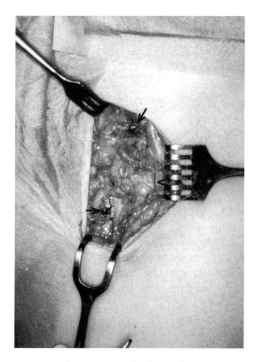

FIGURE 4   The operative findings show the two blue nodes (arrows) and a blue lymphatic duct bypassing the caudal node (arrow head).

Discussion

It is not true that the node closest to the primary tumor is by definition the (only) sentinel node. It is also not so that the hottest node is by definition the (only) sentinel node. The radioactivity content of a node is determined by parameters such as its size and the lymph flow rate. A large second-tier node occasionally accumulates more radioactivity than a small first-echelon node. For these reasons, it is questionable to use the radioactivity content or the sentinel node-to-background ratio to determine whether a node is a sentinel node.

How hot a node appears on the images is not only determined by its radioactivity content. One must also reckon with the inverse square law of physics: A superficial node lies closer to the gamma camera and is depicted brighter than an equally radioactive node that is situated deeper and, as a result, lies further away from the gamma camera.

Case 4: Drainage to Multiple Basins

A 34-year old woman was diagnosed with a melanoma in the midline on the back, at the level of the second lumbar vertebra. The lesion was excised with a 2-mm margin. Histological evaluation revealed a superficial spreading melanoma without ulceration (Clark level III, Breslow thickness 1.3 mm). The patient consented to participate in the international Multicenter Selective Lymphadenectomy Trial and was randomized to undergo wide local excision and sentinel node biopsy [1].

Lymphoscintigraphy

A dose of 97 MBq (2.6 mCi) ^{99m}Tc-nanocolloid in a volume of 0.25 mL was injected intradermally around the biopsy scar. Early imaging revealed drainage in three directions (Fig. 5). Sentinel nodes were visualized in the right groin and in both axillae.

Surgery

The surgeon refrained from sentinel node biopsy. The protocol of the trial in which this patient was enrolled does not permit exploration of more than two lymphatic fields because of the uncertain benefit from sentinel node biopsy in this situation. The patient had been informed of the possibility of drainage to more than two basins. She accepted the proposal to undergo wide local excision only.

Discussion

The French anatomist Marie-Philibert-Constant Sappey (1810–1896) described an imaginary 2-cm-wide line running from the upper margin of the umbilicus

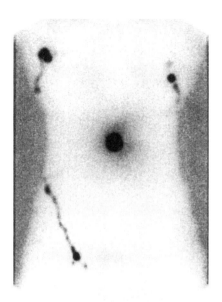

FIGURE 5 The anterior lymphoscintigraphy image obtained 30 minutes after injection of the tracer shows drainage to sentinel nodes in the right groin and both axillae.

around the body to the level of the second lumbar vertebra [2]. Sappey stated that lymph at this line could either flow in a cranial or in a caudal direction. Above this line, lymph drainage typically is to the axilla(e), and below this line to the groin(s).

This patient had her melanoma at the crossing of Sappey's line and the midline, a location where lymphatic drainage is unpredictable. With increasing experience in lymphatic mapping, it is becoming evident that melanomas further away from the midline or Sappey's line also have ambiguous drainage [3,4]. All lymph basins at risk should be surveyed by the nuclear medicine physician. This can be accomplished with spot views or (elegantly) with a whole-body view.

What about the surgeon's decision not to perform sentinel node biopsy? A survival benefit from early nodal basin dissection or early adjuvant systemic treatment has not yet been established [5]. The decision not to perform the operation is therefore justified, particularly because exploring three lymph node basins—and turning the patient on the operating table in between these operations to reinject blue dye on the back—would take an excessive amount of operating room time.

REFERENCES

1. Morton DL, Thompson JF, Essner R, Elashoff R, Stern SL, Nieweg OE, Roses DF, Karakousis CP, Mozillo N, Reintgen D, Wang H, Glass EC, Cochran AJ, the Multicenter Selective Lymphadenectomy Trial Group. Validation of the accuracy in a multicenter-trial of intraoperative lymphatic mapping and sentinel lymphadenectomy for early-stage melanoma. Ann Surg 1999; 230;453–463.
2. Sappey MPC. Anatomie, Physiologie, Pathologie des Vaisseaux Lymphatiques Considerés Chez l'Homme et les Vertebres. 4th ed. Paris: A Delahaye et Lecrosnier, 1888.
3. Uren RF, Howman-Giles RB, Shaw HM, Thompson JF, McCarthy WH. Lymphoscintigraphy in high-risk melanoma of the trunk: predicting draining node groups, defining lymphatic channels and locating the sentinel node. J Nucl Med 1993; 34:1435–1440.
4. Thompson JF, Uren RF, Shaw HM, McCarthy WH, Quinn MJ, O'Brien CJ, Howman-Giles RB. Location of sentinel lymph nodes in patients with cutaneous melanoma: new insights into lymphatic anatomy. J Am Coll Surg 1999; 189:195–204.
5. Nieweg OE, Kapteijn BAE, Thomson JF, Kroon BBR. Lymphatic mapping and selective lymphadenectomy for melanoma: not yet standard therapy. Eur J Surg Oncol 1997; 23:397–398.

Case 5: Lymphatic Lake

A 21-year-old woman presented with a melanoma on the posterolateral aspect of the right arm at midhumeral level. The diagnosis was confirmed on excision biopsy, and the patient was referred for lymphatic mapping using lymphoscintigraphy.

Lymphoscintigraphy

A dose of 5 MBq (0.13 mCi) of ^{99m}Tc antimony sulphide colloid was injected intradermally around the excision biopsy site at three points (total dose, 15 MBq, 0.4 mCi). On the early dynamic image, a single lymphatic vessel was observed passing up to the right axilla (Fig. 6). A bright focus of tracer was observed about half way up the channel between the injection site and the axilla. Tracer was also observed to reach a sentinel node in the right axilla. On the delayed image acquired 2 hours after injection of the radiocolloid, activity was identified in the right axillary sentinel node, but there was no residual activity anywhere along the line of the lymphatic vessel where a bright focus had previously been observed on dynamic imaging.

Surgery

The day after lymphoscintigraphy, the patient was injected immediately preoperatively with patent blue dye around the excision biopsy site on the arm. The patient was then anaesthetized, and an incision was made at the site of the surface mark in the right axilla applied the day before during lymphoscintigraphy. A sentinel node was found at the expected depth beneath the skin, blue stained and ''hot''

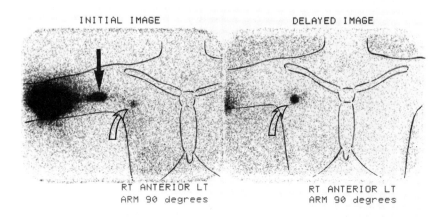

INITIAL IMAGE   DELAYED IMAGE

RT ANTERIOR LT   RT ANTERIOR LT
ARM 90 degrees   ARM 90 degrees

FIGURE 6   On the early dynamic image (left), a single lymphatic vessel is observed passing up to the right axilla from the injection site at midhumeral level. A bright focus of tracer (closed arrow) is observed approximately half way up the channel between the injection site and the axilla. Tracer is also seen reaching a sentinel node in the right axilla (open arrow). On the delayed image acquired 2 hours after injection of the radiocolloid, activity is identified in the right axillary sentinel node (arrow), but there is no residual activity anywhere along the line of the lymphatic vessel.

when examined with a gamma-ray detection probe. No activity whatsoever remained laterally over the course of the lymphatic channel, where the focus of tracer had been noted on dynamic imaging.

Pathology and Follow-Up

The right axillary sentinel node was normal on histological examination, and no evidence of melanoma micrometastasis was found.

Discussion

A lymphatic lake is a focal dilatation of a lymphatic collecting vessel and can occur anywhere along the course of the vessel [1]. Lymphatic lakes do not contain any lymph node tissue and do not retain radiocolloid as lymph nodes do.

Characteristically, they are observed clearly on early dynamic imaging but fade rapidly, typically over a period of 10 to 20 minutes. They are usually not visible on delayed scans performed 2 hours after injection of tracer. Sometimes, however, the washout is slower. If surgery is performed the next day, there will be no activity whatsoever at the site of a lymphatic lake when the area is examined with a probe. We have not seen any lymph node which has behaved in this way.

Lymph nodes retain the majority of their tracer over a 24-hour period when radio-colloids are used for lymphatic mapping.

There is usually only a single lymphatic lake observed along the course of a lymphatic vessel, as in this case; however, they are sometimes multiple [1].

Because lymphatic lakes do not contain lymph node tissue, they do not retain radiocolloid or metastatic melanoma cells and do not need to be removed as part of a sentinel node biopsy procedure. Their importance lies in understanding that they have a characteristic appearance on lymphoscintigraphy so that one can avoid searching for "transient" lymph nodes. It is possible that some reports of tracer passing rapidly and completely through a sentinel node have been caused by misidentification of a lymphatic lake as a sentinel node [2].

REFERENCES

1. Uren RF, Thompson JF, Howman-Giles RB, Lymphatics. In: Lymphatic drainage of the Skin and Breast: Locating the Sentinel Nodes. Uren RF, Thompson JF, Howman-Giles RB, eds. Amsterdam, the Netherlands: Harwood Academic Publishers, 1999, 1–20.
2. Boxen I, McCready D, Ballinger JR. Sentinel node detection and definition may depend on the imaging agent and timing. Clin Nucl Med 1999; 24:390–394.

Case 6: Lymphoscintigraphy After Wide Excision

A dermatologist referred a 44-year-old man after wide excision of a nodular melanoma situated on the lateral side of the right thigh. This was an ulcerated nodular melanoma (Clark level V, Breslow thickness 10.8 mm). The biopsy scar was 11 cm in length and ran in a transverse direction.

Lymphoscintigraphy

A dose of 62.2 MBq (1.7 mCi) ^{99m}Tc-nanocolloid in a volume of 0.30 mL was injected intradermally at four points along on either side of the biopsy scar. Two lymphatic vessels ran from the cranial side of the scar to two separate lymph nodes (Fig. 7). Two other vessels ran from the caudal side of the scar to two other lymph nodes. Therefore, there was a total of four sentinel nodes.

Surgery

Vital dye (1.0 mL) was injected along the entire length of the biopsy wound at either side. A lengthwise incision of 8 cm was made over the right groin. Underneath Scarpa's fascia, a blue lymphatic vessel was identified cranially in the groin. This vessel was followed and found to divide into two vessels going to separate blue nodes. More caudally in the groin, two other blue vessels were observed leading to two other blue nodes. All four nodes received drainage

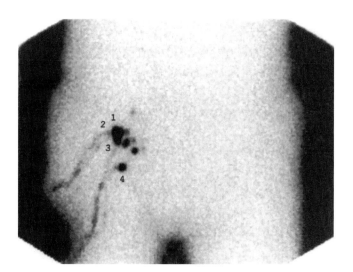

FIGURE 7 The lymphoscintigraphy image shows lymphatic vessels with direct drainage to four sentinel nodes.

directly from the biopsy area and were removed as sentinel nodes. All four were radioactive.

Pathology and Follow-Up

The two nodes that received drainage from the caudal side of the wound contained metastatic disease, the other two were disease-free. An inguinofemoral node dissection was performed and revealed one more tumor-involved lymph node. The patient remained free of the disease 3.5 years later.

Discussion

One end of the scar may drain to another node rather than to the opposite end of the scar; there may be a lymphatic watershed in between. Therefore, it makes sense to administer the tracers along the entire length on either side of the biopsy scar. This patient was treated early in our series. He had undergone a wide excision, and we were confronted with a transverse biopsy scar that was 11 cm in length. It has been shown that the mean number of sentinel lymph nodes removed is increased when lymphatic mapping is performed after wide local excision. Drainage may occur to other nodes than the sentinel node of the original melanoma site. The number of patients in whom two or more basins have to be dissected is also increased, which suggests that more extensive surgery is performed when compared with mapping before wide local excision [1]. Lymphatic mapping and sentinel lymphadenectomy should precede therapeutic wide excision.

REFERENCE

1. Wells KE, Joseph E, Ross M, Cruse CW, Rapaport DP, Glass F, Messina J, Berman C, Cantor A, Reintgen DS. Lymphatic mapping for melanoma before and after wide local excision (abstr). Melanoma Res 1997; 7:S105.

Case 7: Reproducibility of Lymphoscintigraphy

A 49-year-old woman underwent a narrow excision of a melanoma on the left forearm. It was a nodular lesion (Clark level IV, Breslow thickness 2.9 mm). This patient consented to participate in a study on the reproducibility of lympho-scintigraphy.

Lymphoscintigraphy

A dose of 67 MBq (1.8 mCi) ^{99m}Tc-nanocolloid in a volume of 0.30 mL was injected intradermally divided over two doses on either side of the biopsy scar. The first lymphoscintigraphy study showed two sentinel nodes in the left axilla (Fig. 8). Imaging was repeated 2 weeks later on the day before the operation.

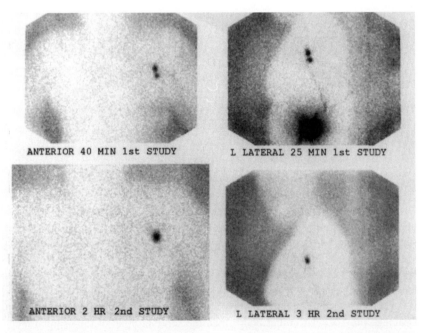

FIGURE 8 The upper lymphoscintigraphy images depict two sentinel nodes in the left axilla. The lower lymphoscintigraphy study was conducted 2 weeks later and shows only one sentinel node.

The second lymphoscintigraphy study was conducted under the same circumstances as the earlier study and was performed by the same investigator using the same agent and the same technique. This time, however, the images showed a single sentinel node in the left axilla (Fig. 8).

Surgery

The operation was performed with the aid of vital dye. One blue lymphatic vessel was identified and traced to a single blue node. The gamma detection probe confirmed that this node was radioactive. Scanning the axilla with the probe, no other radioactive or blue nodes were found. No completion axillary node dissection was performed.

Pathology and Follow-Up

No tumor metastasis was found in the sentinel node. Four years later, the patient remained free of disease.

Discussion

Two studies to date have addressed the reproducibility of lymphoscintigraphy. The first study demonstrated a reproducibility of 88% using ^{99m}Tc-nanocolloid [1]. The second study, in which ^{99m}Tc sulfur colloid was used, demonstrated a reproducibility of 85% [2].

This apparent variability in lymph flow may be one of the reasons for a false-negative sentinel node biopsy results. A number of potential reasons for this limited reproducibility are discussed in Chapter 3 on cutaneous lymphoscintigraphy.

Interobserver variability of lymphoscintigraphy interpretation is limited: In a study of 51 patients, two nuclear medicine physicians agreed on the reading of 83 of the 84 node fields [3].

REFERENCES

1. Kapteijn BAE, Nieweg OE, Valdés Olmos RA, Liem IH, Baidjnath Panday RKL, Hoefnagel CA, Kroon BBR. Reproducibility of lymphoscintigraphy for lymphatic mapping in patients with cutaneous melanoma. J Nucl Med 1996; 37:972–975.
2. Mudun A, Murray DR, Herda SC, Eshima D, Shattuck LA, Vansant JP, Taylor AT, Alazraki NP. Early stage melanoma: lymphoscintigraphy, reproducibility of sentinel node detection, and effectiveness of the intraoperative gamma probe. Radiology 1996; 199:171–175.
3. Uren RF, Howman-Giles RB, Shaw HM, Thompson JF, McCarthy WH. Lymphoscintigraphy in high-risk melanoma of the trunk: predicting draining node groups, defining lymphatic channels and locating the sentinel node. J Nucl Med 1993; 34:1435–1440.

Case 8: Altered Drainage Pattern After Nearby Surgery

A 27-year-old man underwent a narrow excision of a melanoma in the right lateral epigastric region. It was a superficial spreading melanoma (Clark level III, Breslow thickness 1.1 mm). His medical history revealed that a cyst had been excised from underneath the right areola of the breast 12 years previously.

Lymphoscintigraphy

A dose of 63.6 MBq (1.6 mCi) ^{99m}Tc-nanocolloid in a volume of 0.32 mL was injected intradermally around the biopsy scar. Lymphoscintigraphy showed drainage across the midline to one sentinel node in the left axilla (Fig. 9). A second-tier node was depicted a little higher up. There was also drainage to two nodes in the internal mammary chain but not to the ipsilateral axilla.

Surgery

The operation was performed with the aid of vital dye and a gamma-ray detector. Two lymphatic vessels in the left axilla were observed and easily traced to the blue and radioactive sentinel node. The second-tier node was not disturbed. The internal mammary sentinel nodes could not be reached without dividing a rib. The surgeon was not prepared to do that for what he considered to be an experimental procedure.

Pathology and Follow-Up

No tumor metastasis was found in the sentinel node. Two years later, the patient was free of disease.

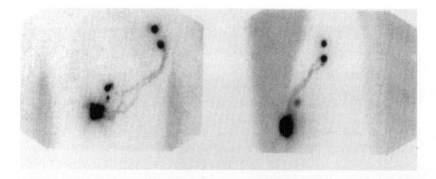

Figure 9   The anterior lymphoscintigraphy image on the left shows drainage to two sentinel nodes in the internal mammary chain and one in the left axilla. The lateral view shows the drainage to the lowermost node in the left axilla.

Discussion

Lymph drainage from the right epigastric region across the midline to the opposite axilla without concomitant drainage to the ipsilateral axilla is unusual. Drainage from the skin to the internal mammary lymph nodes is also rare but occurs via a costal margin node in approximately 20% of patients with melanoma in the superior periumbilical area [1]. The unlikely drainage pattern in this patient can be explained by the prior operation on the ipsilateral breast. Tumors in the epigastric region frequently drain through a lymph vessel that passes underneath the areola. At The Netherlands Cancer Institute, we have noticed a sentinel node in the breast just lateral from the areola in a number of patients.

The lymphatic vessel from the right epigastric region to the right axilla was probably disrupted with the removal of the cyst in that location. Other lymphatic routes developed with the unusual drainage pattern as a result.

REFERENCE

1. JF Thompson, Uren RF, Shaw HM, McCarthy WH, Quinn MJ, O'Brien CJ, Howman-Giles RB. Location of sentinel lymph nodes in patients with cutaneous melanoma: new insights into lymphatic anatomy. J Am Coll Surg 1999; 189:195–204.

Case 9: Popliteal Sentinel Nodes, Flow Imaging

A 67-year-old woman underwent excision with a 2-mm margin of a melanoma on the dorsum of the right foot. Histological examination showed a nodular melanoma (Clark level IV, Breslow thickness 2.6 mm).

Lymphoscintigraphy

A dose of 72 MBq (1.9 mCi) ^{99m}Tc-nanocolloid in a volume of 0.30 mL was injected intradermally around the biopsy scar on the right foot. The first image of the whole leg was obtained 20 minutes later and showed two nodes in the groin and four nodes in the popliteal fossa (Fig. 10).

Surgery

The operation was performed with the aid of vital dye and a gamma-ray detection probe. In the groin, two blue lymphatic vessels were found and led to two blue, radioactive lymph nodes. Both were removed. Subsequently, another dose of blue dye was administered, and the patient was turned over to a prone position. A transverse J-shaped incision was made over the popliteal fossa. No blue ducts were found. The four radioactive nodes were located with the aid of the probe and collected.

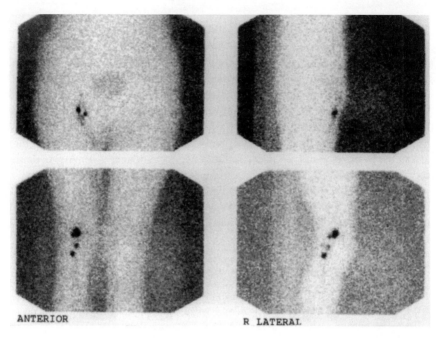

FIGURE 10   Anterior lymphoscintigraphy images (left) and lateral views (right). Two radioactive nodes in the right groin are depicted, and four in the popliteal fossa.

Pathology and Follow-Up

All six lymph nodes were free of disease. Two years later, an in-transit metastasis was removed from the right thigh. No further recurrence has been found during the 1.5 years since.

Discussion

Sentinel nodes are occasionally found in the popliteal fossa [1]. If that happens, the primary lesion is usually situated on the calf. Although the majority of melanomas on the calf drain to sentinel nodes in the groin, the popliteal fossa has to be imaged in patients with a melanoma below the knee.

This patient was treated early after the introduction of lymphatic mapping. No flow images were obtained at that time. As a consequence, it could not be determined whether the nodes in the groin were sentinel (first-tier) nodes or second-tier nodes. The drainage order of the popliteal nodes was also not clarified. The blue dye was not helpful in this case. All radioactive nodes were removed to err on the safe side.

REFERENCE

1.   Thompson JF, Hunt JA, Culjak G, Uren RF, Howman-Giles R, Harman CR. Popliteal lymph node metastasis from primary cutaneous melanoma. Eur J Surg Oncol, in press.

Case 10: Interval Node

A 40-year-old woman presented with a melanoma on the dorsal aspect of the right wrist. After excision biopsy, she was referred for lymphoscintigraphy to define lymphatic drainage pathways and the location of the sentinel lymph nodes.

Lymphoscintigraphy

A dose of 15 MBq (0.4 mCi) of ^{99m}Tc antimony sulphide colloid was injected intradermally around the excision biopsy site. On the early dynamic image, several lymphatic vessels were observed passing up the right arm from the injection sites around the excision-biopsy scar (Fig. 11). Two nodes were observed on the early image, one in the right epitrochlear region and the other an interval node medially in the arm at midhumeral level. These nodes were again evident on the delayed scan performed 2 hours later. However, there were also three small focal

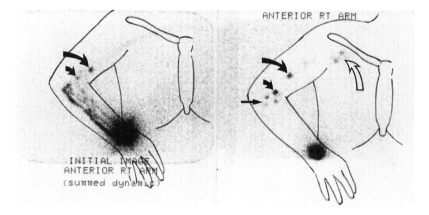

FIGURE 11   On the early dynamic image (left), several lymphatic vessels are observed passing up the right arm from the injection site on the right wrist. Two nodes are observed on this early image, one in the right epitrochlear region (short curved arrow) and the other an interval node medially in the arm (long curved arrow) somewhat higher up. These nodes are again evident on the delayed scan performed 2 hours later (right). There are also three small focal areas of tracer retention (horizontal arrow) that lie over the lateral aspect of the elbow, as well as faint activity in right secondary nodes in the axilla (open curved arrow).

areas of tracer retention overlying the lateral aspect of the elbow, as well as faint activity in right axillary nodes.

Discussion

Interval nodes are nodes that lie between a primary tumor site and a recognized node field somewhere along the course of a lymphatic collecting vessel [1]. They occur in approximately 7% to 22% of patients—depending on the definition of an interval node—and may harbor melanoma metastases, in some cases being the only nodes positive for metastases [2,3]. When they receive tracer directly from a primary tumor site, they are by definition also sentinel nodes and should therefore be removed as part of a sentinel node biopsy procedure.

The definite sentinel nodes in this patient were the right epitrochlear node and the interval node medially in the right arm. The latter area is a common site for an interval node in patients with a melanoma on the forearm. We do not regard the epitrochlear node as an interval node, but rather a node in a recognized node field. Lymphatic lakes are small focal dilatations of the lymphatic collecting vessels, and they do not contain any nodal tissue [4]. The small areas observed laterally over the elbow during lymphoscintigraphy in this patient are most likely lymphatic lakes because, although they were evident during lymphoscintigraphy, the areas did not contain any tracer whatsoever 18 hours later. Lymphatic lakes characteristically are seen clearly on early dynamic imaging but fade rapidly. They are usually not visible on delayed scans performed 2 hours after injection of tracer. Sometimes, however, the washout is slower, as in this patient. We have not observed any lymph node that has behaved in this way. Lymph nodes retain the majority of their tracer over a 24-hour period. The axillary nodes in this patient were second-tier nodes, having received tracer that had already passed through a sentinel node.

REFERENCES

1. Uren RF, Thompson JF, Howman-Giles RB. The sentinel lymph node concept in melanoma. In: Lymphatic Drainage of the Skin and Breast: Locating the sentinel Nodes. Uren RF, Thompson JF, Howman-Giles RB, eds. Amsterdam, the Netherlands: Harwood Academic Publishers, 1999, pp 69–90.
2. Uren RF, Thompson JF, Howman-Giles R, Shaw HM. Interval nodes, the forgotten sentinel nodes in melanoma patients. Arch Surg, in press.
3. Lieber KA, Standiford SB, Kuvshinoff BW, Ota DM, Mansour EG, Polk HC, Jr, Sondak VK. Surgical management of aberrant sentinel lymph node drainage in cutaneous melanoma. Surgery 1998; 124:757–762.
4. Uren RF, Thompson JF, Howman-Giles RB. Lymphatics. In: Lymphatic Drainage of the Skin and Breast: Locating the Sentinel Nodes. Uren RF, Thompson JF, Howman-

Giles RB, eds. Amsterdam, the Netherlands: Harwood Academic Publishers, 1999, pp 1–20.

Case 11: Limited Resolution of the Gamma Camera

A 48-year-old woman with a melanoma (1.2-mm Breslow thickness) on the right forearm had undergone a previous diagnostic excision with a 2-mm margin.

Lymphoscintigraphy

A dose of 67.3 MBq (1.8 mCi) ^{99m}Tc-nanocolloid in a volume of 0.35 mL was injected intradermally around the biopsy scar. The anterior image shows one hot spot in the right axilla to the casual observer (Fig. 12). When the image is examined more carefully and the lateral view is taken into consideration, there may be two sentinel nodes back to back.

Surgery

The operation was performed the next day. One milliliter of patent blue dye was administered around the biopsy site. A 4-cm incision was made along the lower hair line. Two blue lymphatic vessels were observed leading to two adjacent blue nodes. The probe confirmed that both nodes were radioactive. The nodes were freed from the surrounding fatty tissue and collected. Outside the wound, it was confirmed that they were radioactive.

Scanning the wound with the gamma-ray detection probe for remaining radioactivity, the surgeon was surprised to find a definite hot focus right underneath the site where the two sentinel nodes had been removed. Exploring just a little deeper down, a third blue lymphatic channel was uncovered that was traced back to the arm and lead to a third node that was both blue and radioactive.

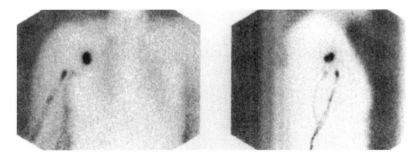

Figure 12 The anterior view obtained after 30 minutes shows one hot spot in the right axilla. The lateral view led to the conclusion that two adjacent sentinel nodes were present.

Instead of the two sentinel nodes that were expected to be present, there were actually three. No completion axillary node dissection was performed.

Pathology and Follow-Up

No tumor metastases were found in the sentinel nodes. Two years later, the patient remained free of disease.

Discussion

Preoperative lymphoscintigraphy indicates the number of sentinel nodes correctly in 83% of the cases [1]. The limited resolution of the gamma camera—discriminating power—is the most prominent cause for inaccurate depiction of the number of sentinel nodes.

Another point illustrated by this case is the value of the gamma detection probe. Without it, the third sentinel node would not have been recovered. After removal of the sentinel node(s), the wound must be scanned to make certain that all sentinel nodes have been identified and collected.

REFERENCE

1. Jansen L, Nieweg OE, Kapteijn BAE, Valdés Olmos RA, Hoefnagel CA, Kroon BBR. Accuracy of lymphoscintigraphy in indicating the number of sentinel lymph nodes in patients with melanoma (abstr). World Federation Surgical Oncology Societies and Society of Surgical Oncology Joint Meeting, San Diego, CA, 1998.

Case 12: False-Negative Sentinel Node Biopsy

A 74-year-old man sought medical attention at another hospital for a mole on the left upper arm that had been present for a number of years. The lesion had recently increased in size and had oozed blood. He was referred for sentinel node biopsy after excision of the suspicious-looking lesion with a margin of 4 mm. The pathologist reported seeing a superficial spreading melanoma with ulceration (Clark level III, Breslow thickness 2.6 mm).

Lymphoscintigraphy

A total of 70 MBq (1.9 mCi) ^{99m}Tc-nanocolloid in a volume of 0.3 mL was injected intradermally divided over four doses around the biopsy scar. The images obtained after 2 hours show one hot spot in the left axilla (Fig. 13). The same result was obtained 5 hours after injection. The location of the node was marked on the skin with indelible ink.

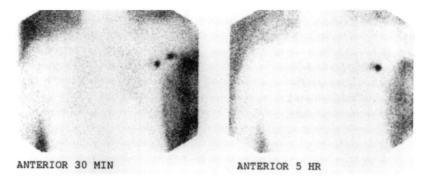

ANTERIOR 30 MIN   ANTERIOR 5 HR

FIGURE 13 The early image shows the sentinel node in the left axilla and radioactivity in the afferent lymphatic vessel with a lymphatic lake. The late view confirms the presence of a single sentinel node.

Surgery

The operation was performed the day after lymphoscintigraphy. A volume of 0.8 mL of patent blue dye was administered divided over two doses, on either side of the biopsy site on left upper arm. A 4-cm incision was made along the lower hair line. A blue lymphatic vessel was found high in the axilla. It was traced to a lymph node that was blue around the entrance of the lymphatic vessel. The gamma detection probe measurements demonstrated that the number of counts in the node was 36 times as high as the number of counts in the remainder of the axilla.

Scanning the wound, another radioactive node was found with a count rate five times as high as the background. This node was not blue. The node was removed and labeled as a nonsentinel node.

Subsequent probe measurements indicated that the count rate had returned to the background level around the axilla. The sentinel node was submitted for frozen section evaluation: no tumor cells. No completing axillary node dissection was performed.

Pathology and Follow-Up

Pathology evaluation included H&E and immunohistochemistry staining (HMB-45, S-100). No tumor cells were found in either node. At a routine follow-up visit 4 months later, the surgeon noted a 2-cm lymph node in the left axilla. Fine-needle aspiration cytology revealed melanoma cells. Left axillary node dissection was conducted. Eighteen lymph nodes were removed, of which 17 contained metastatic melanoma with capsular breech and lymphangioinvasion. A computed tomography scan of the lungs was obtained and showed multiple metastases. After an initial favorable response to systemic treatment, the patient died 8 months later.

Discussion

This is a clear example of a false-negative sentinel node biopsy result. At The Netherlands Cancer Institute, we have had six false-negative sentinel node biopsy results in 200 melanoma patients (sensitivity, 89%) after a median follow-up duration of 32 months [1]. There are several potential reasons for a false-negative sentinel node biopsy result: (1) conceptual failure; (2) technical failure; (3) pathological failure; and (4) biological failure.

The concept of sequential dissemination may not be true in every instance. It is conceivable that occasional tumor cells slip through the sentinel node, lodge in a second-tier node, and proliferate to form a "skip" metastasis. A technical failure was considered unlikely in this case after review of the lymphoscintigraphy images and the technique used. The surgical procedure appears flawless as well.

It is nice for a surgeon to be able to blame a false-negative sentinel node biopsy result on the pathologist. A pathologist makes a limited number of slides from a sentinel node and certainly not the 2,500 or so that are needed to view all the cells in a lymph node. At the Moffit Cancer Center, re-evaluation of six false-negative sentinel nodes revealed metastases in five when reverse-transcriptase polymerase chain reaction was used [2]. In this particular patient, the pathologist was asked to step-section the remainder of the sentinel node, but still no tumor cells were found.

The most likely explanation for the false-negative procedure in this patient is that metastatic disease in the *original* sentinel node blocked drainage to that node. Other compensatory lymphatic vessels opened, and the lymph from the tumor site was diverted to another node that was then identified by the surgeon as a *neo*-sentinel node. This is what can be called a biological failure. One thing that we have modified in our surgical technique since this case is to always palpate the surrounding lymph nodes in the open wound. A rock hard node is removed independent of its color and radioactivity content.

REFERENCES

1. Jansen L, Nieweg OE, Peterse JL, Hoefnagel CA, Valdés Olmos RA, Kroon BBR. Reliability of sentinel node biopsy for staging melanoma. Br J Surg, in press.
2. Haddad F, Shivers S, Costello D, Goscin C, Messina J, Glass F, DeConti R, Berman C, Cruse CW, Wells K, Shons A, Reintgen D. Patterns of recurrence following a negative sentinel lymph node biopsy in 721 patients with stage I or II melanoma (abstr). Eur J Nucl Med 1999; 26(Suppl):S58.

Case 13: Sentinel Node Close to Primary Melanoma Site

A 42-year-old man was referred after excision biopsy of a pigmented lesion on his left midneck. Histological examination had revealed it to be a melanoma 1.8 mm in maximum thickness, invading to Clark level IV.

Lymphoscintigraphy

Preoperative lymphoscintigraphy revealed upward passage of tracer to a single sentinel node in the upper neck with subsequent demonstration of a probable second-tier node more inferiorly (Figs. 14 and 15).

Surgery

At operation, the sentinel node demonstrated on the lymphoscintigram was found without difficulty, being both blue-stained and hot when examined with the gamma-ray detection probe (8978 counts per 10 seconds after removal). The site of the presumed second-tier node was explored, but only a nonblue node that was not hot with the probe was found. When the melanoma site was

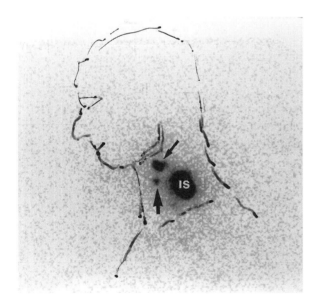

Figure 14 Lymphoscintigram, lateral view (delayed image at 2.5 hours) showing injection site (IS), sentinel lymph node above and anterior to it (small arrow), and second-tier node more inferiorly (large arrow). The second sentinel node found at the time of surgery is not visible because of the bloom around the injection site.

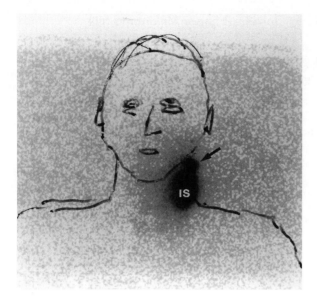

FIGURE 15 Lymphoscintigram, anterior view (delayed image at 2.5 hours) showing injection site (IS) and sentinel lymph node above it (arrow). Neither the second-tier node nor the second sentinel node found at the time of surgery is visible in this projection.

widely excised with a 2-cm clearance margin, however, a second blue-stained sentinel node was found only approximately 1.5 cm from the primary melanoma site. This node was hot when examined with the probe (4161 counts per 10 seconds).

Pathology and Follow-Up

On subsequent histological examination, no evidence of micrometastatic disease was found in either sentinel node. The patient remains well and disease-free after 4 months of follow-up.

Discussion

This case demonstrates the importance of checking carefully beneath a wide excision site for additional sentinel nodes when a primary melanoma site overlies or is in close proximity to a regional lymph node field. The sentinel node close to the primary tumor site was not identified on the preoperative lymphoscintigram because of the radioactive bloom around the tracer injection sites.

A second point demonstrated by this case is that initial lymphatic drainage from primary tumors on the neck can sometimes occur in an upward direction rather than the downward direction that would be expected.

Case 14: Sentinel Node Close to Primary Melanoma Site (II)

A 36-year-old man was diagnosed with a melanoma on the back, over the spina of the right scapula (Clark level III, Breslow thickness 2.5 mm) The lesion had been excised with a narrow margin. The patient was referred for wide local excision and sentinel node biopsy.

Lymphoscintigraphy

A dose of 26 MBq (0.7 mCi) ^{99m}Tc-nanocolloid in a volume of 0.2 mL was injected intradermally around the biopsy scar. One sentinel node was visualized in the right axilla. The lateral view shows one additional hot spot in the supraclavicular fossa, the anterior view shows two hot spots in that field and the right anterior oblique view shows three (Fig. 16).

Surgery

The operation was performed the next day with the aid of blue dye and a gamma-ray detection probe. One milliliter of patent blue dye was administered around the original melanoma site on the right shoulder. A blue, hot node was removed from the right axilla. A repeat dose of 1 ml of blue dye was administered before

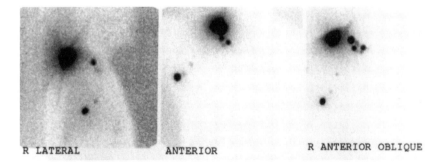

R LATERAL   ANTERIOR   R ANTERIOR OBLIQUE

FIGURE 16   The lateral view shows one supraclavicular node in addition to the node in the right axilla. The anterior view depicts one hot spot in the right axilla and two in the supraclavicular fossa. The right anterior oblique view shows three supraclavicular nodes, one right axillary node, and two second-tier nodes higher up the axilla.

exploring the right supraclavicular fossa. Two blue lymphatic vessels were ob-served converging on one blue radioactive node. No other blue vessels were observed. A second sentinel node was found with the aid of the probe. The third node could not be found. Subsequently, wide local re-excision of the melanoma site was performed with a 2-cm margin.

Pathology and Follow-Up

All three lymph nodes were free of disease by H&E and immunohistochemistry staining (HMB-45, S-100). Six months later, the patient came to the clinic be-cause he felt a lump in the neck. A 1-cm rubbery node was palpated in the right supraclavicular fossa. Fine-needle aspiration cytology revealed melanoma cells. A radical right neck dissection was performed after a search for other sites of disease (including computed tomography scans of chest, neck, and brain; liver ultrasound; bone scintigraphy; blood chemistry) revealed no other tumor loca-tions. Two supraclavicular nodes contained melanoma deposits; the other 28 nodes in the specimen were free of disease. A distant skin metastasis was discov-ered 9 months later. The patient died from brain metastases 1 year after the neck dissection.

Discussion

Some 95% of the injected radioactivity does not travel through the lymphatic system and stays behind at the injection site. This large amount of radioactivity may obscure a nearby sentinel node on the lymphoscintigraphy images. This problem is more often encountered in breast cancer than in melanoma. In mela-noma patients, this occurs mainly in the head and neck area [1–3]. The lateral view showed one supraclavicular sentinel node, the anterior view showed two, and the oblique view showed a third one. Oblique views can be very helpful in tight locations such as this one.

Despite the administration of a second dose of blue dye, only one blue node was recovered from the supraclavicular fossa. A second one was found with the probe. The third node was not found, and this had severe consequences. In retrospect, two mistakes were made. The first one was that the dose of the radio-active tracer was very small. The amount of radioactive ^{99m}Tc diminishes by 50% every 6 hours through physical decay. A dose of 26 MBq (0.7 mCi) is adequate for same-day surgery but insufficient when ^{99m}Tc-nanocolloid is used and the operation is scheduled for the next day.

The second mistake has to do with the scattered gamma rays from the injection site that severely hampered gamma probe identification of the supracla-vicular sentinel nodes in this patient, even with the collimator applied. The wide local excision should have been performed when the blue-dye identification failed. The sentinel node exploration should have been resumed after the removal of the radioactivity at the injection site. Then, the collimator could have been removed, and with the increased sensitivity the sentinel node should have been found easily despite the small amount of radioactivity still present.

REFERENCES

1. Ollila DW, Foshag LJ, Essner R, Stern SL, Morton DL. Parotid region lymphatic mapping and sentinel lymphadenectomy for cutaneous melanoma. Ann Surg Oncol 1999; 6:150–154.
2. Wells KE, Stadelmann WK, Rapaport DP, Hamlin R, Cruse CW, Reintgen D. Parotid selective lymphadenectomy in malignant melanoma. Ann Plast Surg 1999; 43: 1–6.
3. Jansen L, Schraffordt Koops H, Nieweg OE, Doting MHE, Kapteijn BAE, Balm AJM, Vermey A, Plukker JT, Horfnagel CA, Piers DA, Kroon BBR. Sentinel node biopsy for melanoma in the head and neck region. Head Neck 2000; 22:27–33.

Case 15: Tumor-Involved Sentinel Node in the Groin: Superficial and Deep Inguinal Node Dissection?

A 29-year-old man underwent diagnostic excision of a 6.32-mm-thick nodular melanoma on the right buttock (Clark level IV). He was enrolled in the Multicenter Selective Lymphadenectomy Trial and was randomized to undergo wide local excision and sentinel node biopsy.

Lymphoscintigraphy

A dose of 58 MBq (1.6 mCi) ^{99m}Tc-nanocolloid in a volume of 0.30 mL was injected intradermally around the biopsy scar on the right buttock. The dynamic study revealed drainage to a sentinel node in the right groin inferior to Poupart's ligament (Fig. 17). Subsequent scans demonstrated two second-tier nodes higher up and one more caudally. The location of the sentinel node was marked on the skin.

Surgery

The patient was taken to the operating room 24 hours after lymphoscintigraphy. One milliliter of patent blue dye was administered around the biopsy site on the right buttock. The gamma detection probe confirmed that the sentinel node was situated exactly underneath the skin mark placed by the nuclear medicine physician. A 4-cm incision was made over the skin mark, and three lymphatic vessels were identified underneath Scarpa's fascia. The vessels were observed converging on one blue radioactive lymph node. Two efferent blue ducts emerged at the opposite end of the sentinel node and led to a more caudally located second-tier

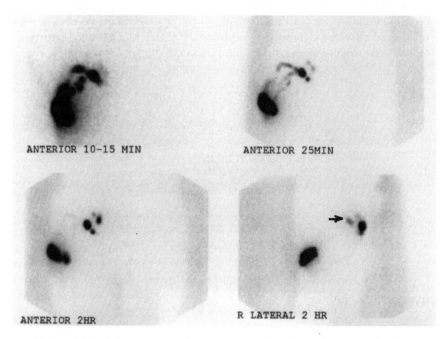

ANTERIOR 10-15 MIN   ANTERIOR 25MIN

ANTERIOR 2HR   R LATERAL 2 HR

FIGURE 17   The dynamic images at 10 minutes after injection of the tracer show drainage to one sentinel node in the right groin inferior from Poupart's ligament. The later images demonstrate two second-tier nodes higher up and one that is situated more caudally. The lateral view demonstrates that one of the second-tier nodes is situated in the deep inguinal area (arrow).

node that was blue and radioactive as well. The blue dye pattern thus showed that this latter node was indeed a second-tier node.

Both nodes were freed from the surrounding tissue. Lymph vessels and blood vessels to and from the nodes were ligated and divided, and the nodes were removed. Subsequently, another second-tier node was collected with the aid of the gamma-ray detection probe. A third second-tier node was not pursued when probe measurements indicated that it was situated above Poupart's ligament.

Pathology and Follow-Up

The sentinel node and the second-tier nodes were step-sectioned and examined with H&E and immunohistochemistry staining (HMB-45, S-100). The sentinel node was found to contain metastatic disease both on H&E and immunohistochemistry staining. The second-tier nodes were free of disease.

A superficial groin dissection was performed 4 weeks later. Frozen-section microscopy of Cloquet's lymph node showed no tumor cells. The remainder of the deep compartment was therefore left undisturbed.

Six lymph nodes were recovered from the specimen and examined with H&E and immunohistochemistry staining. No tumor cells were found.

The patient underwent follow-up evaluation at 3-month intervals and was fine initially. At a follow-up visit 1 year later, history and physical examination were uneventful. The right groin was normal. Blood tests were normal with the exception of the tumor marker S-100: 0.31 µg/L (normal value, <0.16 µg/L).

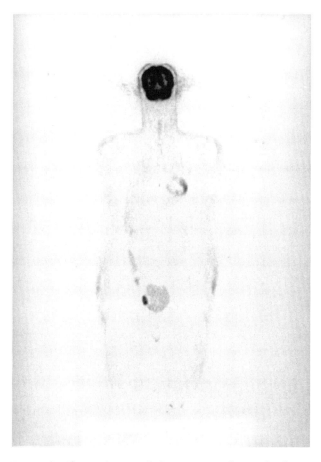

FIGURE 18 The positron emission tomography study shows increased ^{18}F-fluoro-2-deoxyglucose accumulation in an obturator lymph node.

Repeat physical examination was unremarkable again. Chest radiography and liver ultrasound were normal. A positron emission tomography study with the glucose analog ^{18}F-fluoro-2-deoxyglucose was obtained and showed a single hot spot adjacent to the bladder (Fig. 18). Ultrasound confirmed the presence of an enlarged obturator lymph node. An iliac and obturator node dissection was conducted. The 3-cm obturator node was fixed to the surrounding tissues. This node was removed but without margins. Pathological examination revealed the obturator node to be largely replaced by tumor. The disease reached beyond the capsule and the margin was indeed involved. The other 17 nodes were free of disease. Radiotherapy was given to the right groin. Thirteen months later, the patient was clinically disease-free, and the tumor marker level had returned to the normal range.

Discussion

Only some 15% to 21% of the patients with a tumor-involved sentinel node have other nodes in that field involved as well [1–3]. Scintigraphy usually shows drainage of lymph through several superficial lymph nodes before the deep (iliac and obturator) nodes light up. In keeping with the hypothesis of step-wise dissemination, the deep nodes will be free of disease in the majority of patients with a tumor-containing superficial sentinel node. With these thoughts in mind, should a deep (ilio-obturator) node dissection be routinely performed in addition to a superficial inguinal node dissection when the sentinel node contains tumor?

The deep second-tier node visualized on the scintigraphy images of this patient was not removed with the superficial inguinofemoral node dissection. This particular node was most likely the node that proved to be involved later on.

A sensible policy is to perform a deep node dissection when the sentinel node is involved and lymphoscintigraphy shows a second-tier node above Poupart's ligament or when more than one superficial node is involved.

REFERENCES

1. Thompson JF, McCarthy WH, Bosch CMJ, O'Brien CJ, Quinn MJ, Paramaesvaran S, Crotty K, McCarthy SW, Uren RF, Howman-Giles R. Sentinel lymph node status as an indicator of the presence of metastatic melanoma in regional lymph nodes. Melanoma Res 1995; 5:255–260.
2. Gershenwald JE, Thompson W, Mansfield PF, Lee JE, Colome MI, Tseng CH, Lee JJ, Balch CM, Reintgen DS, Ross MI. Multi-institutional melanoma lymphatic mapping experience: the prognostic value of sentinel lymph node status in 612 stage I or II melanoma patients. J Clin Oncol 1999; 17:976–983.
3. Jansen L, Nieweg OE, Peterse JL, Hoefnagel CA, Valdés Olmos RA, Kroon BBR. Reliability of sentinel node biopsy for staging melanoma. Br J Surg, in press.

Case 16: Postoperative Complications

A 46-year-old man was referred with a melanoma on the right calf. There was no evidence of satellite lesions, in-transit metastases, or regional lymphadenopathy. Histological examination showed a superficial spreading melanoma with an intact epidermis (Clark level III, Breslow thickness 1.1 mm). Because the lesion had been excised with a 3-mm margin, a wide local re-excision was planned with sentinel node biopsy.

Lymphoscintigraphy

A dose of 58.2 MBq (1.6 mCi) ^{99m}Tc-nanocolloid in a volume of 0.25 mL was injected intradermally around the biopsy scar on the right calf. Both early and late images showed drainage to a single sentinel node in the right groin.

Surgery

The operation was performed the next morning. One milliliter of patent blue dye was administered around the biopsy site. The sentinel node was identified with the gamma detection probe through the intact skin. A 4-cm longitudinal incision was made somewhat proximal from the node. A blue duct was identified in the subcutaneous tissue and dissected until it was observed entering a blue node. The gamma detection probe showed increased radioactivity in the node compared with the surrounding tissue. Afferent and efferent lymphatic vessels were ligated and divided, and the node was collected. No other blue or radioactive nodes were observed. The subcutaneous cavity tissue was closed with resorbable sutures, and the skin was closed with a running suture. Subsequently, a wide local excision of the primary melanoma site on the calf was performed.

Pathology and Follow-Up

The pathologist found no tumor metastasis in the sentinel node. The patient was discharged the day after the procedure. A few days later, he developed a fluctuating swelling of the wound area in the right groin. The family physician inserted a needle and drained a seroma. The swelling recurred and spontaneously burst through the wound 3 weeks postoperatively. The patient returned to the clinic, where continuous leakage of clear fluid was observed and a lymph fistula was diagnosed. The fistula continued to leak fluid for 4 weeks and then dried up spontaneously. Three years later, the patient remained free of disease.

Discussion

At The Netherlands Cancer Institute, 200 sentinel node biopsies have been performed for melanoma. Despite the policy to ligate lymphatic vessels and to completely obliterate the subcutaneous biopsy cavity, three patients (1.5%) developed a lymph fistula after the operation. The leakage stopped 1 to 2 months later without therapy in all three patients.

Another postoperative complication that is occasionally observed is wound infection. Long-term complications include erysipelas and (slight) edema of the limb. One patient retained the blue dye at the injection site on the back for more than a year before it gradually disappeared. On the whole, however, postoperative morbidity after sentinel node biopsy is low.

BREAST CANCER

Case 1: Normal Drainage Pattern

A 47-year-old woman noticed a lump in her left breast. Physical examination revealed a mobile, firm, 1-cm nodule in the central portion of the breast. No other abnormalities were noted in either breast. There was no axillary lymphadenopathy. Mammography was difficult to interpret because of pronounced density of the normal breast tissue. Ultrasound was suggestive of malignancy. Fine-needle aspiration cytology showed adenocarcinoma cells. The various treatment options were discussed with the patient. She opted for breast-conserving treatment with wide local excision of the tumor, sentinel node biopsy, and postoperative radiotherapy of the breast.

Lymphoscintigraphy

A dose of 90.7 MBq (2.5 mCi) ^{99m}Tc-nanocolloid in a volume of 0.25 mL was injected into the primary breast cancer with a 25-gauge needle. Dynamic (flow) imaging was performed. Anterior and lateral static images were obtained after 30 minutes and after 2 hours. The images showed one lymphatic vessel running to one sentinel node in the left axilla (Fig. 19). The location of the sentinel node was marked on the skin with indelible ink.

Surgery

The operation was performed the next morning with the aid of patent blue dye and a gamma-ray detection probe. One milliliter of patent blue dye was administered in and immediately around the breast cancer when the patient was anesthesized but before sterile draping. A 4-cm incision was made along the lateral margin of the pectoralis major muscle, curving toward the lower hair line. One blue lymphatic duct was observed once Scarpa's fascia was divided and the axillary fat was reached. As the duct was dissected, it followed the typical course in a lateral direction at first and then turned in a medial and cranial direction toward a blue node underneath the pectoralis major muscle at level I. The node

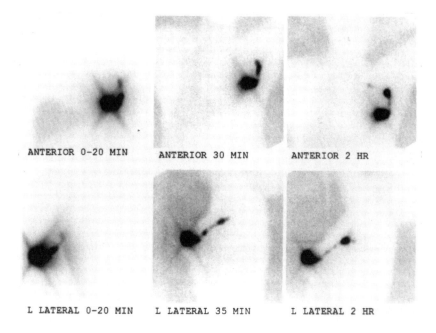

ANTERIOR 0-20 MIN   ANTERIOR 30 MIN   ANTERIOR 2 HR

L LATERAL 0-20 MIN   L LATERAL 35 MIN   L LATERAL 2 HR

FIGURE 19   Anterior and lateral views at various time intervals after injection of ^{99m}Tc-nanocolloid in the breast tumor. A radioactive flood source was placed behind the patient after the earliest images to outline the body contour [2]. The images obtained at 20 minutes after tracer administration show early visualization of the lymphatic vessel. Ten minutes later, the entire lymphatic vessel is visible. Two hours after injection, the sentinel node is depicted.

was identified 6 minutes after the incision had been made. The probe was brought out and it was confirmed that the node was radioactive.

The node was freed from the surrounding fat. Blood vessels and lymphatic vessels to and from the node were ligated and divided. No other blue vessels were observed. The axilla was scanned with the probe for other hot nodes, but none was found. The axillary fat was closed to prevent seroma, and the skin was closed with an intracutaneous running suture. No completion axillary node dissection was performed.

Pathology

No tumor cells were found in the sentinel node at frozen-section microscopy. This was confirmed later when the definitive slides were examined using H&E staining and immunohistochemistry (CAM 5.2).

Discussion

The situation in this patient is as it is encountered in approximately 30% of the patients: one lymphatic vessel with a typical course to one sentinel node. The blue-dye technique was used in this patient, but the probe technique would have been equally effective [1]. The location of this sentinel node is where it is usually found.

The skin mark placed by the nuclear medicine physician is often not of much help in patients with breast cancer. The location of the sentinel node is difficult to mark on the skin because the axilla is fairly deep, and the position of the arm may not be the same during lymphoscintigraphy and during the operation. The accuracy of skin marking can be enhanced by indicating the sentinel node in both the anterior and the lateral projection.

The surgeon had completed a learning phase with one false-negative sentinel node biopsy result in a series of 50 patients in whom completion axillary node dissection was conducted. He was confident enough to omit the axillary node dissection in this patient. This approach had been discussed with the patient at length before the operation. The patient was aware of the benefits and risks and opted for this approach instead of the axillary node dissection that was offered to her as an alternative.

REFERENCES

1. Rutgers EJTh, Jansen L, Nieweg OE, De Vries J, Schraffordt Koops H, Kroon BBR. Technique of sentinel node biopsy in breast cancer. Eur J Surg Oncol 1998; 24:316–319.
2. Valdés Olmos RA, Hoefnage CA, Nieweg OE, Jansen L, Rutgers EJTh, Borger J, Horenblas S, Kroon BBR. Lymphoscintigraphy in oncology: a rediscovered challenge. J Eur J Nucl Med 1999; 26 (Suppl):S2–S10.

Case 2: Lymphoscintigraphy Lateral View

A 46-year old woman discovered a small lump in the left breast. Her surgeon palpated a firm nodule of less than 1 cm in the upper outer quadrant of the breast. Mammography showed a dense tumor with microcalcification extending beyond the lesion. Ultrasound revealed a spiculated mass that was classified as malignant. Fine needle aspiration was performed and showed clusters of adenocarcinoma cells. Because of the fairly large area with microcalcification, mastectomy was thought the best option for this patient. She agreed to undergo a sentinel node biopsy as part of the procedure.

Lymphoscintigraphy

A dose of 63.0 MBq (1.7 mCi) ^{99m}Tc-nanocolloid in a volume of 0.11 mL was injected into the primary breast cancer as a single dose. The anterior images showed a large deposit of radioactivity at the injection site but no drainage (Fig. 20). The lateral view, however, showed a sentinel node in the left axilla. The location of the sentinel node was marked on the skin with indelible ink.

Surgery

The operation was performed the next morning with the aid of patent blue dye and a gamma-ray detection probe. One milliliter of patent blue dye was administered in and around the breast lump. The area around the tumor was massaged for 5 minutes. The location of the sentinel node was identified with the gamma-ray detection probe through the intact skin.

    The lower lateral part of the mastectomy incision was made. A large blue lymphatic duct with a 2-mm diameter was observed and carefully traced to a deep blue lymph node behind the pectoralis major muscle. The node was confirmed to be radioactive and was collected. The wound was scanned for additional hot nodes, but none was found. Because the surgeon was in his learning phase, a modified radical mastectomy was performed with a level I-II axillary node dissection. Some nodes at level III were removed as well.

Pathology and Follow-Up

The primary tumor proved to be a radically excised ductal carcinoma-in-situ with a minimally invasive component. Hormone receptors were present at low levels.

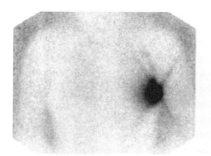 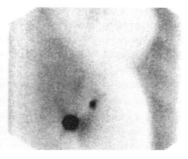

FIGURE 20 The anterior view was obtained 4 hours after administration of ^{99m}Tc-nanocolloid. It shows the radioactivity in the tumor but no drainage. The lateral image was obtained with a hanging-breast technique and shows the sentinel node in the left axilla.

The sentinel node was found to contain tumor cells both with H&E and immuno-histochemistry staining. Two of the 16 other nodes also contained tumor cells. The nodes at level III were free of disease. Radiotherapy was given to the internal mammary node chain, and adjuvant systemic chemotherapy was given, followed by tamoxifen. The patient was free of disease 1 year later.

Discussion

A problem with lymphatic mapping in breast cancer patients is that the injection site and the sentinel node are fairly close to one another. Some 95% of the tracer stays behind at the injection site. This is somewhat less when a tracer with a small particle size is used.

The large number of counts at the injection site may obscure the far smaller number of counts in a lymph node located nearby. Obtaining lymphoscintigraphy views from two angles reduces the risk of missing sentinel nodes. Anterior and lateral views are essential. Oblique views can be helpful [1]. Several techniques have been described to move the breast away from the axilla and improve the

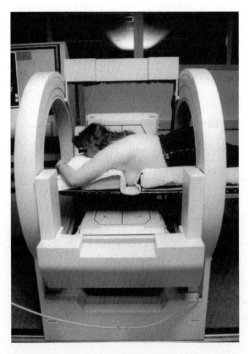

FIGURE 21   Patient positioned for a lateral image with hanging breast.

accuracy of imaging [2,3]. The technique with the patient in a prone position with the breast hanging down is an elegant way to accomplish this (Fig. 21).

Indications for adjuvant radiotherapy to the internal mammary node chain vary from hospital to hospital. In hindsight, radiotherapy to these nodes seems illogical in this patient. One of the great benefits from lymphatic mapping is that this treatment can be restricted to patients who indeed have metastasis in these nodes. Radiotherapy can be avoided in patients who have no drainage to these nodes.

REFERENCES

1. Rutgers EJTh, Jansen L, Nieweg OE, De Vries J, Schraffordt Koops H, Kroon BBR. Technique of sentinel node biopsy in breast cancer. Eur J Surg Oncol 1998; 24:316–319.
2. Glass EC, Haigh PI, Hansen N, Edwards GK, Giuliano AE. Improved identification of axillary sentinel nodes using modified anterior oblique views for lymphoscintigraphy of the breast (abstr). J Nucl Med 1999: 40(Suppl):251P.
3. Valdés Olmos RA, Hoefnage CA, Nieweg OE, Jansen L, Rutgers EJTH, Borger J, Horenblas S, Kroon BBR. Lymphoscintigraphy in oncology: a rediscovered challenge. J Eur Nucl Med 1999; 26(Suppl):S2–S10.

Case 3: Blue Duct Accidentally Divided

A 47-year-old woman noticed a lump in the right breast. Her surgeon observed a skin retraction in the lower inner quadrant and confirmed an underlying suspicious-feeling mass with a 2.5-cm diameter. There was no lymphadenopathy. Ultrasound revealed a spiculated lesion that was classified as malignant. Fine-needle aspiration was performed and showed adenocarcinoma cells. The patient was scheduled for wide local excision and sentinel node biopsy as part of her breast-conserving treatment.

Lymphoscintigraphy

A dose of 97.2 MBq (2.6 mCi) ^{99m}Tc-nanocolloid in a volume of 0.2 mL was injected into the primary breast cancer. The early images showed one lymphatic vessel running to one sentinel node in the right axilla. Later, a second-tier node and a third-tier node became visible as well (Fig. 22). The location of the sentinel node was indicated on the skin with indelible ink.

Surgery

The operation was performed the next morning with the aid of patent blue dye and a gamma-ray detection probe. Patent blue dye (1 mL) was administered divided over four quadrants of the breast cancer. The area around the tumor was

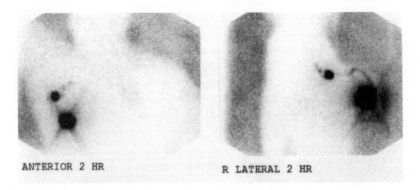

ANTERIOR 2 HR   R LATERAL 2 HR

FIGURE 22   The images obtained at 2 hours after ^{99m}Tc-nanocolloid administration depict the lymphatic vessel, the sentinel node, and second- and third-tier nodes.

massaged for 5 minutes. Twenty minutes after injection of the tracer, a 5-cm incision was made behind the lateral margin of the pectoralis major muscle, curving toward the lower hair line. A blue lymphatic duct was observed, however, it was accidentally divided during the dissection. The remaining stretch of the duct quickly lost its color and could not be traced any further.

Fortunately, the node could be located with the probe. The dissection was continued on in the direction that the probe indicated. The probe was inserted one more time before the node was reached. It was an elongated node that measured $1 \times 1 \times 2$ cm. It was not blue, and it looked and felt normal. The node was collected and submitted for frozen-section analysis. The wound was scanned for additional hot nodes. No other nodes were found, with the exception of second-tier nodes that were left undisturbed. Because a cluster of tumor cells was discovered at frozen-section microscopy, axillary node dissection was performed in addition to wide local excision of the primary lesion.

Pathology and Follow-Up

The definitive pathology slides confirmed the presence of tumor cells in the sentinel node. Ten lymph nodes were recovered from the axillary node dissection specimen. All were free of disease by H&E and immunohistochemistry staining (CAM 5.2). The primary tumor measured 2.1 cm, and it was removed with clear margins. Radiotherapy was administered to the breast. Adjuvant systemic chemotherapy was given as well.

Discussion

Lymphatic mapping requires a very subtle surgical technique [1]. Lymphatic vessels are very fragile and are easily damaged. Once a lymphatic vessel is accidentally divided, the supply of blue dye stops. The remaining stretch quickly loses its color and cannot be traced any further. One needs a considerable amount of luck to find a blue node in the axilla without the lymphatic duct pointing the way. As a rule, the probe will save the day.

It is difficult to say what the best technique is to expose the lymphatic vessel. Some surgeons like to do this with a small blade, others with fine-pointed scissors. There are surgeons who use more robust instruments and spread the overlying tissue so that their assistant can divide it. The electrocautery device can also be used to dissect the lymph vessel. This device provides less "feeling" but has the advantage that it seals the blood vessels. It is of paramount importance to keep the operative field dry because a small amount of blood may obscure a lymphatic vessel that contains just a small amount of dye.

A laparoscope camera can be used to record the operation so that the surgeon can evaluate what went right and wrong.

REFERENCE

1. Rutgers EJTh, Jansen L, Nieweg OE, De Vries J, Schraffordt Koops H, Kroon BBR. Technique of sentinel node biopsy in breast cancer. Eur J Surg Oncol 1998; 24:316–319.

Case 4: Not Every Sentinel Node Is Radioactive

Screening mammography in a 56-year-old woman showed a radiographically malignant lesion in the upper outer quadrant of the right breast. The patient had never noticed an abnormality in her breasts. Physical examination revealed a mobile, firm, 1.5-cm lesion with an irregular surface. Fine-needle aspiration yielded ductal epithelial cells with polymorphic nuclei, consistent with adenocarcinoma. The patient opted for breast-conserving treatment with wide local excision, axillary node dissection, and radiotherapy. She consented to sentinel node biopsy in a learning phase study.

Lymphoscintigraphy

A dose of 53.7 MBq (1.5 mCi) ^{99m}Tc-nanocolloid in a volume of 0.23 mL was injected into the breast cancer. Anterior and lateral lymphoscintigraphy was performed 2 hours after injection and showed no drainage. A repeat study 6 hours after injection showed a similar result (Fig. 23).

Surgery

The operation was performed the next morning. One milliliter of patent blue dye divided over three doses was administered into the tumor. A 4-cm incision along

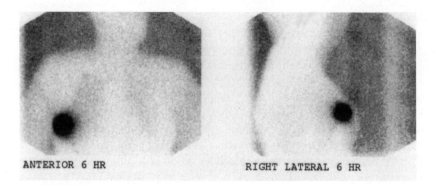

ANTERIOR 6 HR   RIGHT LATERAL 6 HR

FIGURE 23 Anterior and lateral view at 6 hours after injection depict the tumor in the right breast but no lymph node.

the lateral margin of the right pectoralis major muscle was made 3 minutes after administration of the blue dye. A blue lymphatic duct was quickly identified, and the sentinel node was retrieved 6 minutes after the incision was made. The node was evaluated with the gamma-ray detection probe, but no radioactivity was found. After removal of the node, the axilla was scanned for radioactive nodes, but none was found. The operation was continued with wide local excision of the primary tumor and a confirmation level I-II axillary node dissection.

Pathology and Follow-Up

The sentinel node was step-sectioned and examined with H&E and immunohisto-chemistry (CAM 5.2). Both techniques showed a tumor deposit. One of the four-teen nodes in the axillary dissection specimen was also found to be involved. The primary lesion measured 1.6 cm, contained estrogen receptors, and was sur-rounded by clear margins. Radiotherapy was administered, and tamoxifen was prescribed. The patient was free of disease 2 years later.

Discussion

It is not uncommon that no sentinel node is visualized on lymphoscintigraphy. Eleven studies have been published describing results from 739 lymphoscinti-grams. These studies show that a sentinel node is visualized in 75% to 98% of the patients [1]. At The Netherlands Cancer Institute, a sentinel node was visual-ized in 65% of the first series of patients and in 94% in the most recent series of patients. One often hears about a learning phase for the surgeons. Apparently, there is a learning phase for nuclear medicine physicians as well. One of the things that has been learned is that massaging the injection site encourages the flow of the tracer.

Another parameter that may influence lymph drainage is the age of the patient. Apparently, the radioactive tracer travels better in younger patients. Four investigators recently described this finding [2–5].

This particular patient is not a rare case. The blue-dye technique did result in successful identification of the sentinel node in eight of 18 patients in whom the node had not been visualized on the scintigraphy images. In conclusion, it is worthwhile to explore the axilla when no increased uptake is observed on the scans because not every sentinel node is radioactive.

REFERENCES

1. Nieweg OE, Jansen L, Valdés Olmos RA, Rutgers EJTh, Peterse JL, Hoefnage CA, Kroon BBR. Lymphatic mapping and sentinel lymph node biopsy in breast cancer. Eur J Nucl Med 1999; 26(Suppl):S11–S16.
2. Krag D, Weaver D, Ashikaga T, Moffat F, Klimberg VS, Shriven C, Feldman S, Kusminsky R, Gadd M, Kuhn J, Harlow S, Beitsch P. The sentinel node in breast cancer: a multicenter validation study. N Engl J Med 1998; 339:941–946.
3. Makar A, Melis K, van de Weyngaert D, Van Leuven L, Declerco S, Joosens E, Denis L, Kockx M. Identification ratio of the sentinel node in patients with primary breast cancer: a pathological correlation (abstr). Eur J Nucl Med 1999; 26(Suppl):S55.
4. Bourgeois P, Früling J. Aging, lateralisation and lymphoscintigraphy (abstr). Eur J Nucl Med 1999; 26(Suppl):S86.
5. Motomura K, Komoike Y, Inaji H, Koyama H, Kasugai T, Nagumo S. Sentinel node biopsy guided by indocyanin green dye in breast cancer patients (abstr). Eur J Nucl Med 1999; 26(Suppl):S95.

Case 5: Not Every Sentinel Node Is Blue

A 51-year-old woman was referred by her family physician after she had discovered a lump in her left breast. Her surgeon noticed retraction of the skin in the lower outer quadrant of the breast and felt a firm nodule with an irregular surface. The nodule was freely mobile but clearly suspicious of cancer. The radiologist who read the mammograms classified the lesion as malignant. Fine-needle aspiration confirmed the malignant nature of the lesion: adenocarcinoma. The patient preferred mastectomy over breast-conserving surgery. A sentinel node biopsy was planned as part of the procedure.

Lymphoscintigraphy

A dose of 60.4 MBq (1.6 mCi) ^{99m}Tc-nanocolloid in a volume of 0.20 mL was injected into the primary breast cancer. The early images showed no drainage. Later, two radioactive nodes became visible, but lymphatic vessel visualization

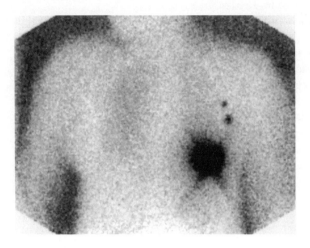

FIGURE 24 Images obtained 4 hours after scintigraphy show two radioactive nodes in the left axilla. Because the order of drainage could not be determined, both nodes are potential sentinel nodes.

was absent (Fig. 24). Because the order of drainage could not be determined, the nuclear medicine physician recommended excision of both nodes. The nodes were marked on the skin.

Surgery

The operation was performed the next morning. The surgeon administered 1.0 mL of vital dye into the breast lesion. The lateral-inferior part of the mastectomy incision was made, and the axilla was entered at the lateral margin of the pectoralis major muscle. At this point, a blue-stained lymphatic duct was identified. The duct was carefully dissected to a blue lymph node. The node was examined with the gamma-ray detection probe. The count rate was 52 counts per second versus a count rate of 18 counts per second for the surrounding normal tissue.

After the node was removed, another lymph node became visible adjacent to where the first node had been situated. This second node was not blue. It was examined with the probe, and a count rate of 42 counts per second was found. This node was removed as sentinel node #2.

The wound was explored for additional blue lymph vessels, but none was found. Subsequently, the wound was explored with the probe, and an increased count rate was found somewhat more cranially. Guided by the probe, a third lymph node was pursued. Like the second sentinel node, this node was radioactive (49 counts per second) but not blue. The node was removed and labeled sentinel node #3. No additional hot or blue nodes were found. A modified radical mastectomy was performed, including Berg level I and II.

Pathology and Follow-Up

The three sentinel nodes were examined with H&E and immunohistochemistry staining. The blue sentinel node #1 was free of disease, whereas sentinel nodes #2 and #3 were both tumor-positive. Nineteen lymph nodes were recovered from the mastectomy specimen. All were examined with H&E and immunohistochemistry, but none was involved with metastatic disease.

The primary tumor was a poorly differentiated invasive ductal carcinoma with a maximum diameter of 1.8 cm and 18 mitoses per 10 high-power fields. Estrogen receptors and progesterone receptors were present. Adjuvant systemic chemotherapy was administered, followed by tamoxifen. One year later, there was no evidence of disease.

Discussion

Cox et al. [1] performed a study in 466 patients with breast cancer and used both ^{99m}Tc sulfur colloid and a vital dye. They found that the sentinel node is both blue and radioactive in 28% of the cases. It is only blue in 32% of the cases and only radioactive in 40% of the cases. A similar study by De Vries et al. [2] using ^{99m}Tc-nanocolloid showed that the sentinel node is both blue and radioactive in 57% of the patients, just blue in 15%, and just radioactive in 28%. These findings indicate that a surgeon needs to have both the blue-dye technique and the probe technique in the repertoire. Without the latter, the surgeon of the patient described here would have missed the two sentinel nodes with metastatic disease.

Some investigators advocate intradermal injection of the dye. It is true that injecting the dye into the overlying skin may visualize a lymphatic vessel and a lymph node more frequently because drainage from the skin is richer than drainage from breast parenchyma. However, injecting the tracer away from the tumor carries the risk that a lymphatic watershed is crossed and that a node is visualized that drains another area of the breast and not the area with the tumor. A finding that supports this train of thought is that drainage to internal mammary lymph nodes is very rarely observed when a tracer is injected intradermally, whereas it is fairly common when the tracer is injected in the parenchyma [3].

REFERENCES

1. Cox CE, Pendas S, Cox JM, Joseph E, Shons AR, Yeatman T, Ku NN, Lyman GH, Berman C, Haddad F, Reintgen DS. Guidelines for sentinel node biopsy and lymphatic mapping of patients with breast cancer. Ann Surg 1998; 226:645–653.
2. de Vries J, Doting MHE, Jansen L, Hoefnagel CA, Valdés Olmos RA, Rutgers EJTh, Kroon BBR, Schraffordt Koops H, Piers DA, Tiebosch ATMG, Nieweg OE. Sentinel

node localisation in breast cancer in two institutions (abstr). Eur J Nucl Med 1999; 26(Suppl):S67.

3. Uren RF, Howman-Giles RB, Thompson JF, Malouf D, Ramsey-Stewart G, Niesche FW, Renwick SB. Mammary lymphoscintigraphy in breast cancer. J Nucl Med 1995; 36:1775–1780.

Case 6: False-Negative Frozen-Section Microscopy

A 57-year-old woman was referred to her physician after a mass was discovered in the left breast. The surgeon noticed a 1.5-cm mass in the upper outer quadrant of the breast. The lesion was classified as malignant on the mammograms. Fine-needle aspiration results were tumor-positive. The axillary lymph nodes were not enlarged. The patient and her surgeon discussed the treatment options and chose wide local excision and sentinel node biopsy.

Lymphoscintigraphy

A total of 67.8 MBq (1.8 mCi) ^{99m}Tc-nanocolloid in a volume of 0.22 mL was injected into the lesion on the day before surgery. The images showed one sentinel node in the left axilla and a few second-tier nodes higher up (Fig. 25). The location of the node was marked on the skin with indelible ink.

Surgery

The operation was performed the next morning with the aid of patent blue dye and a gamma-ray detection probe. Patent blue dye (1 mL) was administered into the breast cancer at the beginning of the operation. A 4-cm incision was made behind the lateral margin of the major pectoralis muscle. A blue lymphatic vessel

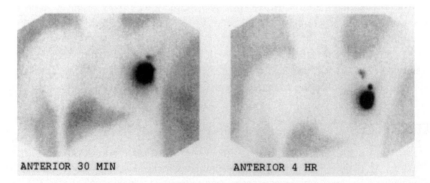

ANTERIOR 30 MIN   ANTERIOR 4 HR

Figure 25   Lymphoscintigraphy shows one sentinel node after 30 minutes. After 4 hours, several faint second-tier nodes are observed as well.

was observed once the axilla was entered, and it was traced to a lymph node at level I. The gamma-ray detection probe confirmed that the node was radioactive. The node measured 1.2 cm and looked and felt normal.

The node was collected and sent to the pathologist for frozen-section analysis. Meanwhile, the axilla was explored, but no additional blue ducts were encountered. The second-tier nodes were identified higher up in the axilla but were not removed. After wide local excision of the primary cancer was performed, the result of the frozen-section microscopy was available: no tumor cells. As a result, no completion axillary node dissection was performed.

Pathology and Follow-Up

The primary tumor was a 1.5-cm invasive ductal carcinoma with both estrogen and progesterone receptors. The tumor was well away from the resection margins. Despite the fact that frozen-section microscopy did not show tumor involvement, immunohistochemistry staining (CAM 5.2) did show a tumor embolus in the marginal sinus of the sentinel lymph node. All possible scenarios had been reviewed with the patient before the operation. The possibility of a false-negative frozen-section result had also been discussed. Nevertheless, she was very upset when the final pathology of the sentinel node was conveyed. Later, she understood and agreed to undergo radiotherapy of the axilla. In this case of minimal dissemination, the multidisciplinary team that treated her was of the opinion that radiotherapy was a safe option. Adjuvant therapy with tamoxifen was also instituted.

Discussion

Frozen-section analysis is, of course, less sensitive than detailed pathology examination that includes step-sectioning and H&E and immunohistochemistry staining. The reliability of intraoperative pathology analysis has been the subject of a number of recent studies. Two investigators presented their results on frozen-sectioning examination in breast cancer and reported a sensitivity of 77% and 87%, respectively [1,2]. At The Netherlands Cancer Institute, the sensitivity is even worse: 70%. The sensitivity of touch imprint cytology seems to be similar: 63% to 86% [1,3,4]. Combining the two techniques does not improve the sensitivity: 77% [5]. The reliability of frozen-section microscopy is even worse in melanoma compared with breast cancer. Several investigators found a sensitivity of approximately 50% [6,7]. Touch imprint cytology is somewhat more sensitive (74%) but still not good enough [8]. A false-negative result is difficult to explain to a patient. Patients experience a false-negative frozen section result as extremely distressing, although that possibility has, of course, been raised ahead of time. The advantage of frozen-section analysis has to be balanced against this disadvantage and against the fact that extra operating room time needs to be reserved (which is not used in >50% of cases).

REFERENCES

1. Van Diest PJ, Torrenga H, Borgstein PJ, Pijpers R, Bleichrodt RP, Rahuser FD, Meijer S. Reliability of intra-operative frozen sections and imprints of sentinel lymph nodes in breast cancer (abstr). Eur J Nucl Med 1999; 26(Suppl):S55.
2. Mayzler O, Goldstein J, Koretz M. Is frozen section examination (FSE) of the sentinel lymph node (SLN) a reliable predictor of histologic status (abstr)? Eur J Nucl Med 1999; 26(Suppl):S56.
3. Keshtgar MRS, Kocjan G, Lakhani SR, Ell PJ. Imprint cytology in sentinel node biopsy in breast cancer: is it reliable (abstr)? Eur J Nucl Med 1999; 26(Suppl):S16.
4. Ku N, Cox C, Reintger D, Smith P, Nicosia S. Role of intraoperative imprint cytology on sentinel nodes in breast cancer (abstr). Eur J Nucl Med 1999; 26(Suppl):S16.
5. Noguchi M, Tsugawa K, Bando E, Miwa K, Yokoyama K, Nakajima K, Michigishi T, Tonami N, Minato H, Nonomura A. Intraoperative examination of sentinel lymph nodes in breast cancer (abstr). Eur J Nucl Med 1999; 26(Suppl):S97.
6. Schraffordt Koops H, Nieweg OE, Tiebosch ATMG, Piers DA, Hoekstra HJ, Kapteijn BAE, Peterse JL, Kroon BBR. Is intra-operative evaluation of frozen sections a reliable method for sentinel nodes in malignant melanoma (abstr)? Melanoma Res 1997; 7(Suppl):S106.
7. Clary BM, Lewis JJ, Brady MS, Busam K, Coit DG. Should frozen section analysis of the sentinel node be performed in patients with melanoma (abstr)? Eur J Nucl Med 1999; 26(Suppl):S68.
8. Messina JL, Ku N, Reintgen DS. Role of touch imprint cytology in pathologic evaluation of sentinel lymph nodes in malignant melanoma (abstr). Eur J Nucl Med 1999; 26(Suppl):S67.

Case 7: False-Negative Sentinel Node Biopsy, Learning Phase

A 43-year-old woman discovered a lump in her left breast at self-examination. At the clinic, her surgeons felt a 2-cm firm lump with an irregular surface in the lower outer quadrant of the left breast. No lymphadenopathy was noted. Mammography and ultrasound were suggestive of carcinoma. Fine-needle aspiration confirmed the presence of adenocarcinoma.

Lymphoscintigraphy

A total of 88 MBq (2.4 mCi) ^{99m}Tc-nanocolloid in a volume of 0.3 mL was injected into the lesion at 8.58 AM on the day before surgery. The images obtained after 4 hours show one hot spot in the left axilla (Fig. 26). The location of the node was marked on the skin with indelible ink.

Surgery

The operation was scheduled for the next morning. However, a conflicting schedule forced the surgeon to postpone the sentinel node exploration until late in the

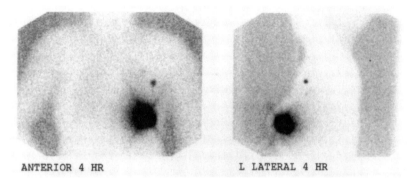

ANTERIOR 4 HR   L LATERAL 4 HR

FIGURE 26 The late anterior and lateral view show one radioactive node in the left axilla 4 hours after administration of the tracer.

afternoon. A volume of 1.0 mL of patent blue dye divided over five portions, was administered into the lesion in the left breast. A 4-cm incision was made along the lower hair line of the left axilla. A blue lymphatic vessel was observed once the axillary fat was reached and dissected. The blue node was identified 6 minutes after the incision was made. The gamma detection probe measurements showed slight uptake in the node: 17 counts per second. The surrounding normal tissue measured eight counts per second. This count rate was substantially lower than expected for the sentinel node. The existence of a second sentinel node was considered, and the search was continued. However, no other blue ducts or nodes with an increased level of radioactivity were found.

The single sentinel node was submitted for pathological evaluation. This case was one of this surgeon's early cases, and a completing axillary node dissection was performed in addition to the wide local excision of the primary tumor.

Pathology and Follow-Up

Pathology evaluation included H&E and immunohistochemistry staining (CAM 5.2). No tumor cells were found in the sentinel node. The axillary node dissection specimen contained 20 nodes. Metastatic disease was found in five of these nodes. The primary tumor was a 1.7-cm invasive ductal carcinoma. The tumor was well away from the resection margins. The breast was treated with radiotherapy. Adjuvant systemic chemotherapy was instituted, followed by tamoxifen. One year later the patient was faring well.

Discussion

At The Netherlands Cancer Institute, we have had two false-negative sentinel node biopsy results in a learning phase of 127 patients with breast cancer (sensitivity, 96%) [1]. The potential reasons for a false-negative sentinel node biopsy result are discussed in melanoma case 12. The most likely explanation for the false-negative results in this patient is the fact that not enough radioactivity was present in the sentinel node for it to be identified with the probe. The dose that was administered was reasonable for detection with a gamma probe within 24 hours, but a considerable longer time lapse was present in this case [2]. The half-life of ^{99m}Tc is 6 hours, which means that every 6 hours the amount of radioactivity decreases by 50%.

Five half-lives passed before this patient was taken to the operating room, which means that some 3% remained of the amount of radioactivity that was originally administered. Most of that was still at the site of injection. Only a small percentage of the tracer ends up in the node. Because of these facts, the probe readings were not very helpful. A reading of eight counts per second in the background tissue and 17 counts per second in a node does not allow reliable measurements. Excision of the primary tumor with the bulk of radioactivity might have given the surgeon a somewhat better chance by removing the background radioactivity that was generated by the injection site. But a count rate in the order of 17 counts per second in a lymph node is still hardly enough for gamma probe detection.

This case led to a few changes in the protocol. Lymphoscintigraphy is performed later in the morning, and a sentinel node operation is now always performed as the first case of the day. When in doubt about the identification of the sentinel node, there is a low threshold to convert the operation to an axillary node dissection, and the patient is informed of this policy before the operation.

This false-negative sentinel node biopsy result happened during the surgeon's learning phase, and an axillary node dissection was performed. Therefore, no harm was done. How long should a surgeon's learning phase be [3–6]? Estimates run from nine to 100 cases, depending on which expert is being asked. A number of factors play a role: the (statistical) end point to be achieved, prior training (teaching course), guidance by an expert, patient population, expertise in the Department of Nuclear Medicine, expertise in the Department of Pathology, dexterity, etc.

REFERENCES

1. de Vries J, Doting MHE, Jansen L, Hoefnage CA, Valdés Olmos RA, Rutgers EJTh, Kroon BBR, Schraffordt Koops H, Piers DA, Tiebosch ATMG, Nieweg OE. Sentinel node localisation in breast cancer in two institutions (abstr). Eur J Nucl Med 1999; 26(Suppl):S67.
2. Thompson JF, Niewind P, Uren RF, Bosch CM, Howman-Giles R, Vrouenraets BC. Single-dose isotope injection for both preoperative lymphoscintigraphy and intraoperative sentinel lymph node identification in melanoma patients. Melanoma Res 1997; 7:500–506.

3. Cody HS, 3rd, Hill AD, Tran KN, Brennan MF, Borgen PI. Credentialing for breast lymphatic mapping: how many cases are enough? Ann Surg 1999; 229:723–726.
4. Morton DL, Giuliano AE, Reintgen DS, Roses DF, Ross MI, Thompson JF. Lymphatic mapping and sentinel node biopsy in patients with breast cancer and melanoma (2). Contemp Surg 1998; 53:281–298.
5. Giuliano AE. See one, do twenty-five, teach one: the implementation of sentinel node dissection in breast cancer. Ann Surg Oncol 1999; 6:520–521.
6. Cox CE, Bass SS, Boulware D, Ku NK, Berman C, Reintgen DS. Implementation of new surgical technology: outcome measures for lymphatic mapping of breast carcinoma. Ann Surg Oncol 1999; 6:553–561.

Case 8: Lymphoscintigraphy Provides a Road Map for the Surgeon

A 79-year-old patient had been treated for a right breast cancer 8 years previously. At a routine follow-up visit, the surgeon noticed a 1.5-cm lump in the upper outer quadrant of the left breast. Mammography showed a possibly malignant lesion that had not been present in earlier studies. Fine-needle aspiration confirmed that the lesion was malignant. A modified radical mastectomy was planned. The patient consented to sentinel node biopsy before modified radical mastectomy.

Lymphoscintigraphy

A dose of 51 MBq (1.4 mCi) ^{99m}Tc-nanocolloid in a volume of 0.20 mL was administered into the breast lesion. The late anterior image (4 hours after injection) showed one faint hot spot in the right subclavicular area (Fig. 27). No other not spots were observed. The location was marked on the skin with indelible ink.

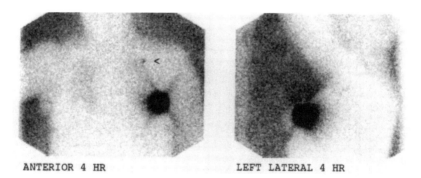

ANTERIOR 4 HR   LEFT LATERAL 4 HR

FIGURE 27 Anterior and lateral lymphoscintigraphy images obtained 4 hours after administration of the tracer. Faint uptake is observed at the infraclavicular level (arrow head). There is no increased uptake in the axilla.

Surgery

The operation was performed the next day. The gamma detection probe could not locate the sentinel node through the intact skin. One milliliter of patent blue dye was administered into the lesion before preparing and draping the left breast. The cranial flap for the mastectomy was partially raised, and the pectoralis major muscle fibers were split to get to level III of the axilla. No blue duct was observed in this area. After massaging the breast tissue from the tumor in the direction of the subclavicular fossa, a tiny lymphatic vessel stained blue. This vessel was traced to a lymph node that was barely 2 mm in diameter. The gamma-ray detection node demonstrated a modestly increased count rate over the node. The node was removed from the operative field and submitted for pathological evaluation before the modified radical mastectomy was completed.

Pathology and Follow-Up

The sentinel node was shown to contain a small cluster of tumor cells in the marginal sinus. The 18 nodes recovered from the mastectomy specimen were examined with immunohistochemistry and proved to be free of disease. The primary tumor measured 2.2 cm and was removed with adequate margins. Hormone receptors were demonstrated, and tamoxifen was prescribed. Two years later, the patient was clinically disease-free.

Discussion

Metastasis at level III is rare without involvement of the lower levels of the axilla. Several studies showed an incidence of 0.4% to 3% in breast cancer patients [1–4]. For some time, the term "skip" metastasis has been used to describe such isolated metastases at level III. These were thought to result from tumor cells that passed through level I and II nodes to finally lodge at level III. However, lymphoscintigraphy demonstrated direct drainage to level III twice in a series of 113 patients with breast cancer [5]. Drainage to supraclavicular nodes was observed in 20% of upper quadrant lesions [6]. With our current knowledge of lymphoscintigraphy, we can assume that these "skip" metastases are the result of direct drainage to level III nodes.

This case demonstrates the value of preoperative lymphoscintigraphy. Without lymphoscintigraphy, the sentinel node in this patient would not have been found because the blue duct was not visible from the incision in the axilla, and the small amount of radioactivity in the node prevented its detection with the gamma-ray detection probe before the incision was made. The direct approach through the pectoralis major muscle provides better exposure of level III of the axilla than the approach through the lower axilla.

REFERENCES

1. Rosen PP, Lesser ML, Kinne DW, Beattie EJ. Discontinuous or ''skip'' metastases in breast carcinoma: analysis of 1228 axillary dissections. Ann Surg 1983; 197:276–283.
2. Danforth DN Jr, Findlay PA, McDonald HD, Lippman ME, Reichert CM, d'Angelo T, Gorrell CR, Gerber NL, Lichter AS, Rosenberg SA, deMoss ES. Complete axillary lymph node dissection for stage I-II carcinoma of the breast. J Clin Oncol 1986; 4: 655–662.
3. Boova RS, Bonanni R, Rosato FE. Patterns of axillary nodal involvement in breast cancer: predictability of level one dissection. Ann Surg 1982; 196:642–644.
4. Veronesi U, Rilke F, Luini A, Sacchini V, Galimberti V, Campa T, Dei Bei E, Greco M, Magni A, Merson M, Quagliuolo V. Distribution of axillary node metastases by level of invasion. An analysis of 539 cases. Cancer 1987; 59:682–687.
5. Jansen L, Nieweg OE, de Vries J, Valdés Olmos RA, Jager PL, Doting MHE, Piers DA, Rutgers EJTh, Hoefnagel CA, Kroon BBR. Lymphoscintigraphy to identify unusual locations of sentinel lymph nodes in patients with breast cancer (abstr). J Nucl Med 1999; 40(suppl):70.
6. Uren RF, Howman-Giles RB, Thompson JF, Malouf D, Ramsey-Stewart G, Niesche FW, Renwick SB. Mammary lymphoscintigraphy in breast cancer. J Nucl Med 1995; 36:1775–1780.

Case 9: Sentinel Node in the Internal Mammary Chain

A 39-year-old woman noticed retraction of the nipple of the left breast. She had no history of breast disease and was otherwise healthy. Her physician felt a firm nodule in the upper inner quadrant of the breast. The lesion was not fixed to skin or muscle, had an irregular surface, and measured 3 × 4 cm. There were no enlarged lymph nodes in the left axilla. Mammography suggested a malignancy, and fine-needle aspiration cytology revealed well differentiated tubular adenocarcinoma. The treatment options were discussed with the patient, and she opted for simple mastectomy with sentinel node biopsy.

Lymphoscintigraphy

A dose of 72.2 MBq (2.0 mCi) ^{99m}Tc-nanocolloid in a volume of 0.30 mL was injected into the breast tumor on the day before the operation. The images showed two overlapping hot spots in the axilla (Fig. 28). There was also one sentinel node in the left internal mammary chain with several second-tier nodes.

Surgery

The operation was performed the next day. Patent blue dye (1 mL) was administered into the tumor in the left breast. A 4-cm incision was made along the lateral

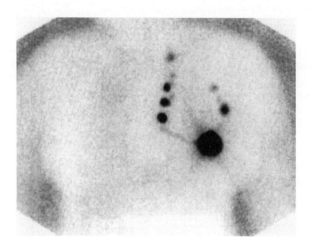

FIGURE 28   The late anterior view shows one hot spot in the right axilla and another that is less bright. A sentinel node and several second-tier nodes are depicted in the ipsilateral internal mammary node chain.

mammary fold so that it could be encompassed in the mastectomy incision. Two blue lymphatic ducts were observed coming from the breast and leading to two adjacent axillary nodes. The probe confirmed that both nodes were radioactive. The nodes were removed and submitted for frozen-section analysis.

Subsequently, the probe was used to find the location of the internal mammary sentinel node. It was identified in the third intercostal space. The upper medial part of the mastectomy incision was made, and a flap was raised. A blue lymph vessel was identified and followed in a medial direction until it disappeared between the pectoralis muscle fibers toward the fourth intercostal space. The muscle fibers were split in a transverse direction, and the intercostal muscles were freed from the fifth rib. The blue duct was observed passing underneath the fourth rib without entering a lymph node. Next, the third intercostal space was opened. A branch from the internal mammary artery caused troublesome bleeding and was clipped. On top of the pleura, a blue lymph node was observed with a diameter of just 3 mm. The node was removed from the underlying pleura after the probe showed it to be radioactive. The nodes higher up the chain were not removed.

Frozen-section examination showed that one of the axillary sentinel nodes contained metastatic disease. The operation was continued with a modified radical mastectomy, including level I, II, and some level III nodes.

Pathology and Follow-Up

H&E and immunohistochemistry staining revealed a 1-cm metastasis in each axillary sentinel node. The internal mammary sentinel node contained a 1-mm micrometastasis. The mastectomy specimen contained 16 lymph nodes, one of which contained a micrometastasis. The primary tumor measured 1.7 cm and was removed with clear margins. The tumor was both estrogen and progesterone receptor–positive. Radiotherapy was administered to the left internal mammary node chain and the left chest wall. Adjuvant chemotherapy was also given, and thereafter tamoxifen.

Discussion

Drainage to internal mammary lymph nodes is reported in up to 38% of patients with breast cancer [1–5]. Dissemination to these nodes is common: approximately 30% in patients with primary operable breast cancer [6,7]. Most of these patients have drainage to both the axilla and the internal mammary chain. Urban found metastases limited to the internal mammary chain in only 4% of the patients in whom they performed radical extended mastectomy in the 1950s [7]. Cody described Urban's last series of patients and found that 11% had metastases in the internal mammary nodes only and not in the axilla [7].

Whether the internal mammary chain nodes should be treated locally and, if so, how they should be treated is a subject of long-standing controversy. Excision and radiotherapy have not convincingly been shown to improve the survival rate when routinely applied [8–10]. A limited survival benefit was observed in patients with axillary metastasis and a medial or central location of the primary cancer [7,11]. This is understandable because these patients have the greatest incidence of tumor-positive nodes in the internal mammary chain. Treatment of these nodes could theoretically serve to prevent a locoregional recurrence, but that is a rare event [12]. Should a sentinel node in the internal mammary chain be pursued? The potential benefit of biopsy of sentinel nodes in the internal mammary chain is that it may be a more sensitive tool to select patients for adjuvant radiotherapy than tumor location or axillary lymph node status. Positive internal mammary nodes are an indication for systemic therapy [13]. The internal mammary node status is indeed an important prognostic factor for the presence of distant metastases [7,11].

On the other hand, retrieval of an internal mammary chain node is difficult, and the survival benefit of adjuvant regional or systemic treatment in this situation is probably small. If one decides to perform a biopsy of sentinel nodes in the internal mammary node chain, the radiolabeled tracer should be injected deep in the breast because these nodes are rarely observed when the tracer is administered in the skin or in the subareolar lymphatic plexus.

Finding internal mammary sentinel nodes is technically challenging. The blue dye technique often cannot be used because the lymph vessel usually runs underneath the pectoralis major muscle and underneath the intercostal muscles. Identification with the probe is also difficult because of the proximity of the injection site; the cancer is usually located in a medial quadrant. Excision of the primary tumor will remove the bulk of the radioactive tracer, assuming that the tracer is administered in or immediately adjacent to the lesion in a small volume. Another problem is that the relatively large probe is difficult to manipulate in the narrow intercostal space. The node is sometimes not located in the intercostal space but behind a rib, where it is hidden from view. The sentinel node sits on top of the fragile pleura. When the pleura is accidentally damaged during the procedure, a vacuum drain is left in the thoracic cavity. The drain is removed the next day.

REFERENCES

1. Dixon JM, Dobie V, Chetty U. The importance of interpectoral nodes in breast cancer. Eur J Cancer 1993; 29A:334–336.
2. Lacour J, Lê MG, Hill C, Kramar A, Contesso G, Sarrazin D. Is it useful to remove internal mammary nodes in operable breast cancer? Eur J Surg Oncol 1987; 13:309–314.
3. Uren RF, Thompson JF, Howman-Giles RB. Patterns of lymphatic drainage in breast cancer. In: Lymphatic Drainage of the Skin and Breast: Locating the Sentinel Nodes. Uren RF, Thompson JF, Howman-Giles RB, eds. Amsterdam, the Netherlands: Harwood Academic Publishers, 1999, pp 147–158.
4. Jansen L, Nieweg OE, de Vries J, Valdés Olmos RA, Jager PL, Doting MHE, Piers DA, Rutgers EJTh, Hoefnagel CA, Kroon BBR. Lymphoscintigraphy to identify unusual locations of sentinel lymph nodes in patients with breast cancer (abstr). J Nucl Med 1999; 40(Suppl):70.
5. Byrd DR, Dunnwald LK, Mankoff DA, Anderson BO, Moe RE, Yeung RS, Eary JF. Internal mammary lymph node drainage in sentinel node lymphoscintigraphy for breast cancer (abstr). J Nucl Med 1999; 40(Suppl):138P.
6. Urban JA, Baker HW. Radical mastectomy in continuity with en bloc resection of the internal mammary lymph-node chain: a new procedure for primary operable cancer of the breast. Cancer 1952; 5:992–1008.
7. Cody HS 3rd, Urban JA. Internal mammary node status: a major prognosticator in axillary node-negative breast cancer. Ann Surg Oncol 1995; 2:32–37.
8. Lacour J, Lê MG, Hill C, Kramar A, Contesso G, Sarrazin D. Is it useful to remove internal mammary nodes in operable breast cancer? Eur J Surg Oncol 1987; 13:309–314.
9. Lacour J, Lê MG, Caceres E, Koszarowski T, Veronesi U, Hill C. Radical mastectomy versus radical mastectomy plus internal mammary dissection: ten year results of an international cooperative trial in breast cancer. Cancer 1983; 51:1941–1943.
10. Arriagada R, Lê MG, Mouriesse H, Fontaine F, Dewar J, Rochard F, Spielmann

M, Lacour J, Tubiana M, Sarrazin D. Long-term effect of internal mammary chain treatment: results of a multivariate analysis of 1195 patients with operable breast cancer and positive axillary nodes. Radiother Oncol 1988; 11:213–222.

11.   Urban JA. Management of operable breast cancer: the surgeon's view. Cancer 1978; 42:2066–2077.

12.   Recht A, Pierce SM, Abner A, Vicini F, Osteen RT, Love SM, Silver B, Harris JR. Regional nodal failure after conservative surgery and radiotherapy for early-stage breast carcinoma. J Clin Oncol 1991; 9:988–996.

13.   Donegan WL. The influence of untreated internal mammary metastases upon the course of mammary cancer. Cancer 1977; 39:533–538.

Case 10: Sentinel Node in the Contralateral Internal Mammary Node Chain, Immunohistochemistry

A 60-year-old woman was diagnosed with a 1-cm breast cancer in the upper outer quadrant of the right breast. Wide local excision and sentinel node biopsy were scheduled.

Lymphoscintigraphy

A dose of 88.4 MBq (2.4 mCi) ^{99m}Tc-nanocolloid in a volume of 0.31 mL was injected into the breast tumor on the day before the operation. The dynamic study obtained during 20 minutes after injection showed a lymphatic vessel running toward the right axilla and another vessel running in a medial direction. After 30 minutes, one sentinel node in the right axilla and another in the contralateral internal mammary node chain were visualized (Fig. 29). A second-tier node was later visualized in both fields. The location of the sentinel nodes was marked on the skin.

Surgery

The operation was performed the next day. One milliliter of patent blue dye was administered into the tumor in the right breast. A 4-cm incision was made along the lateral margin of the right pectoralis major muscle. A blue lymphatic duct was identified at the lateral margin of the underlying muscle and dissected until it was observed entering a blue lymph node. The probe confirmed that the node was radioactive. Frozen-section analysis revealed no tumor involvement.

Subsequently, a 5-cm transverse incision was made over the left parasternal skin mark. The pectoralis major muscle fibers were split, and the intercostal muscles were freed from the lower (fourth) rib. A 3-mm lymph node was observed underneath. The node was not blue. The node was removed from the underlying pleura after the probe showed it to be radioactive. Wide local excision of the primary tumor was performed with a 1-cm margin.

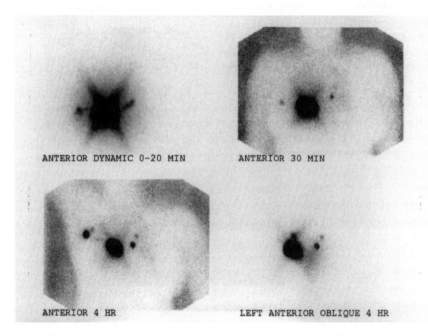

ANTERIOR DYNAMIC 0-20 MIN   ANTERIOR 30 MIN

ANTERIOR 4 HR   LEFT ANTERIOR OBLIQUE 4 HR

FIGURE 29 The dynamic anterior lymphoscintigraphy view obtained during the first 20 minutes shows lymphatic vessels running in a medial direction and in a lateral direction from the site of tracer administration. The images obtained after 30 minutes show a sentinel node in the right axilla and another in the contralateral internal mammary node chain. The late images also depict a second-tier node in each field. An additional left anterior oblique view was obtained to visualize the ipsilateral internal mammary node chain, but no other hot spots were observed.

Pathology and Follow-Up

Evaluation by the pathologist revealed a 0.8-cm, estrogen receptor–positive ductal breast cancer that had been removed with tumor-free margins. The axillary sentinel node was confirmed to be free of disease when examined with H&E and immunohistochemistry. H&E staining of the internal mammary node did not reveal tumor cells. However, metastatic disease was found when the node was examined with immunohistochemistry (CAM 5.2).

At the institution where this patient was treated, adjuvant systemic treatment is not given to a patient with a 0.8-cm tumor without lymph node involvement. Therefore, she received adjuvant systemic treatment with tamoxifen solely as a consequence of the removal of the contralateral internal mammary chain sentinel node. She was also referred to a radiotherapist for adjuvant radiotherapy to the internal mammary node chain, but the radiotherapist believed that this was not indicated.

Discussion

Lymph drainage from breast cancer across the midline is unusual. Occasionally, metastases are found in the contralateral axilla, but dissemination to the contralateral internal mammary node chain is rare. It was not observed by Uren et al. in a series of 92 patients [1].

Three recent studies describe internal mammary chain sentinel nodes [1–3]. The incidence in the Dutch study was 15%, the incidence in the U.S. study was remarkably similar: 18%. In the Australian series, the internal mammary drainage was observed in 34% of patients [1]. Direct drainage across the midline to the opposite internal mammary chain was not mentioned in these studies. Internal mammary nodes can be removed without additional morbidity [2].

Pathologists have several techniques to increase the sensitivity of sentinel node evaluation beyond that of routine H&E staining. Immunohistochemistry staining is widely available and improves the ability to detect metastatic disease by some 20%. Knowledge of the tumor status of a sentinel node in the internal mammary chain enhances the accuracy of staging. This case demonstrates that the pursuit of such a node may lead to the decision to treat a patient with adjuvant systemic treatment that would otherwise not have been given.

Although scientific evidence from clinical studies is lacking, it seems to make sense to treat a patient with a tumor-involved internal mammary node with adjuvant radiotherapy. Nodes higher up the parasternal chain may be involved as well. The decision of the radiotherapist not to treat this patient is therefore questionable. The tumor status of an internal mammary sentinel node has the potential to become the most important—if not only—indication for radiotherapy to this lymph node field in the future.

REFERENCES

1. Uren EF, Thompson JF, Howman-Giles RB. Patterns of lymphatic drainage in breast cancer. In: Lymphatic Drainage of the Skin and Breast: Locating the Sentinel Nodes. Uren RF, Thompson JF, Howman-Giles RB, eds. Amsterdam, the Netherlands: Harwood Academic Publishers, 1999, pp 147–158.
2. Jansen L, Nieweg OE, de Vries J, Valdés Olmos RA, Jager PL, Doting MHE, Piers DA, Rutgers EJTh, Hoefnagel CA, Kroon BBR, Lymphoscintigraphy to identify unusual locations of sentinel lymph nodes in patients with breast cancer (abstr). J Nucl Med 1999; 40(Suppl):70.
3. Byrd DR, Dunnwald LK, Mankoff DA, Anderson BO, Moe RE, Yeung RS, Eary JF. Internal mammary lymph node drainage in sentinel node lymphoscintigraphy for breast cancer (abstr). J Nucl Med 1999; 40(Suppl):138P.

Case 11: Sentinel Node in Interpectoral Fossa (Rotter's Sentinel Node)

A 50-year-old woman sought medical attention 4 weeks after discovering a lump in the left breast. Her surgeon noticed a 1.5-cm firm nodule in the upper inner quadrant. Physical examination was otherwise unremarkable. The radiologist reported seeing a malignant lesion on the mammograms and ultrasound. Fine-needle aspiration was performed and showed clusters of large atypical epithelial cells consistent with adenocarcinoma. The diagnosis and the various treatment options were discussed with the patient. She preferred simple mastectomy and sentinel node biopsy over breast-conserving treatment.

Lymphoscintigraphy

A dose of 95.1 MBq (2.6 mCi) ^{99m}Tc-nanocolloid in a volume of 0.2 mL was injected into the primary breast cancer. Dynamic (flow) images showed no drainage. Anterior and lateral static images were obtained after 30 minutes and after 4 hours and showed two nodes with tracer accumulation in the left axilla (Fig. 30). The order of drainage could not be determined.

Surgery

The operation was performed the next morning. One milliliter of patent blue dye was administered in three doses into the breast cancer. The breast was gently massaged. The lateral-inferior part of the mastectomy incision was made, and the axillary fat was exposed. A blue lymphatic vessel was observed and traced

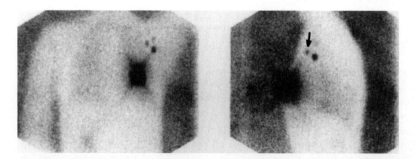

Figure 30 Anterior and lateral static views obtained 4 hours after ^{99m}Tc-nanocolloid administration show two radioactive nodes, one in the left axilla, the other between the pectoralis muscles (arrow). The latter node is located more ventrally than the average axillary sentinel node.

to a blue node. The gamma-ray detection probe showed that the count rate was 10 times as high as the count rate in the surrounding normal tissue. The node was collected. The other node could not be located, neither through visualizing a blue duct nor with the aid of the probe.

The surgeon decided to perform the simple mastectomy next and then—with the bulk of the radioactivity removed—try again to locate the other radioactive node. During the mastectomy, a blue lymphatic vessel was observed running in a lateral direction and disappearing between the pectoralis major muscle fibers.

The background count rate had decreased fourfold after mastectomy. That proved to be enough to trace the other sentinel node. It was located deep between the pectoralis major and pectoralis minor muscle. The blue lymphatic vessel was observed emerging from the pectoralis major muscle and entering the node. The node measured just 0.5 cm; it was both blue and radioactive. It was removed and sent to the pathology laboratory. No frozen-section microscopy was performed because it was too small. No axillary node dissection was performed.

Pathology

No tumor cells were found in either node with H&E and immunohistochemistry (CAM 5.2).

Discussion

In one series, a sentinel node between the pectoralis muscles was found in two of 113 patients with breast cancer [1], and in one of 92 patients with breast cancer in another series [2]. This location is difficult to determine beforehand examining the lymphoscintigraphy images. In retrospect, one of the hot nodes may be located somewhat more anteriorly than is usual on the lateral view.

The larger tracer volumes and the popularity of injection over greater areas of the breast may explain why Rotter's sentinel nodes are rarely described. They may be obscured by the radioactivity at the injection site. Something that is surprising in patients with a Rotter's sentinel node is how deeply the node is located in between the muscles. The lymphatic vessel reaches the node through the pectoralis major muscle.

It makes sense to pursue a Rotter's sentinel node because it may contain metastatic disease in the absence of an involved node in the axilla [3]. Most of the radioactivity stays behind at the injection site, and its scattered radiation may obscure a sentinel node with little accumulation of the tracer. Wide local excision or simple mastectomy will remove the troubling radioactivity and facilitate sentinel node retrieval, as this case demonstrates.

REFERENCES

1. Jansen L, Nieweg OE, de Vries J, Valdés Olmos RA, Jager PL, Doting MHE, Piers DA, Rutgers EJTh, Hoefnagel CA, Kroon BBR. Lymphoscintigraphy to identify unusual locations of sentinel lymph nodes in patients with breast cancer (abstr). J Nucl Med 1999; 40(Suppl):70.
2. Uren RF, Thompson JF, Howman-Giles RB. Patterns of lymphatic drainage in breast cancer. In: Lymphatic Drainage of the Skin and Breast: Locating the Sentinel Nodes. Uren RF, Thompson JF, Howman-Giles RB, eds. Amsterdam, the Netherlands: Harwood Academic Publishers, 1999, pp 147–158.
3. Jansen L, Nieweg OE, Valdés Olmos RA, Rutgers EJTh, Peterse JA, De Vries J, Doting MHE, Kroon BBR. Improved staging of breast cancer through lymphatic mapping and sentinel node biopsy. Eur J Surg Oncol 1998; 24:445–446.

Case 12: Sentinel Node in the Breast Parenchyma

A 49-year-old woman was diagnosed with a lump in the left breast at a routine check-up. Mammography was performed and demonstrated a 2-cm malignant-looking lesion in the lower outer quadrant with microcalcifications. Fine-needle aspiration revealed atypical epithelial cells with large polymorphic nuclei consistent with adenocarcinoma. The various treatment options were discussed with the patient, and she opted for simple mastectomy and sentinel node biopsy.

Lymphoscintigraphy

A dose of 81.1 MBq (2.2 mCi) ^{99m}Tc-nanocolloid in a volume of 0.2 mL was injected into the primary breast cancer. Dynamic (flow) images showed no drainage. Anterior and lateral static images were obtained and showed one sentinel node in the breast parenchyma and a hot node in the left axilla after 2 hours (Fig. 31). Whether the latter node was a first-tier node receiving drainage directly from the primary tumor or a second-tier node receiving drainage from the intraparenchymal node was unclear because the lymphatic vessels were not depicted.

Surgery

The operation was performed the next morning with the aid of patent blue dye and a gamma-ray detection probe. Patent blue dye (1 mL) was administered into the breast cancer. The axillary node was pursued first. The lateral-inferior part of the mastectomy incision was made, and the axilla was entered. A blue lymphatic vessel was observed and was traced to the node. The node was collected. When the surgeon attempted to trace the lymphatic vessel closer to the injection site to find out if it originated in the intraparenchymal node, the vessel was accidentally divided and lost. As a result, it could not be determined whether the node

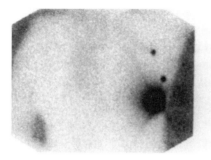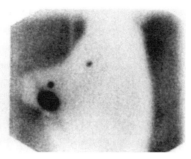

FIGURE 31 Anterior and lateral static views obtained 2 hours after ^{99m}Tc-nanocolloid administration show one sentinel node in the breast parenchyma and another hot node in the left axilla.

that had been removed was a sentinel node or a second-tier node. We decided to err on the safe side and submit the node as a sentinel node.

Attention then shifted to the intraparenchymal node. No blue duct was observed in the area where the node was expected to be. Scattered radiation from the injection site prevented its identification using the gamma-ray detection probe. An attempt was made to solve the problem after performing the simple mastectomy. Outside the patient, the surgical specimen was then explored with the gamma detection probe, but again to no avail. The next step was to excise the breast cancer with its overwhelming amount of radioactivity from the specimen. This was still not enough to identify the sentinel node. The last step was to bring out the probe with the greatest diameter and remove its collimator to increase sensitivity. That move finally enabled identification of the sentinel node. The node was indeed situated close to where the primary tumor had been and measured 2 × 4 mm. It was entirely blue with dye, although 2.5 hours had elapsed since the administration of the dye.

Pathology

No tumor cells were found in the sentinel nodes at frozen-section microscopy. This was later confirmed when the definitive slides were examined using H&E and immunohistochemistry (CAM 5.2). This meant that no completion axillary node dissection was performed.

Discussion

Sentinel nodes are occasionally found in the breast parenchyma. This situation was encountered in three of 113 patients with breast cancer treated at The Netherlands Cancer Institute and the University of Groningen [1], and in nine of 92 patients treated by Uren et al. [2]. Sentinel nodes in the breast have also been described in melanoma [3].

Finding a sentinel node close to the site where the tracer was administered is a considerable challenge. Most of the radioactivity stays behind at the injection site, and its scattered radiation overwhelms the far smaller number of gamma rays emitted from the sentinel node. Applying the collimator to the probe provides side shielding and an additional sense of direction that enables retrieval of the axillary node, but that approach is not good enough to find an intraparenchymal node. The next option is to get rid of the troublesome injection site. In this case, that meant performing the mastectomy. Subsequently, the radioactive tumor can be excised from the surgical specimen. With the source of interference for the probe gone, the collimator and side shielding can be removed to increase the working surface of the probe crystal. As a result, more gamma rays reach the probe, and its sensitivity is increased. This facilitates the detection of a single weak source.

In patients scheduled for breast-conserving surgery, the wide local excision can be performed before an intraparenchymal node is pursued. Injection of a small volume of the tracer into the primary tumor prevents the spread of the radioactive tracer over a wide area. This is advantageous when one is confronted with a nearby sentinel node, because wide local excision will remove the entire injection site and facilitate subsequent probe detection of the node.

REFERENCES

1. Jansen L, Nieweg OE, de Vries J, Valdés Olmos RA, Jager PL, Doting MHE, Piers DA, Rutgers EJTh, Hoefnagel CA, Kroon BBR. Lymphoscintigraphy to identify un- usual locations of sentinel lymph nodes in patients with breast cancer (abstr). J Nucl Med 1999; 40(Suppl):70.
2. Uren RF, Thompson JF, Howman-Giles RB. Patterns of lymphatic drainage in breast cancer. In: Lymphatic Drainage of the Skin and Breast: Locating the Sentinel Nodes. Uren RF, Thompson JF, Howman-Giles RB, eds. Amsterdam, the Netherlands: Har- wood Academic Publishers, 1999, pp 147–158.
3. Bianchi C, Habib FA, Morita E, SPL Leong. Identification of bilateral breast sentinel lymph nodes draining primary melanoma of the back by preoperative lymphoscintig- raphy and intraoperative mapping. Clin Nucl Med 1999; 24:501–503.

Case 13: Sentinel Nodes in Multiple Node Fields

A 56-year-old woman presented with a 2-cm tumor in the upper outer quadrant of her left breast. Fine-needle biopsy confirmed the clinical diagnosis of breast carcinoma. Preoperative mammary lymphoscintigraphy was performed before sentinel node biopsy.

Lymphoscintigraphy

^{99m}Tc antimony sulphide colloid (7 MBq [0.2 mCi] in 0.2 mL/injection) was injected into the breast tissue at four points around the tumor. Tracer was observed flowing to a sentinel node in the left axilla and via a separate discrete channel to a node in the medial left supraclavicular fossa (Fig. 32). A third discrete channel was observed passing to a sentinel node in the left internal mammary chain. This latter channel crossed the center line of the left breast, as did the channel passing to the medial left supraclavicular fossa. This patient thus had three sentinel nodes in three different node fields.

Discussion

Using appropriate small-particle radiocolloids, lymphatic drainage is observed crossing the center line of the breast in approximately half of the patients with breast cancers that lie completely in the inner or outer quadrant [1]. Lymphatic drainage to the axilla or internal mammary chain cannot be predicted on the basis of the location of the cancer in the breast.

Drainage to the internal mammary chain is observed in 40% to 45% of patients with breast cancer when small particle–sized colloids are used [1]. This is in contrast to a reported incidence of 8% when larger particles such as filtered

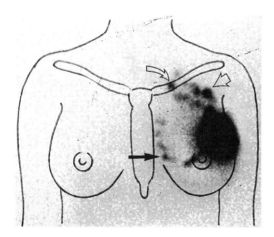

FIGURE 32 The four injection sites in the left breast are observed as a single focus of activity in this exposure setting. Tracer is observed flowing to a sentinel node in the left axilla (open short arrow) and via a separate channel to a node in the left supraclavicular fossa (curved open arrow). A third discrete channel is observed passing in a curvilinear fashion to a third sentinel node in the left internal mammary chain (horizontal arrow).

sulphur colloid are used [2]. It would therefore seem that if drainage to the internal mammary nodes is to be detected in all patients, small particle–sized colloids should be used.

Some investigators observe drainage to sentinel lymph nodes outside the axilla in approximately half of the patients with breast cancer. If a sentinel node biopsy is performed only on sentinel nodes in the axilla, the node status of the patient may be incorrectly assessed in these patients. Logic suggests that the true node status of patients with breast cancer will only be determined by biopsy of all sentinel nodes, regardless of their location.

REFERENCES

1. Uren RF, Thompson JF, Howman-Giles RB. Lymphatics. In: Lymphatic Drainage of the Skin and Breast: Locating the Sentinel Nodes. Uren RF, Thompson JF, Howman-Giles RB, eds. Amsterdam, the Netherlands: Harwood Academic Publishers, 1999, pp 147–158.
2. Krag D, Weaver D, Ashikaga T, Moffat F, Klimberg VS, Shriver C, Feldman S, Kusminsky R, Gadd M, Kuhn J, Harlow S, Beitsch P. The sentinel node in breast cancer: a multicenter validation study. N Engl J Med 1998; 339:941–946.

OTHER NEOPLASMS

Case 1: Carcinoma of the Vulva

A 68-year-old woman was diagnosed with squamous cell carcinoma of the right labium minus. The lesion measured 1.0×1.5 cm. Examination of the groins revealed no lymphadenopathy (T1N0). She was scheduled for vulvectomy and sentinel node biopsy as part of her gynecologist's learning phase. Subsequent completing bilateral inguinal node dissection was planned.

Lymphoscintigraphy

A dose of 74.4 MBq (2.0 mCi) ^{99m}Tc-nanocolloid in a volume of 1.0 mL was injected intradermally at five points around the carcinoma on the right side of the vulva. Lymphoscintigraphy showed a sentinel node in the right groin and a second-tier node higher up (Fig. 33). There was no drainage to the left groin. The location of the sentinel node was indicated on the skin with ink.

Surgery

The operation was performed the next day. One milliliter of patent blue dye was administered around the lesion. The location of the sentinel node could be identified with the probe. The point with the highest number of counts coincided with the skin mark that had been placed by the nuclear medicine physician.

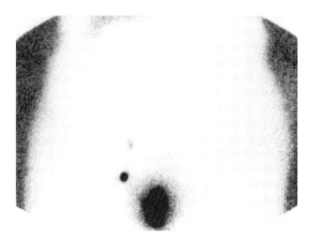

FIGURE 33   The anterior view was obtained 2 hours after injection of the tracer around the carcinoma on right side of the vulva. The image shows a sentinel node in the right groin and a second-tier node higher up. No uptake is noted in the contralateral groin.

A 4-cm transverse incision was made over the node. A blue node was quickly identified in the deep layer of subcutaneous tissue. The probe confirmed that it was indeed the radioactive node. The surrounding tissue was divided, and the node was submitted for pathological evaluation. No other hot or blue nodes were identified. The operation was resumed with excision of the carcinoma and bilateral superficial inguinofemoral node dissection.

Pathology and Follow-Up

Histological evaluation revealed that the primary cancer was 1.6 cm in diameter and that the excision margins were free of disease. The sentinel node was largely replaced by squamous cell carcinoma, but the capsule was not breached. One of the seven other nodes on the right side was also involved. Four nodes on the left side were free of disease. The patient was faring well without evidence of disease 3 years later.

Discussion

No clear-cut guidelines exist for the management of lymph nodes in patients with stage I vulvar carcinoma. It is controversial whether lymph node dissection should be performed and, if so, to what extent.

Seven investigators recently reported on lymphatic mapping in patients with carcinoma of the vulva [1–7]. The sentinel node was identified in 113 of 118 patients (98%). The sentinel node was tumor-positive in 25 of 86 patients (29%). None of these seven investigators reported a false-negative result. Several investigators have reported early experience in cervical cancer and endometrial cancer [4,8,9]. It will be interesting to learn where these developments will lead us.

REFERENCES

1. Levenback C, Burke T, Wolf J, Bodurka-Bevers D, Bevers M, Gershenson D. Intraoperative lymphatic mapping of the vulva: relationship between sentinel node identification with blue dye and tumor location (abstr). Eur J Nucl Med 1999; 26(Suppl):S69.
2. De Cicco C, Sideri M, Bartolomei M, Grana C, Maggioni A, Bocciolone I, Mangioni C, Paganelli G. Can sentinel node biopsy avoid complete groin dissection in early vulvar cancer (abstr)? Eur J Nucl Med 1999; 26(Suppl):S69.
3. De Hullu JA, Verheijen RHM, Hollema H, Piers DA, Schraffordt Koops H, Pijpers HJ, Van Diest PA, Aalders JG, Van der Zee AGJ. Multiple sectioning and immunohistochemical staining in detection of metastases in sentinel lymph node (SLN)S in squamous cell cancer (SCC) of the vulva (abstr). Eur J Nucl Med 1999; 26(Suppl):S70.
4. Makar A, Melis K, Van den Weyngaert D, Van Leuven L, Declercq S, Joosens E, Gerris J, Kockx M. Sentinel node mapping in vulva and endometrium cancers (abstr). Case reports. Eur J Nucl Med 1999; 26(Suppl):S88.
5. DeCesare SL, Fiorica JV, Grendys E, Reintgen D, Hoffman MS, Puleo C, Berman C, Cavanagh D. Intraoperative lymphoscintigraphy for identification of the sentinel lymph nodes in vulvar cancer (abstr). Eur J Nucl Med 1999; 26(Suppl):S88.
6. Delval D, Scharlaeken F, Lecart C. Conservative radioguided surgery in a case of stage II vulvar cancer (abstr). Eur J Nucl Med 1999; 26(Suppl):S88.
7. Levavi H, Sabah G, Levy T, Neri A, Ovadia J, Ben-Refael Z, Gutman H. Sentinel node in patients with vulvar cancer: intra-operative identification and prognosis (abstr). Eur J Nucl Med 1999; 26(Suppl):S89.
8. Verheijen R, Pijpers HJ, Burger C, Wüst M, Kenemans P. Sentinel node detection in cervical carcinoma: a pilot study (abstr). Eur J Nucl Med 1999; 26(Suppl):S69.
9. Dargent D, Martin X, Mathevet P. Laparoscopic identification of the sentinel node in cervical cancer (abstr). Eur J Nucl Med 1999; 26(Suppl):S69.

Case 2: Merkel's Cell Carcinoma

A 34-year-old woman was examined at another hospital with a 3 × 4 cm tumor in the right thigh. The tumor was attached to the skin and had developed in the scar of a cut that she suffered 22 years earlier. Physical examination revealed no other abnormalities. Excision with a narrow margin was performed. Pathological evaluation revealed a neuroendocrine tumor of the skin (Merkel's cell carcinoma) that involved the excision margin. A computed tomography scan of the chest was normal. She was then referred for further treatment. Sentinel node biopsy was planned in addition to wide local re-excision and radiotherapy.

Lymphoscintigraphy

A dose of 42.8 MBq (1.2 mCi) ^{99m}Tc-nanocolloid in a volume of 0.2 mL was injected intradermally at four sites around the biopsy scar. Lymphoscintigraphy showed two lymphatic vessels and one elongated hot spot in the right groin (Fig. 34). The hot spot was marked on the skin.

Surgery

The operation was performed the next day. One milliliter of patent blue dye was administered around the biopsy site. A 3-cm incision was made over the skin mark in the right groin. Two blue lymphatic vessels were observed leading to two blue nodes that were 1 cm apart. The probe confirmed that both nodes were radioactive, and both were collected. Wide excision of the original tumor site was performed.

Pathology and Follow-Up

The sentinel nodes were free of disease. No residual tumor was recognized in the re-excision specimen. Radiotherapy was not performed in view of the favorable pathology result. The patient remained free of disease 5 years later.

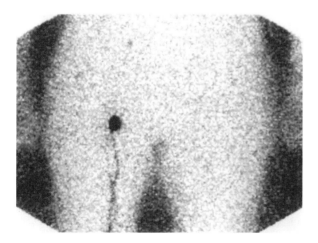

FIGURE 34   Two lymphatic vessels are observed leading to one elongated hot spot in the right groin.

Discussion

A number of different tumor types originating in mucous membranes, epidermis, dermis, and subcutis have the tendency to disseminate to lymph nodes and constitute potential indications for lymphatic mapping. Squamous cell carcinoma is the most obvious candidate, Merkel's cell carcinoma is another.

Merkel cell carcinoma is a high-grade malignant neuroendocrine carcinoma of the skin. It is believed that the carcinoma originates from Merkel's cells because the ultra structure of the tumors is strikingly similar to that type of epidermal sensory cells. The tumor disseminates to the regional lymph nodes in 55% of the patients [1]. Therefore, Merkel's cell carcinoma seems to be an excellent indication for lymphatic mapping. Three studies on lymphatic mapping have been published [2–4]. Two of a series of 12 patients demonstrated metastatic disease in their sentinel lymph nodes, and complete dissection of the involved nodal basin revealed additional positive nodes [2]. The node-negative patients received no further surgical therapy, with no evidence of recurrent local or regional disease at a maximum of 26 months of follow-up evaluation (median, 10.5 months).

REFERENCES

1. Hitchcock CL, Bland KI, Laney RG, 3rd, Franzini D, Harris B, Copeland EM 3rd. Neuroendocrine (Merkel cell) carcinoma of the skin: its natural history, diagnosis, and treatment. Ann Surg 1988; 207:201–207.
2. Messina JL, Reintgen DS, Cruse CW, Rappaport DP, Berman C, Fenske NA, Glass LF. Selective lymphadenectomy in patients with Merkel cell (cutaneous neuroendocrine) carcinoma. Ann Surg Oncol 1997; 4:389–395.
3. Wasserberg N, Feinmesser M, Schachter J, Fenig E, Gutman H. Sentinel-node guided lymph-node dissection for Merkel cell carcinoma. Eur J Surg Oncol 1999; 25:444–446.
4. Bilchik AJ, Giuliano A, Essner R, Bostick P, Kelemen P, Foshag LJ, Sostrin S, Turner RR, Morton DL. Universal application of intraoperative lymphatic mapping and sentinel lymphadenectomy in solid neoplasms. Cancer J Sci Am 1998; 4:351–358.

Case 3: Clear Cell Sarcoma

A 67-year-old woman was referred because of a 3-cm mass on the sole of the right foot. Apart from mild hypertension, she was in a good general physical condition, and examination was otherwise unremarkable. An incisional biopsy showed the tumor to be a clear cell sarcoma. The plan was to perform sentinel node biopsy and wide local excision.

Lymphoscintigraphy

A dose of 73.0 MBq (2.0 mCi) ^{99m}Tc-nanocolloid in a volume of 0.25 mL was injected intradermally at four sites around the tumor. Lymphoscintigraphy showed drainage to one sentinel node in the right groin (Fig. 35).

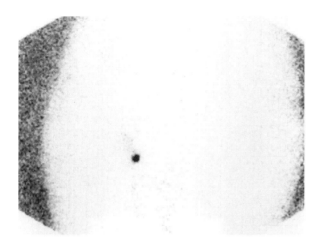

FIGURE 35 The anterior image obtained shows a single sentinel node in the right groin.

Surgery

Once the patient was asleep on the operating table, 1 mL of patent blue dye was administered in the skin around the tumor. One blue, radioactive inguinal node was collected. Subsequently, the tumor on the right foot was excised with a 2-cm margin. The defect was covered with a split skin graft.

Pathology and Follow-Up

Histological evaluation of the sentinel node revealed no tumor cells. The margins of the sarcoma specimen were clear but narrow. Postoperative radiotherapy (50 Gy) was given. There have been no signs of recurrence since the operation. Four years later, the patient was alive and well.

Discussion

Clear cell sarcoma is a separate soft tissue sarcoma entity. Because of its biology and the presence of intracellular melanin, it has been suggested that this tumor should be regarded as a melanoma. However, a distinct chromosomal translocation sets it apart from melanoma. Clear cell sarcoma shares with melanoma a tendency to spread to lymph nodes, which is uncommon in most types of soft tissue sarcoma. Lymph node metastases have been described in 11 of a series of 40 patients (27.5%) [1].

Other sarcoma types that have a tendency the spread to lymph nodes are epitheloid sarcoma, embryonal rhabdomyosarcoma, and angiosarcoma. Management strategies may differ in patients with such types of soft tissue sarcoma [2], and the specific dissemination pattern suggests that they may benefit from lymphatic mapping and sentinel node biopsy.

REFERENCES

1. Mazeron JJ, Suit HD. Lymph nodes as sites of metastases from sarcomas of soft tissue. Cancer 1987; 60:1800–1808.
2. Pisters PW. Combined modality treatment of extremity soft tissue sarcomas. Ann Surg Oncol 1998; 5:464–472.

Case 4: Squamous Cell Carcinoma of the Penis

A 79-year-old man was referred because of a squamous cell carcinoma on the ventral part of the glans of the penis measuring 3.0 × 3.8 cm. There were no enlarged lymph nodes in the groins. He was scheduled to undergo sentinel node biopsy and partial amputation of the penis.

Lymphoscintigraphy

A dose of 60.6 MBq (1.6 mCi) ^{99m}Tc-nanocolloid was injected intradermally at four sites around the tumor. The anterior image showed drainage to two adjacent hot spots in the left groin and to one sentinel node in the right groin (Fig. 36). There was also a second-tier node visualized on the right side. The lateral view demonstrated that this latter node was a deep (iliac) node.

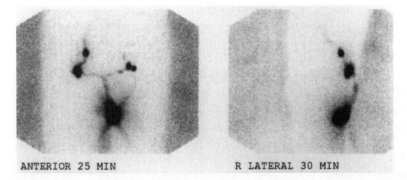

ANTERIOR 25 MIN   R LATERAL 30 MIN

FIGURE 36   Two adjacent hot spots are visible in the left groin, and one sentinel node is visible in the right groin. There is also a second-tier node on the right side. The lateral view demonstrates that this latter node is a deep (iliac) node.

Surgery

The radioactive nodes could be identified with the probe through the intact skin. One milliliter of patent blue dye was administered in the skin around the tumor. One blue, radioactive sentinel node was collected on the right side, and two blue radioactive nodes were recovered on the left side. The right iliac node was not pursued. Subsequently, a partial amputation of the penis was performed. No completion inguinal node dissection was performed.

Pathology and Follow-Up

Histological evaluation showed a well-differentiated T2 squamous cell carcinoma that had been removed with clear margins. The sentinel nodes were examined with H&E and immunohistochemistry staining (pankeratin) and were free of disease. One year later the patient was alive and without evidence of disease.

Discussion

The treatment of patients with penile squamous cell carcinoma and positive lymph nodes is a straightforward regional node dissection, whereas the treatment of patients with clinically normal inguinal nodes is surrounded by controversy. Although it can be argued that early removal of involved nodes is beneficial, elective lymph node dissection results in overtreatment of 80% of the patients [1]. Elective inguinal node dissection should usually be performed on both sides and results in a considerable incidence of postoperative morbidity [2].

Sentinel node biopsy was performed in a recent study of 55 patients with squamous cell carcinoma of the penis [3]. Lymphoscintigraphy revealed bilateral drainage in 43 patients (78%). The sentinel node was always identified and contained metastatic disease in 11 patients (20%). No elective lymph node dissection was performed. After a median follow-up duration of 22 months, two patients returned with involved inguinal nodes after a tumor-free sentinel node had been removed (sensitivity, 85%). The investigators concluded that lymphatic mapping and sentinel node biopsy can be used to select patients with penile cancer who may benefit from inguinal node dissection. And so the sentinel node biopsy returns to the tumor type in which it had originally been described in 1977 [4].

REFERENCES

1. Persky L, deKernion J. Carcinoma of the penis. CA Cancer J Clin 1986; 36:258–273.
2. Johnson DE, Lo RK. Complications of groin dissection in penile cancer: experience with 101 lymphadenectomies. Urology 1984; 24:312–314.

3. Horenblas S, Jansen L, Meinhard W, Hoefnagel CA, de Jong D, Nieweg OE. Detection of occult metastasis in squamous cell carcinoma of the penis using a dynamic sentinel node procedure. J Urol 2000; 163:100–104.
4. Cabañas RM. An approach for the treatment of penile carcinoma. Cancer 1977; 39: 456–466.

19

The Future of Lymphatic Mapping and Sentinel Lymphadenectomy

Bin B. R. Kroon and Omgo E. Nieweg
The Netherlands Cancer Institute, Amsterdam, the Netherlands

Liesbeth Jansen
Gelre Hospital, Lukas Site, Apeldoorn, the Netherlands

Emiel J. Th. Rutgers
The Netherlands Cancer Institute and Antoni Van Leeuwenhoek Hospital, Amsterdam, the Netherlands

INTRODUCTION

Although the procedure of lymphatic mapping and sentinel lymphadenectomy is said to be one of the major developments in surgical oncology this decade [1,2], many technical aspects still need further refinement. Indications for the procedure also have to be further clarified. For example, which tumor types are most suitable? Are there certain subgroups within these tumor types that may benefit in particular?

MELANOMA
Is There an Indication for Sentinel Lymphadenectomy?

For more than a century, the value of elective lymph node dissection in patients with melanoma has been debated [3–6]. Now that the method of lymphatic mapping and sentinel lymphadenectomy offers the opportunity to reliably identify regional nodes with microscopic involvement [1], this debate has shifted to the issue of ''selective'' lymph node dissection (i.e., completion removal of regional lymph node basin only if there is microscopic involvement of the sentinel node). Several retrospective studies have provided evidence suggesting that this approach has a beneficial effect. Patients who underwent node dissection at the stage of microscopic involvement had a survival advantage of approximately 20%, compared to patients who underwent dissection of clinically detected involved nodes [7]. In addition, a prospective randomized trial of the WHO Melanoma Program showed that patients with truncal melanoma, whose microscopically involved nodes were removed electively, fared significantly better than those who underwent delayed dissection for palpable nodes [8].

A definite answer with respect to the value of the procedure can only be expected to come from a randomized prospective study. Fortunately, such a study is ongoing in the form of the Multicenter Selective Lymphadenectomy Trial that was initiated by the person who first described the method, D. L. Morton [9]. In this trial, patients with a melanoma 1 mm or greater in thickness according to Breslow or level IV or greater according to Clark are randomized between wide excision of the primary lesion only, versus wide excision plus sentinel node biopsy followed by a completing regional node dissection in case of microscopic involvement of this node. As endpoints, the possible survival benefit of the latter approach will be balanced against acute and possible long-term side effects of the diagnostic procedure. Long-term side effects may consist of the trapping of tumor cells that are ''in-transit'' between the primary tumor and the regional lymph node basin. Also, unpredictable lymphatic spread due to alterations in lymph flow patterns, and hematogenous spread may occur as well as an increase in the rate of regional recurrence [10].

The identification of a subgroup of patients (definable by Breslow thickness or by other prognostic variables) for which sentinel lymphadenectomy possibly will lead to benefit may be another outcome of the above-mentioned trial. At present, the lower limit of thickness to perform a sentinel lymphadenectomy varies between 0.75 mm and 1.5 mm, whereas most investigators do not set an upper limit. Interesting conclusions in this regard were drawn in a report on a mathematical model that was generated to predict sentinel node involvement [11]. This model was based on two significant predictors for positive sentinel nodes: Breslow thickness and age. These two factors emerged after a multivariate analysis using stepwise logistic regression of age, gender, Clark level, Breslow thickness, presence of ulceration, location, and number of nodal basins. In individual patients, this model can be used for counseling purposes regarding the likelihood of metastatic disease in the sentinel nodes. It can also be used routinely to identify subgroups of patients who will have the most to gain from the procedure. Better noninvasive staging procedures, both for regional and systemic disease, may also further refine the selection of patients for sentinel node biopsy. Currently available noninvasive regional staging procedures are ultrasound, combined with aspiration cytology [12,13], computed tomography (CT) scanning [14], magnetic resonance imaging (MRI), and positron emission tomography (PET). Promising results on the use of sonography have been published. Until now, the use of monoclonal antibodies for the detection of regional metastases has lacked sensitivity [15]. Results regarding the prediction of the occurrence of hematogenous metastasis, however, are encouraging. Multimarker reverse transcriptase–polymerase chain reaction (RT-PCR) techniques have been developed to detect malignant melanoma cells in the blood and lymph nodes [16–18]. The presence of specific tumor markers for melanoma, such as the new sensitive immunoluminometric assay, LIA-mat®Sangtec® 100 (S-100), seems to be a useful prognostic parameter for hematogenous spread [19].

Extent of Completion Lymph Node Dissection

A question that remains is: Is it always necessary to clear the entire lymphatic basin after the removal of an involved sentinel node? In the series reported so far, an additional 10–20% of involved nodes were found in the definitive regional node dissection specimen [1,20–22]. An interesting observation was made by the group from Moffitt Cancer Center in Tampa [23]. In a series of 88 patients, they found that all those with involved nodes beyond the positive sentinel node(s) had a primary melanoma thickness of greater than 1.5 mm in thickness. These results suggest that the disease in sentinel-node-positive patients with a primary tumor of less than 1.5 mm in thickness may be confined to the sentinel node and, therefore, that they may not necessarily require further lymph node dissection.

Sentinel Lymphadenectomy as a Selection Criterion for Adjuvant Treatment Strategies

It has been suggested that patients with a relatively low tumor burden may benefit most from adjuvant treatment strategies [24]. If effective schedules should become available, for instance in the form of interferon-alpha in a tolerable dose [25] or a vaccine [26], micrometastasis detected by sentinel lymphadenectomy may prove to be an attractive selection criterion for these adjuvant treatments.

In this respect, the relevance of the RT-PCR technique for the detection of tyrosinase or other specific markers for the presence of melanoma cells in the sentinel lymph node has to be elucidated [9,27]. In one report, RT-PCR positivity in histologically negative sentinel nodes was associated with a recurrence rate of 10.6%, compared to a rate of 2.3% in RT-PCR-negative patients [28]. This suggests that RT-PCR is of practical value in melanoma staging and therefore could be a selection criterion for entering patients in adjuvant treatment schedules.

Technical Aspects

Although lymphoscintigraphy is a well-established procedure in lymphatic mapping and plays a crucial role in localizing sentinel nodes preoperatively, little is known about its sensitivity. In this regard, reproducibility of lymphoscintigraphy with a technetium-99m (^{99m}Tc)-labeled nanocolloid (Nanocoll®, Sorin Radiofarmaci S.r.I., Saluggia, Italy) was studied by Kapteijn et al. [29]. In 25 patients, two scintigraphic studies were performed in an identical manner, with a 2–4-week interval. The basins identified to be at risk for metastasis correlated between the two studies. However, in three patients (12%), there was a difference in the number of sentinel nodes depicted on the first and second scans. The number of unidentified sentinel nodes can be reduced by combining lymphoscintigraphy and mapping with patent blue [30,31]. However, efforts should be made to achieve optimal reproducibility of lymphoscintigraphy, both to increase the reliability of the method and to avoid removing nonsentinel nodes from the lymphatic basin.

Another poorly settled issue of lymphoscintigraphy is the choice of the radiopharmaceutical, especially with respect to particle size. An antimony sulfur colloid, human serum albumin, and a sulfur colloid, all labeled with ^{99m}Tc (which comes close to the ideal radionuclide), have been compared in patients with truncal melanoma [32]. There was no significant difference in the number of drainage basins identified by these three radiopharmaceuticals. Further comparative studies with regard to the number of identified sentinel and nonsentinel nodes are desirable to establish the best radiopharmaceutical, especially regarding its biological properties.

BREAST CANCER

Technical Aspects

The procedure of lymphatic mapping and sentinel lymphadenectomy is more difficult to perform in patients with breast cancer than in patients with melanoma. The injection site, for instance, of the tracers cannot always be determined as precisely as it can for melanoma, due to deeper tumor localization. This may result in reduced sensitivity and selectivity of the method. Injections into [33] and around [34–36] the breast tumor have been applied; some authors have even advocated injections into the subcutaneous tissue [37] or into the skin overlying the tumor [38]. The theoretical rationale for these latter two sites is based on the fact that the embryologic origin of the mammary gland is an appendix of the skin. An interesting observation in this regard is that a radiopharmaceutical injected around the tumor and blue dye injected intradermally both drained to the same axillary nodes [38]. The absence of internal mammary drainage after intracutaneous injection, however, casts doubt on the validity of the intracutaneous approach. Refined studies on lymphatic drainage patterns of the breast are clearly needed. Concern has been expressed that intradermal injection may lead to a blue tattoo, caused by retarded dissipation of the dye from the injection site [39].

Breast edema after axillary node dissection and postoperative irradiation could be promoting factors for this suggested sequel. A clear advantage of subcutaneous and cutaneous applications is fast drainage to the axillary nodes, which is said to never fail. In our experience, axillary drainage after intratumoral injection of the ^{99m}Tc nanocolloid failed in about 6% of the patients.

Another complicating factor in lymphatic mapping for patients with breast cancer is the short distance between an injection site in the upper, outer quadrant and the axilla, and between a medial injection site and the parasternal lymph node area. This may cause problems in discriminating the radioactivity of the sentinel node from the radioactivity at the injection site. Excising the radioactive tumor area before performing sentinel lymphadenectomy might help to reduce shine through activity from the injection site, but such a policy may interfere with the blue dye lymphatic mapping part of the procedure. The abandonment of the blue dye technique in sentinel lymphadenectomy in patients with breast cancer with reliance only on the radioactive tracer, as advocated in one study [37], has provoked criticism [40]. It was stated that with radioactivity alone, sentinel nodes cannot always reliably be discriminated from second-tier nodes.

Preoperative lymphatic mapping by lymphoscintigraphy will prove to be indispensable because it points out sentinel nodes that cannot be found with the probe at the time of operation. These nodes can be localized in the axilla and outside the axilla. It can therefore be predicted that the combination of preoperative lymphoscintigraphy and intraoperative use of both a gamma detection probe and a vital dye will become the standard technique to stage the regional lymph node basins in breast cancer patients.

Other questions related to performing lymphoscintigraphy in breast cancer patients which must be answered in the future are the following: What is the best radiopharmaceutical? What is the optimal dose of radioactive tracer? What is the optimal volume to be injected?

Indications

Now that sentinel lymphadenectomy has developed into a reliable method in patients with breast cancer, prospective randomized trials are in progress to determine the value of the procedure. These trials compare standard axillary dissection in all patients with sentinel node biopsy followed by axillary dissection only in node-positive patients. Relevant endpoints of these trials include local control, survival, morbidity, quality of life, and economic aspects. Some investigators question, however, whether these prospective studies are necessary for the implementation of a new diagnostic procedure. Another interesting trial option that could be addressed, once sentinel node biopsy has evolved into a standard procedure, is the performance of a axillary clearance versus irradiation of the axilla in sentinel-node-positive patients, and even the option of a wait and see policy (combined with adjuvant treatment) in patients with minute nodal metastasis could be studied.

Further research is also required to prove the validity of lymphatic mapping and sentinel lymphadenectomy after excising the primary tumor. The same applies to using the method on nonpalpable malignant breast lesions.

As for melanoma, improvements in imaging techniques, such as ultrasound combined with aspiration cytology [41], CT scanning [42], MRI [43], and PET [44], may decrease the number of patients who have to undergo sentinel lymphadenectomy in the future. Ultimate refinement in the detection of micrometastases may come from the search for specific tumor-seeking agents, such as monoclonal antibodies [45]. Lack of selectivity of these agents, however, is still a limiting factor, and tumor deposits smaller than 3 mm cannot be detected by the other mentioned imaging techniques. The same holds true for the tumor tracer sestamibi [46]. Other possible developments, such as greater insights into the characteristics of the primary tumor, or the finding of a reliable tumor marker in the blood, eventually could outweigh the importance of the axillary lymph node status [47].

Improved Staging by Sentinel Lymphadenectomy

With the introduction of sentinel lymphadenectomy, pathologists now only have to examine one or a few nodes instead of a whole dissection specimen. As a result, upstaging of a certain percentage of patients will occur due to optimal histological, immunological, and molecular biological analysis. What this means in terms of indications for adjuvant treatment and in terms of survival will probably become evident in the near future.

Lymphatic mapping will also provide data on drainage patterns from the breast to the parasternal lymph node chain. Biopsy of sentinel nodes located in this region will elucidate the impact of parasternal lymph node metastasis on prognosis and will refine the indications for parasternal surgery and irradiation, adjuvant chemotherapy, and hormone treatment strategies [48].

OTHER TUMORS

It is likely that the procedure of lymphatic mapping and sentinel lymphadenectomy also will be a valuable new tool in the management of penile carcinoma [49,50], the tumor for which Cabañas was the first to investigate the concept of selective lymphatic drainage [51]. Promising results have also been reported for vulvar carcinoma [52]. At present, it is only possible to speculate about the value of lymphatic mapping and sentinel lymphadenectomy for gastrointestinal and pulmonary tumors. Preliminary results in colorectal cancer, however, are not encouraging [53]. For the reliable application of the method to these tumors, more sophistication of endoscopic (and laparoscopic?) techniques is necessary. The lack of easy and reliable follow-up procedures to monitor nondissected lymph node areas in these tumors, in case of a negative sentinel node, poses a major problem.

SUMMARY

The procedure of lymphatic mapping and sentinel lymphadenectomy is valuable for the staging of melanoma patients. However, a prospective randomized study is necessary to prove whether the early detection and excision of melanoma micrometastases to the regional lymphatics leads to improved regional control and better survival. Such a trial also has to monitor acute and possible long-term side effects. The impact of adjuvant treatment at the stage of lymphatic micrometastasis also has to be investigated prospectively.

Sentinel node biopsy is similarly of value in the staging and early regional treatment of patients with breast cancer. Several technical problems, however, have to be solved in this tumor and a uniform method of performing the procedure should be adopted.

Advancements of noninvasive imaging techniques to detect regional lymph node metastases may decrease the number of patients that will need to undergo sentinel lymphadenectomy. The same holds true as we gain greater insight into the prognostic characteristics of the primary tumor. For the more distant future, it even may be anticipated that sentinel lymphadenectomy could become an obsolete procedure, when more sophisticated tumor markers and improved molecular biology techniques will become available for detecting circulating tumor cells in the blood.

REFERENCES

1. DI Morton, D-R Wen, JH Wong, JS Economou, LA Cagle, FK Storm, LJ Foshag, AJ Cochran. Technical details of intraoperative lymphatic mapping for early stage melanoma. Arch Surg 127:392–399, 1992.
2. OE Nieweg, BAE Kapteijn, JF Thompson, BBR Kroon. Lymphatic mapping and selective lymphadenectomy for melanoma: not yet standard therapy. Eur J Surg Oncol 23:397–398, 1997.
3. U Veronesi, J Adamus, DC Bandiera, O Brennhovd, E Caceres, N Cascinelli, F Claudio, RL Ikonopisov, VV Javorski, S Kirov, A Kulakowski, J Lacour, F Lejeune, Z Mechl, A Morabito, I Rode, S Sergeev, E Van Slooten, K Szczygiel, NN Trapeznikov, RI Wagner. Delayed regional lymph node dissection in stage I melanoma of the skin of the lower extremities. Cancer 49:2420–2430, 1982.

4. AS Coates, CI Ingvar, K Petersen-Schaefer, HM Shaw, GW Milton, CJ O'Brien, JF Thompson, WH McCarthy. Elective lymph node dissection in patients with primary melanoma of the trunk and limbs treated at the Sydney Melanoma Unit from 1960 to 1991. J Am Coll Surg 180:402–409, 1995.

5. CM Balch, S-J Soong, AA Bartolucci, MM Urist, CP Karakousis, TJ Smith, WJ Temple, MI Ross, WR Jewell, MC Mihm, RL Barnhill, HJ Wanebo. Efficacy of an elective regional lymph node dissection of 1–4 mm thick melanomas for patients 60 years of age and younger. Ann Surg 224:255–266, 1996.

6. BBR Kroon, A Jonk. Elective lymph node dissection in melanoma: still a controversial issue. Neth J Surg 43:129–132, 1991.

7. CM Balch. The role of elective lymph node dissection in melanoma: Rationale, results, and controversies. J Clin Oncol 6:163–172, 1988.

8. N Cascinelli, A Moribato, M Santinami, RM MacKie, F Belli, on behalf of the WHO Melanoma Programme. Immediate or delayed dissection of regional nodes in patients with melanoma of the trunk: A randomized trial. Lancet 351:793–796, 1998.

9. DL Morton. Management of regional lymph nodes in melanoma patients. Melanoma Res 7(Suppl 1):S22, 1997.

10. R Essner, DL Morton. Elective lymph node dissection. In: FJ Lejeune, PK Chaudhuri, TK Das Gupta, eds. Malignant Melanoma. Medical and Surgical Management. New York: McGraw-Hill, 1994, pp. 205–214.

11. E Joseph, D Rapaport, F Glass, J Messina, CW Cruse, C Berman, R Deconti, G Lyman, A Cantor, DS Reintgen. Generation of mathematical model to predict sentinel node involvement in malignant melanoma. Melanoma Res 7(Suppl 1):S78, 1997.

12. L Prayer, H Winkelbauer, N Gritzmann, F Winkelbauer, M Helmer, H Pehamberger. Sonography versus palpation in the detection of regional lymph node metastases in patients with malignant melanoma. Eur J Cancer 26:827–830, 1990.

13. CR Rossi, A Seno, A Vecchiato, M Foletto, A Tregnaghi, A De Candia, L Rubaltelli, C Montesco, M Lise. The impact of ultrasound scanning in the staging and follow-up of patients with clinical stage I cutaneous melanoma. Eur J Cancer 33:200–203, 1997.

14. MWM Van den Brekel, FA Pameijer, W Koops, FJM Hilgers, BBR Kroon, AJM Balm. Computed tomography for the detection of neck node metastases in melanoma patients. Eur J Surg Oncol 24:51–54, 1998.

15. LM Lamki, AA Zukiwski, LJ Shanken, SS Legha, RS Benjamin, CE Plager, DF Salk, RW Schroff, JL Murray. Radio-imaging of melanoma using ^{99m}Tc-labeled Fab fragment reactive with a high molecular weight melanoma antigen. Cancer Res 50(Suppl):904–908, 1990.

16. DSB Hoon, Y Wang, PS Dale, AJ Conrad, P Schmid, D Garrison, Ch Kue, LJ Foshag, AJ Nizze, DL Morton. Detection of occult melanoma cells in blood with a multiple-marker polymerase chain reaction assay. J Clin Oncol 13:2109–2116, 1995.

17. DSB Hoon, T Okamoto, C Kuo, AJ Conrad, P Schmid, DL Morton. Detection of metastatic melanoma in blood by multimarker RT-PCR: correlation to clinical stage and recurrence of disease. Melanoma Res 7(Suppl 1):S56, 1997.

18. X Wang, W Li, SC Shivers, DS Reintgen. Early detection of circulating melanoma cells in peripheral blood by RT-PCR. Melanoma Res 7(Suppl 1):S56, 1997.

19. EM Rankin, CM Korse, JMG Bonfrer. The prognostic value of circulating protein S-100β in malignant melanoma patients. Melanoma Res 7(Suppl 1):S87, 1997.

20. JF Thompson, WH McCarthy, CMJ Bosch, CJ O'Brien, MJ Quinn, S Paramaesvaran, K Crotty, SW McCarthy, RF Uren, R Howman-Giles. Sentinel lymph node status as an indicator of the presence of metastatic melanoma in regional lymph nodes. Melanoma Res 5:255–260, 1995.

21. DJ Krag, SJ Meijer, DL Weaver, BW Loggie, SP Harlow, KK Tanabe, EH Laughlin, JC Alex. Minimal access surgery for staging of malignant melanoma. Arch Surg 130:654–658, 1995.

22. BAE Kapteijn, OE Nieweg, IH Liem, WJ Mooi, AJM Balm, SH Muller, JL Peterse, RA Valdés Olmos, CA Hoefnagel, BBR Kroon. Localizing the sentinel node in cutaneous melanoma: gamma probe detection versus blue dye. Ann Surg Oncol 4: 156–160, 1997.

23. LF Glass, J Messina, J Glass, E Joseph, R Deconti, CW Cruse, D Rapaport, C Berman, N Fenske, DS Reintgen. The results of complete lymph node dissections in 88 melanoma patients with positive sentinel nodes. Melanoma Res 7(Suppl 1):S104, 1997.

24. A Barth, DL Morton. Role of adjuvant therapy in melanoma management. Cancer 75:726–734, 1995.

25. JM Kirkwood, JM Strawderman, MS Ernstoff, TJ Smith, EC Borden, TH Blum. Interferon-α.2b adjuvant therapy of high-risk resected cutaneous melanoma: The Eastern Cooperative Oncology Group Trial EST 1684. J Clin Oncol 14:7–17, 1996.

26. DL Morton, LJ Foshag, DSB Hoon, JA Nizze, LA Wanek, PHC Chang, DG Davtyan, RK Gupta, R Elashoff, RF Irie. Prolongation of survival in metastatic melanoma after active specific immunotherapy with a new polyvalent melanoma vaccine. Ann Surg 216:463–482, 1992.

27. DS Reintgen, AJ Conrad. Detection of occult melanoma cells in sentinel lymph nodes and blood. Semin Oncol 24(Suppl 4):S4-11–S4-15, 1997.

28. W Li, SC Shivers, X Wang, E Joseph, DS Reintgen. RT-PCR of sentinel lymph node metastases in malignant melanoma patients. Melanoma Res 7(Suppl 1):S34, 1997.

29. BAE Kapteijn, OE Nieweg, RA Valdés Olmos, IH Liem, RKL Baidjnath Panday, CA Hoefnagel, BBR Kroon. Reproducibility of lymphoscintigraphy for lymphatic mapping in cutaneous melanoma. J Nucl Med 37:972–975, 1996.

30. BAE Kapteijn, OE Nieweg, SH Muller, IH Liem, CA Hoefnagel, EJTh Rutgers, BBR Kroon. Validation of gamma probe detection of the sentinel node in melanoma. J Nucl Med 38:362–366, 1977.

31. JJ Albertini, CW Cruse, D Rapaport, K Wells, M Ross, R DeConti, CG Berman, K Jared, J Messina, G Lyman, F Glass, N Fenske, DS Reintgen. Intraoperative radiolymphoscintigraphy improves sentinel lymph node identification for patients with melanoma. Ann Surg 223:217–224, 1996.

32. P Sharkey, C Berman, DS Reintgen. Comparison of radiopharmaceuticals utilized in lymphoscintigraphy. Melanoma Res 7(Suppl 1):S87, 1997.

33. BAE Kapteijn, OE Nieweg, JL Peterse, EJTh Rutgers, BBR Kroon. Sequential lymphatic dissemination of breast cancer. Eur J Surg Oncol 22:399, 1996.

34. JJ Albertini, GH Lyman, Ch Cox, T Yeatman, L Balducci, N Ku, S Shivers, C

Berman, K Wells, D Rapaport, A Shons, J Horton, H Greenberg, S Nicosia, R Clark, A Cantor, DS Reintgen. Lymphatic mapping and sentinel node biopsy in the patient with breast cancer. JAMA 276:1818–1822, 1996.

35. AE Giuliano, PS Dale, RR Turner, DL Morton, SW Evans, DL Krasne. Improved axillary staging of breast cancer with sentinel lymphadenectomy. Ann Surg 222: 394–401, 1995.

36. R Pijpers, S Meijer, OS Hoekstra, GJ Collet, EFI Comans, RPA Boom, PJ Van Diest, GJJ Teule. Impact of lymphoscintigraphy on sentinel node identification with technetium-99m-colloidal albumin in breast cancer. J Nucl Med 38:366–368, 1997.

37. U Veronesi, G Paganelli, V Galimberti, G Viale, S Zurrida, M Bedoni, A Costa, C De Cicco, JG Geraghty, A Luini, V Sacchini, P Veronesi. Sentinel node biopsy to avoid axillary dissection in breast cancer with clinically negative lymph nodes. Lancet 349:1864–1867, 1997.

38. PJ Borgstein, S Meijer, R Pijpers. Intradermal blue dye to identify sentinel lymph node in breast cancer. Lancet 349:1668–1669, 1997.

39. AE Giuliano. Intradermal blue dye to identify sentinel lymph node in breast cancer. Lancet 350:958, 1997.

40. OE Nieweg, J De Vries, L Jansen, H Schraffordt Koops, BBR Kroon. Sentinel node biopsy in breast cancer. Lancet 350:808, 1997.

41. CI Perre. Breast cancer diagnostic and staging aspects. Thesis. University of Amsterdam, 1996.

42. RJ Isaacs, JM Ford, SG Allan, GV Forgeson, S Gallagher. Role of computed tomography in the staging of primary breast cancer. Br J Surg 80:1137, 1993.

43. HT Turoglu, NA Janjan, MK Thorsen, KA Shaffer, PS Ritch, RM Hansen, AP Walker, M Gai, BD Collier. Imaging of regional spread of breast cancer by internal mammary lymphoscintigraphy, CT and MRI. Clin Nucl Med 17:482–484, 1992.

44. OE Nieweg, EE Kim, W-H Wong, WF Broussard, SE Singletary, GN Hortobagyi, RS Tilbury. Positron emission tomography with fluorine-18 deoxyglucose in the detection and staging of breast cancer. Cancer 71:3920–3925, 1993.

45. L Biassoni, M Granowska, MJ Caroll, F McNeill, R Howell, D Ellison, A Granowski, SJ Mather, RA Carpenter, KE Britton. Primary breast cancer: Tc-99m SM3, antistripped mucin core protein monoclonal antibody in assessment of axillary node involvement. Eur J Nucl Med 22:35, 1995.

46. CI Perre, JE Rütter, PA Vos, P De Hooge. Technetium-99-m-sestamibi uptake in axillary lymph node metastases in breast cancer patients. Eur J Surg Oncol 23:142–144, 1997.

47. WL McGuire, GM Clark. Prognostic factors and treatment decisions in axillary node negative breast cancer. N Engl J Med 326:1756–1761, 1992.

48. L Jansen, OE Nieweg, RA Valdés Olmos, EJTh Rutgers, JL Peterse, J de Vries, MH Doting, BBR Kroon. Improved staging of breast cancer through lymphatic mapping and sentinel node biopsy: A case report. Eur J Surg Oncol 24:445–446, 1998.

49. BAE Kapteijn. Biopsy of the sentinel node in melanoma, penile carcinoma and breast carcinoma. The case for lymphatic mapping. Thesis. University of Amsterdam, 1997.

50. S Horenblas. Diagnosis and treatment of penile cancer, new strategies. Eur Urol Today 6:3–4, 1995.

51. RM Cabañas. An approach for the treatment of penile carcinoma. Cancer 39:456–466, 1977.
52. C Levenback, TW Burke, M Morris, A Malpica, KR Lukas, DM Gershenson. Potential applications of intraoperative lymphatic mapping in vulvar cancer. Gynecol Oncol 59:216–220, 1995.
53. JJA Joosten, LJA Stroble, EDM Bruggink, CAP Wauters, M Pruszezynski, Th Wobbes, TJM Ruers. Intraoperative lymphatic mapping and the sentinel node concept in colorectal cancer. Eur J Nucl Med 26(suppl):S74.

Index

About the Editors

OMGO E. NIEWEG is a staff member in the Department of Surgery, The Netherlands Cancer Institute, Amsterdam. Dr. Nieweg is the author or coauthor of over 400 papers, journal articles, and presentations, and is a member of the Society of Surgical Oncology (U.S.A.), the European Society of Surgical Oncology, and the Dutch Societies of Nuclear Medicine and Surgery. He received the M.D. (1976) and Ph.D. (1983) degrees from the University of Groningen, the Netherlands.

RICHARD ESSNER is Assistant Director of Surgical Oncology, John Wayne Cancer Institute at Saint John's Health Center, Santa Monica, California, and Clinical Professor of Surgery, University of Southern California, Los Angeles. The author or coauthor of over 100 scientific papers, articles, and lectures, he is an editor of the *Journal of Surgical Oncology*, a Fellow of the American College of Surgeons, and a member of the Society of Surgical Oncology and the American Association of Cancer Research. He received the B.A. degree (1981) from Emory University, Atlanta, Georgia, and the M.D. degree (1985) from the Emory University School of Medicine, Atlanta, Georgia.

DOUGLAS S. REINTGEN is Professor of Surgery at the University of South Florida and Program Leader of Cutaneous Oncology at the H. Lee Moffitt Cancer Center and Research Institute, Tampa, Florida. The author, coauthor, or coeditor of over 600 scientific articles, papers, book chapters, and lectures, he is an editor-in-chief of melanoma.net and breastdoctor.com and senior editor of the Oncology section for YourDoctor.com, serves on the editorial board of the *Journal of the*

Skin Cancer Foundation, and is a member of the American Association for Cancer Research, the American College of Surgeons, and the World Health Organization. He received the B.A. degree (1975) from Duke University, Durham, North Carolina, and the M.D. degree (1979) from Duke University Medical Center, Durham, North Carolina.

JOHN F. THOMPSOM is Executive Director of the Sydney Melanoma Unit, Sydney Cancer Centre, Royal Prince Alfred Hospital, Australia, and Professor of Surgery (Melanoma and Surgical Oncology) at the University of Sydney, Australia. The author or coauthor of over 250 peer-reviewed scientific articles, book chapters, papers, and monographs, he is an associate editor of the *European Journal of Surgical Oncology*, a member of the editorial board of the *Annals of Surgical Oncology*, a Fellow of the American College of Surgeons, vice president of the International Society for Regional Cancer Therapy, and a member of the Royal Australasian College of Surgeons and the Society of Surgical Oncology. He received the B.Sc. (1968), M.B.B.S. (1971), and M.D. (1997) degrees from the University of Sydney, Australia.